DNA
VACCINES

DNA VACCINES

Technical Design Report

DESIGN OF A GENE TO ERADICATE HIV

by

Lane B. Scheiber II, MD

Lane B. Scheiber, ScD

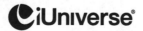

DNA VACCINES
DESIGN OF A GENE TO ERADICATE HIV

iUniverse books may be ordered through booksellers or by contacting:

iUniverse
1663 Liberty Drive
Bloomington, IN 47403
www.iuniverse.com
1-800-Authors (1-800-288-4677)

ISBN: 978-1-5320-1721-6 (sc)
ISBN: 978-1-5320-1722-3 (e)

Library of Congress Control Number: 2017903200

Print information available on the last page.

iUniverse rev. date: 09/12/2017

Courier Gene Technology
Changing the Global Approach to Medicine Series, Volume 5

VIR*e*SOFT Developers of Medically Therapeutic RNA Vector Technologies, Medical Vector Therapy, Molecular Virus Killers, Quantum Gene, Executable Gene, Genetic Reference Tables, Prime Genome, Prime Genomic Cube, Genomic Keycode, Essential Equation 4 Life, Dandelion Rift, the Tritron, the Quadsitron, the Quadsistor, Fourth Generation Biologics and Molecular Gene Activators, Embedded DNA Vaccines, Theory of the Quadsitron Ether, Theory to Unify GLEAM (Gravity, Light, Electrons, Atoms, Magnetism).

MedStar Labs, Inc.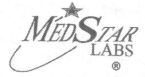

CHANGING THE GLOBAL APPROACH TO MEDICINE, Volume 1
New Perspectives on Treating AIDS, Diabetes, Obesity, Aging, Heart
Attacks, Stroke, and Cancer
by Lane B. Scheiber II, MD and Lane B. Scheiber, ScD

CHANGING THE GLOBAL APPROACH TO MEDICINE, Volume 2
Medical Vector Therapy
Also introducing the Quantum Gene and the Quadsistor
by Lane B. Scheiber II, MD and Lane B. Scheiber, ScD

CHANGING THE GLOBAL APPROACH TO MEDICINE, Volume 3
Cellular Command and Control
Also introducing the Prime Genome and the Tritron
by Lane B. Scheiber II, MD and Lane B. Scheiber, ScD

FOURTH GENERATION BIOLOGICS: Molecular Virus Killers
Changing the Global Approach to Medicine Series, Volume 4
by Lane B. Scheiber II, MD and Lane B. Scheiber, ScD

IMMORTALITY: QUATERNARY MEDICINE CODE
by Anthony Scheiber

CURSE OF THE SNOW DRAGON
by Anthony Scheiber

THE HUMAN COMPUTER
by Anthony Scheiber

EARTH PRO: The Rings of Sol
by Anthony Scheiber

DEDICATION

Thanks to our wives, Karin and Mary Jane,
for all of their love and support, without which this
effort could never have been accomplished.

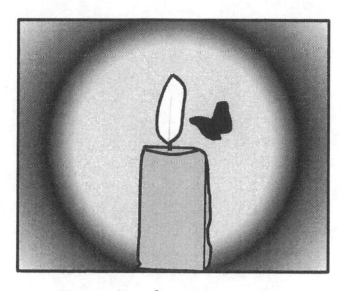

Tenacity for Discovery

Like a moth
drawn to a flame,
we
tirelessly
seek the truth,
The time is now to venture
beyond 1859,
and
embrace
the
core implementer
TERRA.HOLOMETABOLOUS.PROGRAMME

TERRA.HOLOMETABOLOUS.PROGRAMME

The Bio Program Responsible for the Complete
Biologic Metamorphosis of the Earth

ECOMETABOLOUS

The Process Where the Earth Was
Completely Transformed from an Arid
Inhospitable Toxic Stormy Oceanless
Volcanic Planet to
72% of the Planet Surface Covered with
Water, an Atmosphere of 79% Nitrogen,
20% Oxygen, and Numerous Multi-layered
Ecosystems Inhabiting Every Possible
Edge and Depth of the Surface of the Globe.

EVOLUTION

The Observation that since arrival Terra.
Holometabolous.Programme
Has Shaped the Environment and Dynamically
Adapted Life to Optimally Survive Given
the Parameters of the Prevailing Natural
Conditions at Any Given Time in Earth's History

PREFACE

The Next Generation of the Central Dogma of Microbiology

'Dawn of the DNA Programmer'

Contemporary computers work with a machine code of ones and zeros. In essence, the digital computer programmer utilizes sequences of ones and zeros to generate representations of data and command instructions. From digital computer to digital computer the ones and zeros that comprise the primary language that drives computer technology represents the same physical entity. The primary language of the digital computer, referred to as machine language, is physically represented by either a transistor that is OFF with a voltage output of 0.3 mV or a transistor that is ON with a voltage output of 5 mv. Digital computer programs work in a single dimensional plane where the computer programs are constructed of sequences of ones and zeros. The arrangements of ones and zeros in computer code represent changes to the voltage output of transistors represented in the heart of the computer's central processor, the accompanying microchips and memory devices.

A biologic DNA programmer faces a multi-dimensional process. Instead of programming in ones and zeros, the machine language of the deoxyribonucleic acid (DNA) is a quaternary code. The DNA is comprised of four elements referred to as nucleotides: adenine, cytosine, guanine, and thymine. A fifth nucleotide is utilized when DNA is converted to ribonucleic acid (RNA). When RNA is generated by transcribing the DNA, the thymine nucleotide is replaced by the nucleotide uracil. In addition to a base four DNA code, there is a sixty-four code language to represent twenty amino acids.

Amino acids represent the building blocks of proteins. The human body can generate approximately 30,000 differing proteins. Proteins comprise the brick and mortar to construct individual cells. In the larger picture, proteins provide the means to build, operate and maintain the many complex structures comprising a multicellular organism such as the human body.

The arrangement of the nucleotides comprising the DNA quaternary code provides the data necessary to construct the 30,000 individual proteins. A unit of three nucleotides is termed a codon. A codon codes for an amino acid. Stringing codons together into sequences allows for amino acids to be merged together to construct proteins. Given there are four nucleic acids that comprise the DNA, the differing combinations of the four nucleotides allows for sixty-four possible codons. Except for the amino acid methionine, the amino acids are represented by at least two codons. Three amino acids arginine, leucine and serine are represented by six different codons.

Amino acids represent differing molecules. The base of the molecule is generally the same amongst the amino acids comprising an amino group (NH_2), carboxyl group (COOH) and a carbon atom. Amino acids are generically represented as $NH_2CHRCOOH$ where the R represents a side chain. The side chains differ amongst the amino acids conferring different molecular properties to the amino acids. Given the differing configurations of the side chains the twenty amino acids, an amino acid may be classified as: nucleophilic, hydrophobic, aromatic, acidic, amide or basic.

In addition to amino acids being assembled together to generate proteins to produce a wide variety of differing cellular structures, amino acids can be sequenced together to produce proteins that are capable of transferring from the cytoplasm where they are constructed to the inner chamber of the nucleus and bond to specific sequences of nuclear DNA.

DNA provides the template from which RNAs are generated. The RNA carries the codon code utilized to sequence amino acids to generate proteins. Refined RNA molecules migrate from the nucleus to the cytoplasm of the cell. Once in the cytoplasm, translation of the RNA results in production of proteins. Certain proteins, termed nuclear proteins, are able to act as feedback signals by entering the nucleus of the cell that generated the protein and effect function of the DNA.

In the case of some hormones, such as thyroid hormone, the nuclear protein is generated and excreted by one cell, to enter another cell, migrate to the nucleus of the target cell and generate a response in the target cell by effecting a change in the transcription of the target cell's DNA. Once a nuclear protein enters the nucleus of the cell, the nuclear protein seeks out a specific sequence of DNA and binds to the sequence, or the nuclear protein binds to and reconfigures a protein that is already bound to the DNA. Both forms of nuclear proteins regulate transcription of a specific gene embedded in the DNA.

Where the digital computer programmer writes computer programs in terms of base two: comprised of zeros and ones, the DNA programmer must think in terms of base four: comprised of zeros, ones, twos and threes. The DNA programmer must also consider the composition of the four nucleotides arranged into codons and the physical characteristics and behavior of the twenty amino acids when it comes to the molecules being nucleophilic, hydrophobic, aromatic, acidic, amide and basic.

This text steps through the concepts of designing a nucleotide sequence to be embedded into the nuclear DNA of a vulnerable human cell, so as to fortify the cell against invasion by the HIV genome by providing the human cell the means to effectively repel the HIV genome if HIV's RNA is inserted into the cell. Once perfected, such technology will be able to be expanded to treat a wide variety of challenging medical conditions. Such a strategy would afford medical therapy to target most virus genomes and many bacterial pathogens. The principles of this therapy could also be expanded to target onco genes, which contribute to the development of cancer and neutralize lethal inherited pathologic genes, which result in inherited disease states.

This text does not represent the efforts of the first DNA programmers. The final pages of this text provide analysis of HIV-1 HXB2 genome, which is constructed with a Base-3/Base-4 frame-shifting bio-programming data compression technique. The HIV genome represents a computer technology far more complex/efficient than current digital computer technology. This is explicit evidence DNA programmers have previously participated in the design/construct of the genomic programming responsible for the biology/ecology abundantly thriving across the surface of planet Earth.

TABLE OF CONTENTS

POST SCRIPTS

PROPOSALS TO DEVELOP DNA VACCINES
UTILIZING A VIRTUAL LAB

CHAPTER 1

OVERVIEW
OBJECTIVE: DESIGN A GENE TO SILENCE THE HIV GENOME TO ERADICATE AIDS

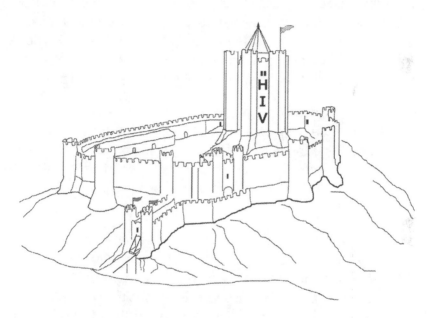

The Human Immunodeficiency Virus (HIV) is believed to have originated in non-human primates in West-central Africa and to have transferred to humans in the early 1900's. Well-documented cases of HIV in humans did not become apparent until about 1959. It is believed that the virus first arrived in the United States in about 1966. HIV spreads by a number of means and has expanded into a worldwide epidemic. There are approximately 35 million people currently living with HIV, more than a million in the US alone. HIV is the underlying cause of Acquired Immunodeficiency Syndrome (AIDS). Tens of millions of people have died of AIDS-related causes since the beginning of the epidemic. There exist means to slow down HIV's replication process, but currently there is no cure to eradicate HIV virion production from an infected body.

The Human Immunodeficiency Virus (HIV) genome embeds its genetic coding into the nuclear genome of the human T-Helper cell. Once the HIV genome becomes inserted into the T-Helper cell's nuclear DNA, in essence HIV is protected by at least two layers of shielding. Embedded HIV genome is likened to a king in a castle. HIV is protected by the exterior membrane of the T-Helper cell and the interior membrane of the nucleus; similar to a king in a castle protected by the exterior walls of the castle and the interior keep of the castle. To successfully go after HIV and eradicate the virus's genetic footprint, one needs to target the HIV virus as it resides embedded in the nuclear DNA of the T-Helper cell. The act of eradicating HIV is similar to breaching the exterior walls of a castle and pursuing HIV into the interior chambers of the keep of the castle.

There are four zones of targeting a virus such as HIV. Zone-One is the extracellular environment. Zone-Two is the cytoplasmic environment inside the cell membrane excluding the nucleus of the cell. Zone-Three refers to the cytoplasmic environment inside the nucleus of the cell. Zone-Four refers to viral genetics embedded in the nuclear DNA.

The aim of this effort is to develop a strategy to make cells defensible against pathologic viruses. To accomplish this task involves designing a molecule that is capable of seeking out the genome of a virus such as HIV and neutralizing the viral genome's capacity to be transcribed. If a viral genome cannot be transcribed, then the life-cycle of the virus is terminated and the viral genome is no longer a threat to the cell or the body as a whole. Studying the mechanism used by the nuclear machinery of a cell to transcribe a gene provides clues to targets that can be exploited. The architecture of the transcription machinery also provides potential molecules that can be modified to seek out the exploitable nuclear targets.

To take on such a challenge as to target HIV as it exists embedded in the nuclear DNA of the T-Helper cell one must take aim at a specific target in the HIV genome that is unique to HIV and not found in the remaining human genome. HIV contains a twenty-five character unique identifier existing between the TATA box and the Transcription Start Site. This unique identifier is a biologic target specific to HIV, not found in the human genome, which can be exploited to act as an inimitable antiviral therapeutic target.

The Transcription Factor IIIA (TFIIIA) molecule is a protein that is utilized in the assembly of a transcription complex used in association with Polymerase III to read rRNA genes and viral genes. The TFIIIA molecule is comprised of nine zinc finger loops, which are utilized to bind to neighboring structures. Five of the zinc finger loops (1-5) bind directly to nuclear DNA. The remaining four zinc finger loops (6-9) bind to other proteins required in the assembly of a transcription complex. Manipulation of the binding characteristics of the zinc finger loops that bind to the DNA allows for the construct of TFIIIA molecules that will target unique identifiers of viral genomes. By constructing amino acid sequences in the zinc finger loops of a modified TFIIIA molecule that will permanently bind to a specific segment of viral DNA or RNA offers the means of neutralizing intracellular viral genomes.

By reverse engineering the mRNA required to generate the modified TFIIIA molecule and then reverse engineering the gene to produce then the gene intended to produce the mRNA, an embeddable DNA vaccine aimed at repelling a specific intracellular viral genome becomes possible. Using means similar to how the HIV genome is transported to a T-Helper cell, a therapeutic embeddable DNA vaccine could be delivered to vulnerable cells in the body; once inserted into a human cell, the DNA vaccine would be inserted into the nuclear DNA of the cell. The embeddable DNA vaccine would then lay dormant until the cell was threatened by a specific viral infection.

The model of targeting and neutralizing pathologic viral genomes by generating modified TFIIIA molecules to seek out a genomic unique identifier specific to the viral genome can be expanded to include treatment of numerous other disease states. Cancer causing genes and pathologic genes associated with the development of genetic disorders, such as Huntington's Chorea, can be targeted and neutralized in a similar manner as described above. Any disease state where a unique identifier is definable, could be treated by designing a modified TFIIIA molecule or similar protein to seek out and bind to the unique identifier in an effort to prevent the genome from being transcribed, thus neutralizing the threat be it infection, cancer or genetic disorder. The number of therapeutic molecules that are possible as a result of this approach are limited only by the number of disease states that involve a pathologic DNA or RNA sequence.

CHAPTER 2

BRIEF REVIEW OF THE HIV VIRION AND LIFE CYCLE

The Human Immunodeficiency Virus (HIV) is believed to have originated in non-human primates in West-central Africa and to have transferred to humans in the early 1900's. Well-documented cases of HIV in humans did not appear until about 1959. It is believed that the virus arrived in the United States in about 1966. HIV spreads by a number of means and has expanded into a worldwide epidemic. There are approximately 35 million people currently living with HIV, more than a million in the US alone. HIV is the underlying cause of Acquired Immunodeficiency Syndrome (AIDS). Tens of millions of people have died of AIDS-related causes since the beginning of the epidemic. There exist means to slow down HIV's replication process, but currently there is no cure to eradicate HIV virions production from an infected body.

In Volume III of this series a unique identifier for the HIV genome was reported. This discovery gave rise to the concept that HIV could be stopped by attacking the HIV genome at the DNA level. This led to an effort to determine a cure for those infected with the virus. In Volume IV of this series, a Transcription Factor IIIA molecule was modified to take advantage of HIV's unique identifier. The Transcription Factor IIIA's binding sites were modified to seek out and permanently bind to HIV's twenty-five nucleotide that act as the viral genome's unique identifier.

The primary function of a virus is to generate copies of itself. The ill effects that are experienced when one is infected by a virus may simply be related to the presence of the virus and the type of host cell the virus virion interacts with to effect replication. Some viruses, such as Ebola virus, possess elaborate means to cause a state of illness in its victim.

HUMAN IMMUNODEFICIENCY VIRUS

The Human Immunodeficiency Virus (HIV) virion is comprised of an outer coat made of a shell wrapped with an outer envelope. Mounted on the outer envelope are glycoprotein 120 (gp120) probes and glycoprotein 41 (gp41) probes. See Figure 1. The HIV virion uses the gp120 probes to seek out its host, a human T-Helper cell. The gp120 attaches to a CD4+ cell surface receptor on a T-Helper cell. Once the gp120 probe has made contact with a CD4+, a conformational channel change occurs in the gp120 probe, which allows the gp41 probe to become exposed and intercept the surface of the T-Helper cell. The gp41 probe interacts with either a CCR5 or CXCR4 cell-surface receptor on the exterior of the T-Helper cell. Once the gp41 probe successfully makes contact with the surface of the T-Helper cell, the gp41 probe's action facilitates in the opening of an access port in the exterior membrane of the T-Helper cell. With an access port open, the HIV virion injects the HIV RNA genome and proteins that it carries into the T-Helper cell. The proteins are used to facilitate the conversion of the HIV RNA genome to a DNA genome and in the insertion of the HIV DNA genome into the cell's nuclear DNA.

The HIV virion carries in its core two RNA strands and three different modifier enzymes. Each RNA strand is a positive stranded RNA approximately 9719 nucleotides in length. The three different proteins include an integrase enzyme, a reverse transcriptase enzyme and a protease enzyme. Once the HIV virion's genetic material has been inserted into the cytoplasm in the interior of a T-Helper cell, the reverse transcriptase and protease enzymes convert the HIV RNA to double stranded DNA (dsDNA). The integrase enzyme transports the HIV dsDNA into the nucleus of the T-Helper cell and inserts the HIV's dsDNA into the T-Helper cell's nuclear DNA. Once HIV's genetic material is integrated into the T-Helper cell's nuclear DNA it lays dormant until activated. HIV's genome may sit dormant for years, thus the virus is classified as a latent virus.

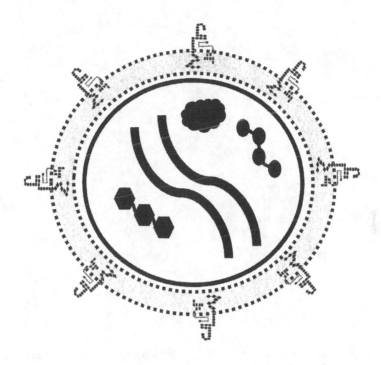

Figure 1 Illustration of an HIV virion

The life cycle of the Human Immunodeficiency Virus is presented in Figure 2. When triggered by the cell replication process, the HIV DNA genome takes command of the T-Helper cell's biologic machinery to produce numerous copies of the HIV virion. Upon release, the HIV virion becomes enveloped with the exterior of membrane of the T-Helper cell and seeks another T-Helper cell to infect.

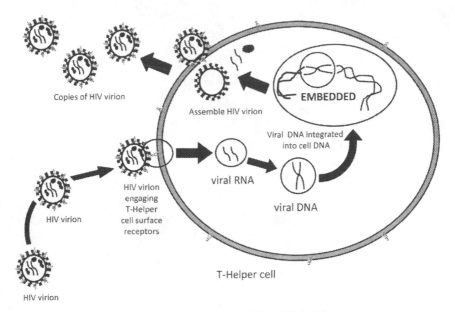

Figure 2 Life cycle of the HIV virion

HIV is a one dimensional virus, attacking the T-Helper cell, a second-line immune defender. Slowly HIV works to reduce the number of T-Helper cells resulting in the immune system becoming dysfunctional. AIDS occurs when the immune system weakens to the point the body becomes susceptible to other pathogens. Pathogens that infect a body in which the immune system has become compromised are generally referred to as opportunistic infections. HIV may not be the primary cause of death in some individuals, it may be the presence of one or more opportunistic infections that lead to a fatal outcome.

CHAPTER 3

BASIC GENETICS

THE CELL

A 'eukaryote' refers to a nucleated cell. Eukaryotes comprise nearly all animal and plant cells. A human eukaryote or nucleated cell is comprised of an exterior lipid bilayer plasma membrane, cytoplasm, a nucleus, and organelles. The exterior plasma membrane defines the perimeter of the cell, regulates the flow of nutrients, water and regulating molecules in and out of the cell, and has embedded into its structure receptors that the cell uses to detect properties of the environment surrounding the cell membrane. The cytoplasm acts as a filling medium inside the boundaries of the plasma cell membrane and is comprised mainly of water and nutrients such as amino acids, oxygen, and glucose.

The nucleus, organelles, and ribosomes are suspended in the cytoplasm. Organelles include the Golgi apparatus, mitochondria, smooth endoplasmic reticulum and vacuoles. See Figure 3. The Golgi apparatus constructs molecules and packages these molecules in a vacuole. Vacuoles act as cytoplasmic storage vessel for chemicals and a variety of proteins including hormones and enzymes. The mitochondria act as the powerhouse of the cell converting glucose into ATP, a form of utilizable chemical energy. The smooth endoplasmic reticulum constructs complex protein molecules.

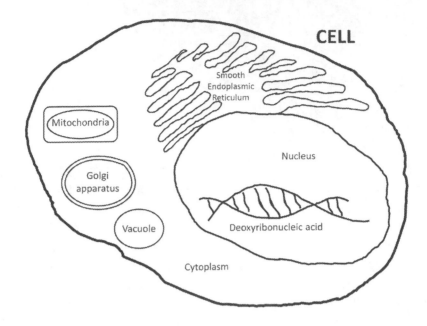

Figure 3   Basic cell design

The nucleus contains the majority of the cell's genetic information in the form of double stranded deoxyribonucleic acid (DNA). Human DNA is divided into 46 subunits referred to as chromosomes. The chromosomes are subdivided into information files referred to as genes. Genes undergo the process of transcription, which results in the production of messenger RNAs. Messenger RNAs migrate into the cytoplasm and undergo the process of translation to produce proteins.

Organelles generally carry out specialized functions for the cell and include such structures as the mitochondria, the endoplasmic reticulum, storage vacuoles, lysosomes and Golgi complex (sometimes referred to as a Golgi apparatus).

Suspended in the cytoplasm, but also located in the endoplasmic reticulum and mitochondria are cellular structures referred to as ribosomes. Ribosomes are complex macromolecules comprised of ribosomal ribonucleic acid (rRNA) molecules and ribosomal proteins that combine and couple to a messenger ribonucleic acid (mRNA) molecule. The rRNAs and the ribosomal proteins congregate to form a macromolecule structure that surrounds a mRNA molecule. Ribosomes decode genetic information in a mRNA molecule in a process refers to as translation to manufacture proteins to the specifications of the instruction code physically present in the mRNA molecule. More than one ribosome may be attached to a single mRNA at a time.

Proteins are comprised of a series of amino acids bonded together in a linear strand, referred to as a chain. The term 'protein' also refers to marcomolecules that may be comprised of one or more similar or differing strands of amino acids bonded together. Insulin is a protein structure comprised of two strands of amino acids; one strand comprised of 21 amino acids long and the second strand comprised of 30 amino acids. The two amino acid strands comprising the insulin molecule are linked by two disulfide bridges. There are an estimated 30,000 different proteins the cells of the human body may manufacture.

The human body is comprised of approximately 240 different cell types, many with specialized functions requiring unique combinations of proteins and protein structures such as glycoproteins (a protein combined with a carbohydrate) to accomplish the required task or tasks a specialized cell is designed to perform. Forms of glycoproteins are known to be utilized as cell-surface receptors.

On the surface of a eukaryote cell are cell surface receptors. Some of the receptors are functional as in the insulin receptor that regulates the cell's capacity to absorb glucose. Other cell surface receptors act as a means of communications. Differing combinations of cell surface receptors and markers act as the means to identify cells. The immune system of a multi-celled organism needs to know which cells are suppose to be present in the body of the organism and which cells may be acting as foreign invaders of the body. Some cell surface receptors are utilized as means to open pathways through the cell membrane.

ELEMENTS OF THE DNA

For purposes of this text, there are several general definitions. A 'ribose' is a five carbon or pentose sugar ($C_5H_{10}O_5$) present in the structural components of ribonucleic acid, riboflavin, and other nucleotides and nucleosides. A 'deoxyribose' is a deoxypentose $C_5H_{10}O_4$) found in deoxyribonucleic acid.

A 'nucleoside' is a compound of a sugar usually ribose or deoxyribose with a nitrogenous base by way of an N-glycosyl link. A 'nucleotide' is a single unit of a nucleic acid, composed of a five-carbon sugar (either a ribose or a deoxyribose), a nitrogenous base and a phosphate group. There are two families of 'nitrogenous bases', which include: pyrimidine and purine.

A 'pyrimidine' is a six-member ring made up of carbon and nitrogen atoms; the members of the pyrimidine family include: cytosine (c), thymine (t) and uracil (u). A 'purine' is a five-member ring fused to a pyrimidine type ring; the members of the purine family include: adenine (a) and guanine (g). See Figure 4. A 'nucleic acid' is a polynucleotide which is a biologic molecule such as ribonucleic acid (RNA) or deoxyribonucleic acid (DNA) that facilitates the reproduction of organisms.

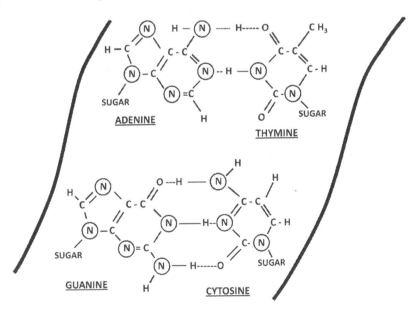

NUCLEOTIDES

Figure 4 Illustration of the four nucleotides comprising DNA

A 'ribonucleic acid' (RNA) is a linear polymer of nucleotides formed by repeated riboses linked by phosphodiester bonds between the 3-hydroxyl group of one and the 5-hydroxyl group of the next. RNAs are a single strand macromolecule comprised of a sequence of nucleotides. These nucleotides are generally referred to by their nitrogenous bases, which include: adenine, cytosine, guanine and uracil. RNAs are subset into different types, which include messenger RNA (mRNA), transport RNA (tRNA), ribosomal RNA (rRNA) and a variety of small RNAs.

A ribosome is a complex comprised of rRNAs and proteins. The ribosome is responsible for the correct positioning of a mRNA and charged tRNA to facilitate the proper alignment and bonding of amino acids into a strand to produce a protein. A 'charged' tRNA is a tRNA that is carrying an amino acid. Ribosomal RNA (rRNA) represents a subset of RNAs that form part of the physical structure of a ribosome. Small RNAs include snoRNA, U snRNA, and miRNA. The snoRNAs modify precursor rRNA molecules. U snRNAs modify precursor mRNA molecules. The miRNA molecules modify the function of mRNA molecules.

A 'deoxyribose' is a deoxypentose ($C_5H_{10}O_4$) sugar. Deoxyribonucleic acid (DNA) is comprised of three basic elements: a deoxyribose sugar, a phosphate group and nitrogen containing bases. DNA is a macromolecule made up of two chains of repeating deoxyribose sugars linked by phosphodiester bonds between the 3-hydroxyl group of one and the 5-hydroxyl group of the next; the two chains are held antiparallel to each other by weak hydrogen bonds. DNA strands contain a sequence of nucleotides, which include: adenine, cytosine, guanine and thymine. Adenine is always paired with thymine of the opposite strand, and guanine is always paired with cytosine of the opposite strand; one side or strand of a DNA macromolecule is the mirror image of the opposite strand. Nuclear DNA is regarded as the medium for storing the master plan of hereditary information including information regarding the construct and maintenance of an organism.

Genes are considered segments of the DNA that represent units of inheritance.

Chromosomes exist in the nucleus of a cell and consist of a DNA double helix bearing a linear sequence of genes, coiled and recoiled around aggregated proteins, termed histones. The number of chromosomes varies from species to species. Most Human cells carries twenty two pairs of chromosomes plus two sex chromosomes; two 'x' chromosomes in women and one 'x' and one 'y' chromosome in men.

Chromosomes carry genetic information in the form of units, which are referred to as genes. The entire nuclear genome, forty-six chromosomes, is comprised of 3 billion base pairs of nucleotides. As an example, the human genome is considered to be comprised of 30,000 genes, approximately one gene for each protein the human body constructs. It is possible one gene directs the construct of more than one protein. Viral genomes harbor the templates to produce multiple proteins.

The instruction codes necessary to assemble the estimated 30,000 proteins into intracellular and extracellular structures has yet to be deciphered.

CONSTRUCT OF A GENE

Current gene theory is derived from Gregor Mendel (1822-1884), who discovered the basic principles of heredity by breeding garden peas at the abbey where he resided, while teaching at Brunn Modern School. Gregor Mendel built and documented a model of inheritance, often referred to as Mendelian genetics, which has acted as the foundation of modern genetics. Gregor Mendel documented changes in characteristics of the plants he grew and described the physical traits as being related to 'heritable factors'. Over time Mendel's term 'heritable factor' has been replaced by the terms 'gene' and 'allele'. Much of what the current term 'gene' describes remains related to and distinctly linked to the physical traits of the live organisms they describe.

Per J. K. Pal, S.S. Ghaskabi, *Fundamentals of Molecular Biology*, 2009: 'The central dogma of molecular biology...states that the genes present in the genome (DNA) are transcribed into mRNAs, which are then translated into polypeptides or proteins, which are phenotypes.' 'Genome, thus, contains the complete set of hereditary information for any organism and is functionally divided into small parts referred to as genes. Each gene is a sequence of nucleotides representing a protein and/or a RNA. The genome of a living organism may contain as few as 500 genes as in case of Mycoplasma, or as many as an estimated 30,000 genes as in case of human beings.' Viruses, being intracellular pathogens, are comprised of genomes which contain far fewer genes. In the case of Ebola virus, there are only seven genes comprising the genome.

As a matter of comparison, current computer technology utilizes the binary numeric language. Every task a computer performs is related to the language of 'zeros' and 'ones'. Transistors that comprise the inside of computer chips are either turned 'off' representing a 'zero' or turned 'on' representing a 'one'. At the core of all computer programs is the machine language of 'zeros' and 'ones'. The most sophisticated central processing unit (CPU) in the world only reads and processes the language of 'zeros' and 'ones'. All text, all pictures, all video, all sound and music is diluted down to the form of 'zeros' and 'ones', and consequently all of the computing and storage power of a computer is performed by the computer language of 'zeros' and 'ones' referred to as machine language.

The nucleus of a biologically active cell arguably possesses the most sophisticated and well-organized processing power in the world. To run such a powerful processing unit, a form of biologic computer language would seem to be a necessary foundation by which to transfer stored information from the DNA to the remainder of the biologically active portions of a cell as needed. Given that the DNA comprising the chromosomes and mitochondrial DNA are both comprised of four different nucleotides including adenosine, cytosine, guanine and thymine, and RNA is comprised of four nucleotides including adenosine, cytosine, guanine and uracil (uracil in place of thymine), it appears evident the biologic computer language used by a cell's genome is an information language derived from base-four mathematics. Instead of current computer technology utilizing binary computer code comprised of 'zeros' and 'ones', the DNA and RNA in a biologically active cell utilize an information language comprised of 'zeros', 'ones', twos' and 'threes' to store and transfer information, which represents a base-four language or quaternary language.

The above definitions of a 'gene' refer to genes residing in a specific place or locus on a chromosome. Identifying that a gene is present in a particular location is obvious to the human observer, but from a functional standpoint for cell biology this does not necessarily help a cell find or use the information stored in the nucleotide sequence of a particular gene. To rely on location alone, as a means of identifying a gene, would put the function of the entire genome at peril of failure if even a single base pair of nucleotides were added or deleted from the genome.

The current understanding of the actual biologic structure of a gene is far more elaborate than the standard definition of a gene leads a casual reader to believe; this knowledge has evolved greatly since Gregor Mendel's work in the 19th century. A gene appears to be comprised of a number of segments loosely strung together along a particular section of DNA. In general, there are at least three global segments associated with a gene that include: (1) the Upstream 5' flanking region, (2) the transcriptional unit and (3) the Downstream 3' flanking region. See Figure 5. The term 'upstream' refers to DNA sequencing that occurs prior to the Transcription Start Site (TSS) if viewed from the 5' end to the 3' end of the DNA; while the term 'downstream' refers to DNA sequencing located after the TSS.

NUCLEAR DNA QUANTUM GENE

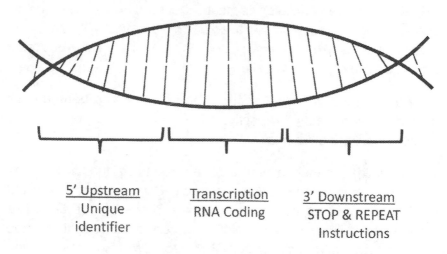

5' Upstream
Unique
identifier

Transcription
RNA Coding

3' Downstream
STOP & REPEAT
Instructions

Figure 5 Basic structure of a gene

The Upstream 5' flanking region of a gene is comprised of the 'enhancer region', the 'promoter-proximal region', and 'promoter region'.

The 'transcriptional unit' begins reading the gene at a location designated the TSS, which is located in a site called the 'initiator region' (inR), which may be described in a general form as Py_2CAPy_5. The transcription unit is comprised of the combination of segments of DNA nucleotides to be transcribed into RNA and spacing units known as 'introns' that are not transcribed or if transcribed are later removed post transcription, such that they do not appear in the final RNA molecule. In the case of a gene coding for a mRNA molecule, the transcription unit will contain all three elements of the mRNA, which includes: (1) the 5' noncoding region, (2) the translational region and (3) the 3' noncoding region.

The Downstream 3' flanking region contains DNA nucleotides that are not transcribed and may contain what has been termed an 'enhancer region'. An enhancer region in the Downstream 3' flanking region may promote the gene previously transcribed to be transcribed again.

An 'enhancer region' may or may not be present in the Upstream 5' flanking region. If present in the Upstream 5' flanking region, the enhancer region helps facilitate the reading of the gene by encouraging formation of the transcription mechanism. An enhancer may be 50 to 1500 base pairs in length occupying a position upstream from the transcription start site.

On either side of the DNA sequencing comprising a gene and its flanking regions, may be inactive DNA, which act as boundaries, termed 'insulator elements'.

The 'transcription mechanism', also referred to as 'the transcription machinery' or the 'transcription complex' (TC) in humans, is reported to be comprised of over forty separate proteins that assemble together to ultimately function in a concerted effort to transcribe the nucleotide sequence of the DNA into RNA. The transcription mechanism includes elements such as 'general transcription factor Sp1', 'general transcription factor NF1', 'general transcription factor TATA-binding protein', 'TF$_{II}$D', 'basal transcription complex', and a 'RNA polymerase protein' to name only a few of the approximately seventy proposed elements that may combine to form a transcription complex. The elements of the transcription mechanism function as (1) a means to recognize the location of the start of a gene, (2) as proteins to bind the transcription mechanism to the DNA such that transcription may occur and (3) as means of transcribing the DNA nucleotide coding to produce a RNA molecule or a precursor RNA molecule.

There are at least three RNA polymerase proteins, which include: RNA polymerase I, RNA polymerase II, and RNA polymerase III. RNA polymerase I tends to be dedicated to transcribing genetic information that will result in the formation of rRNA molecules. RNA polymerase II tends to be dedicated to transcribing genetic information that will result in the formation of mRNA molecules. RNA polymerase III appears to be dedicated to transcribing genetic information that results in the formation of tRNAs, small cellular RNAs and viral RNAs.

The 'promoter proximal region' is located upstream from the TSS and upstream from the core promoter region. See Figure 6. The 'promoter proximal region' includes two sub-regions termed the GC box and the CAAT box. The 'GC box' appears to be a segment rich in guanine-cytosine nucleotide sequences. The GC box binds to the 'general transcription factor Sp1' of the transcription mechanism. The 'CAAT box' is a segment which contains the nucleotide sequence 'ggccaatct' located approximately 75 base pairs (bps) upstream from the transcription start site (TSS). The CAAT box binds to the 'general transcription factor NF1' of the transcription mechanism.

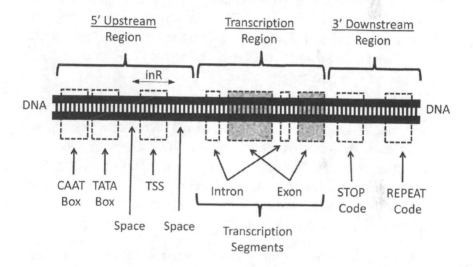

Figure 6 Detailed structure of a gene

e 'core promoter' region is considered the shortest sequence within which RNA polymerase II can initiate transcription of a gene The core promoter may include the inR and either a TATA box or a 'downstream promoter element' (DPE). The inR is the region designated Py_2CAPy_5 that surrounds the transcription start site (TSS). The TATA box is located 25 base pairs (bps) upstream from the TSS. The TATA box acts as a site of attachment of the $TF_{II}D$, which is a promoter for binding of the RNA polymerase II molecule. The DPE may appear 28 bps to 32 bps downstream from the TSS. The DPE may act as an alternative site of attachment for the $TF_{II}D$ when the TATA box is not present.

The transcription mechanism or transcription complex appears to be comprised of different elements depending upon whether rRNA is being transcribed versus mRNA or tRNA or small cellular RNA or viral RNA. The proteins that assemble to assist RNA Polymerase I with transcribing the DNA to produce rRNA appear different from the proteins that assemble to assist RNA polymerase II with transcribing the DNA to produce mRNA and from the proteins that assemble to assist RNA polymerase III with transcribing the DNA to produce tRNA, small cellular RNA or viral RNA. A common protein that appears to be present at the initial binding of all three types of RNA polymerase molecules is TATA-binding protein (TBP). TBP appears to be required to attach to the DNA, which then facilitates RNA polymerase to bind to the promoter along the DNA. TBP assembles with TBP-associated factors (TAFs). Together TBP and 11 TAFs comprise the complex referred to as $TF_{II}D$.

Upstream from the TATA box is the 'initiator element', which may be considered as part of the 'core promoter' region. The initiator element is a segment of the nuclear DNA that binds the basal transcription complex. The basal transcription complex is comprised of a number of proteins that make initial contact with the DNA prior to the RNA polymerase binding to the transcription mechanism. The basal transcription complex is associated with an activator.

An activator is a protein comprised of three components. The three components of the activator include: (1) DNA binding domain, (2) Connecting domain, and (3) Activating domain. When the activator's DNA binding domain attaches to the DNA at a specific point along the DNA, the activator's activating domain then causes the other elements of the transcription mechanism to assemble at this location. Generally, the assembly of the other proteins occurs downstream from where the activator's DNA binding domain attached to the DNA. There is evidence that the activator is associated with the activity of small RNAs.

The design of the cell is so complex, all of its functions so diverse and intricate that some form of practical order is necessitated. The genes must be ordered in some fashion, especially in a human, where there are at least 30,000 different genes used by the cells. Some estimates put the total number of genes present in the human nuclear DNA genome to be closer to 100,000. If no means of order existed as to how the genes could be identified, then 'random circumstance' would dictate a cell locating a particular portion of genetic information that it requires, at any given time. Randomness tends to favor the occurrence of random events rather than a purposeful order. A 'random circumstance' approach to any living cell would tend to favor failure of the cell rather than survival of the cell.

TRANSCRIPTION: DECODING OF DNA PRODUCES RNA

The majority of the cell's DNA comprises the chromosomes, which are double stranded helical structures located in the nucleus of the cell. DNA in a circular form, can also be found in the mitochondria, the powerhouse of the cell, the organelle that converts glucose into energy molecules termed adenosine triphosphate (ATP). ATP molecules are utilized to provide energy for cellular chemical reactions. DNA represents the genetic information a cell needs to manufacture the materials it requires to sustain life and to replicate. Genetic information is stored in the DNA by arrangements of four nucleotides referred to as: adenine, thymine, guanine and cytosine. DNA represents instruction coding, that in the process known as transcription, the DNA's genetic information is decoded by transcription protein complexes referred to as polymerases (or polymerase complex), to produce ribonucleic acid (RNA). RNA is a single strand of genetic information comprised of coded arrangements of four nucleotides: adenine, uracil, guanine and cytosine. In a RNA, 'uracil' takes the place of 'thymine', thymine being present in the DNA. Several different types of RNAs have been identified, which include messenger RNAs (mRNA), transport RNAs (tRNA) and ribosomal RNAs (rRNA).

TRANSLATION: DECODING OF RNA PRODUCES PROTEIN

Proteins are comprised of a series of amino acids bonded together in a linear strand. Messenger RNAs (mRNA) are created by transcription of DNA to act as the blueprints to generate proteins. See Figure 7. Messenger RNA generated by transcription of nuclear DNA, migrate out of the nucleus of the cell, and are utilized as protein manufacturing templates by ribosomes. Different mRNAs code for different proteins. As previously mentioned, there are as many as 30,000 varieties of proteins, therefore there are at least 30,000 different mRNA molecules.

A ribosome is a protein complex that manufactures proteins by deciphering the instruction code located in a mRNA molecule. When a specific protein is needed, pieces of the ribosome complex bind around the strand of mRNA that carries the specific instruction code that will generate the required protein. The ribosome traverses the mRNA strand and deciphers the genetic information coded into the sequence of nucleotides that comprise the mRNA molecule.

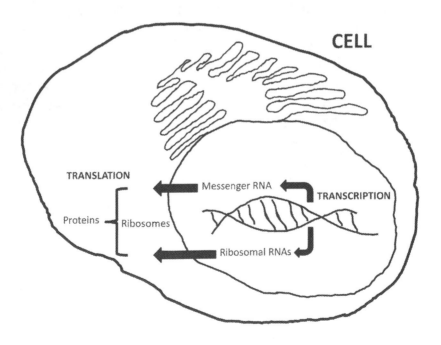

Figure 7 Process of transcription to translation

The construct of a ribosome is macromolecule comprised of ribosomal RNA (rRNA) molecules and ribosomal proteins. Ribosomal RNAs and ribosomal proteins are often designated with a number measured in Svedberg (S) units, which represents the sediment coefficient. The sediment coefficient is influenced by both molecular weight of the molecule and surface area of the molecule. In humans there are generally recognized at this time two mitochondrial rRNAs identified as 12S rRNA and 16S rRNA, and there are generally recognized four rRNAs that reside in the cytoplasm of a cell identified as 5S rRNA, 5.8S rRNA, 18S rRNA and 28S rRNA. There may be other rRNAs, as of yet unidentified, that reside in some of the other structures in the cell that engage in manufacturing of macromolecules, such as the smooth endoplasmic reticulum, the rough endoplasmic reticulum and the Golgi complex.

In eukaryotes, in the cytoplasm, the ribosome complex is referred to as an 80S ribosome. Generally, two ribosomal proteins and two rRNA molecules comprise a ribosome complex. This 80S ribosome is comprised of one 'dome-shape' 60S ribosomal protein and one 'cap-shaped' 40S ribosomal protein.

In the forms of life referred to as vertebrates (Humans are classified as a form of vertebrate), of the four rRNAs that reside in the cytoplasm of a eukaryote cell, the 18S rRNA is found in and helps comprise the physical structure of the 40S protein subunit of the ribosome complex and the 5S rRNA, 5.8S rRNA, and 28S rRNA molecules are found in and help comprise the physical structure of the 60S protein subunit of the ribosome complex.

The rRNA molecules are thought to provide at least three different functions for the ribosome complex. The rRNA molecules are thought to: (1) assist with identification of the messenger RNA to be translated, (2) act as an enzyme to facilitate the production of the protein molecule being translated, and (3) possibly cause folding at certain locations in the three dimensional structure of the protein being generated as the ribosome complex decodes the mRNA molecule.

Transport RNAs (tRNA) are constructed in the nucleus or in the mitochondria, and are coded for one of the 20 amino acids the cells of the human body use to construct proteins. Once a tRNA is created by transcription of the DNA, the tRNA seeks out the type of amino acid it has been coded for and attaches to that specific amino acid. The tRNA then delivers the amino acid it carries to a ribosome that is waiting for that specific amino acid. Proteins are manufactured by the ribosomes binding together sequences of amino acids. The order by which the amino acids are bonded together is dictated by the way the mRNA is constructed and how the ribosome interprets the information encoded in the string of nucleotides present in the mRNA strand.

A sequence of three nucleotides present in a mRNA molecule represents a unit of information referred to as a codon. Codons code for all of the 20 amino acids used to construct protein molecules and also for START and STOP commands. In the process known as translation, the ribosome decodes the codons present in the mRNA, initiating the protein manufacturing process at a START codon, then interfacing with tRNAs carrying the amino acids that match the sequence of codons in the mRNA as the ribosome traverses the length of the mRNA molecule. The ribosome functions as a protein factory by taking amino acids delivered by tRNAs and binding the amino acids together in the order dictated by the sequence of codon instructions coded into the mRNA template as directed by the manner of the nucleic acid arrangement in the mRNA molecule. Protein synthesis ceases when a ribosome encounters a STOP code. Once complete, the protein molecule is released by the ribosome.

CHAPTER 4

ANALYSIS OF THE mRNA STRUCTURE OF THE HBX2 STRAIN OF THE HIV-1 GENOME

We have studied the HIV-1 genome for many years as we consider it to be an excellent teaching tool. The detail about it including how it enters the T-Helper cell, becomes attached to the cell's DNA and reproduces to form new HIV-1 virions has given us a new perspective on the role of viruses and their impact on the evolution of life forms[1]. We have always been fascinated by the diagrams used to illustrate the positions of the genes in the HIV-1 genome. For example, when one looks at a gene map of the HIV genome like the one in Reference 1 (Landmarks), shown here as Figure 8, one gets the feeling that Nature just jumbled the genes together into the genome. The fact that some genes overlap others and some have parts at distant locations gives rise to the feeling that this is never going to work. However, we know that that is not true and, in fact, it turns out to be very interesting.

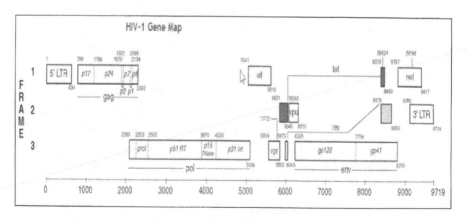

Figure 8 Landmarks of the HIV-1 Genome
Gene Map for HXB2 Strain

---

[1] See Volumes 2 and 3 of Changing the Global Approach to Medicine.

As we sought to improve our understanding of the HIV genome at the DNA level we came across Reference 2 (Ocwieja) which describes the layout of the mRNAs for the HIV-189.6 strain of the virus. As an aid to understanding the material in the reference, we decided to try to apply the techniques therein to the HBX2 strain of HIV-1, which we have been working with (Reference 2, NCBI). As we attempted to apply the techniques, we realize that we must keep in mind two issues. Reference 2 (Ocwieja) contains a great deal of laboratory results and these results show that there are many possible combinations of mRNAs that the cells might use to create the required HIV-1 proteins. Thus, it became our objective to simply identify a representative and consistent set of mRNAs that makes some sense. Attempting to identify the best or optimum set is beyond the scope of this effort.

Material

The specific code we have been working with is referred to as GenBank K03455.1 (NCBI, 3). An abbreviated and annotated version of the code can be found in the Appendix. Additional material is available in the references, especially in the Supplemental Tables of Reference 2 (Ocwieja).

Analysis

1. Overview

We have previously discussed the HBX2 strain of the HIV-1 virus in some detail[2]. Here we merely make note of the location of the TATA box starting at 427 position and the 25 nucleotide sequence ID directly following the TATA box as shown in the Appendix. As noted in the Appendix, Reference 3 (NCBI) has the transcription start site (TSS) beginning at position 455, but Reference 4 (Excel), which elaborates on the data in the genome, indicates the mRNA starts at 456. Our results are not sensitive to the position of the TSS as both lead to the same results.

---

[2] Volumes 2 and 3 of Changing the Global Approach to Medicine.

2. Approach

When the HIV genome is read by the polymerase II it produces a pre-mRNA which is then used to create a number of mRNAs which are used to produce the HIV proteins. Reference 2 (Ocwieja) specifies that the mRNAs have two forms, spliced and unspliced. We examine the unspliced version first and then proceed to those that are spliced. For the unspliced version, we will use the data in reference 3 (NCBI) in the analyses. For the spliced versions we will describe the degree to which we are able to apply the techniques in reference 2 (Ocwieja) to the HBX2 strain.

3. Unspliced mRNA

The unspliced form of the HIV mRNA, which we refer to as mRNA1, is used to produce the proteins in the gag and pol groups. The data in the reference sequence (Reference 3, NCBI) specifies that the start codon for the gag group, which is an ATG, is located in positions 790-92 and that the stop codon for the group is in positions 2290-92 which is a TAA stop code. We note that this stop codon is followed by a second stop codon just one codon away, at locations 2296-98. This stop codon is a TAG; we refer to this mRNA as mRNA1a.

Further, the data in the reference sequence (Reference 3, NCBI) specifies that the start codon for the pol group, which is a ATG, is located in positions 2358-60 and that the stop codon for the group is in positions 5094-96, which is a TAG stop code. We refer to this mRNA as mRNA1b.

Both of these groups of proteins are translated as sets without internal stop codons.

4. Spliced mRNAs

The remainder of the HIV proteins are produced from mRNAs that have undergone splicing. To understand how the each of these proteins is produced we must understand how each of the mRNAs is spliced together. Here we utilize the data in Reference 2 (Ocwieja).

As a first step we identify the location of the initial splice site of the first intron. From Supplementary Table 5 of Reference 2 (Ocwieja) (Note: Supplementary tables are referenced, but not presented in this text.) we see that all of the HIV-1$_{89.6}$ mRNAs have the same initial set of code. For those that are spliced, that initial set ends at a position identified as D1. Supplemental Table 3 in Reference 2 (Ocwieja) specifies that D1 has a splice site code sequence of tg|GTgagt where the left most 'g' is at the 742 position, the symbol "|" indicates the splice site cut (i.e., the separation of the exon and the intron), and G, at the 743 position, represents the first base of the intron being removed.

Examining the HXB2 data in the appendix, we note that this same splice code sequence appears in this version with the donor 'g' base in position 743. From this we conclude that all of the spliced mRNAs have the same nucleotides in their 456-743 positions. It is noted that this removes the gag and pol groups start codons from being involved in any of the remaining mRNAs. Part of the task in the following is to locate the start and stop codons for each of the proteins in each of the spliced mRNAs.

Next we extract the data from the supplemental tables for the remainder of the proteins[3]. This data is shown in Table 1. The Splice Position Ref is shown as it is the key to relating the protein in Supplemental Table 5 (not shown here) to the Splice Position and Splice Site Sequence in Supplemental Table 3 (not shown here). In the data shown in the Splice Site Sequence column, the G on the left side of the separator "|" is the end of the intron that is removed. We will now attempt to locate these splice sites in the HXB2 strain.

Protein	Splice Position Ref	Splice Position[4]	Splice Site Sequence
Vif	A1	4912	cgggtttattacAG|g
Vpr	A2	5389	tgattgttttcAG|a

---

[3] There are many choices here, but as stated in the beginning, our objective is simply to identify a representative and consistent set of mRNAs that makes some sense.

Tat	A3	5776	tttattcatttcAG	a
Rev	A4c	5935	ctttcattgccaAG	c
Vpu	A5	5975	atctcctatggcAG	g
Env	Unclear	-	-
Nef	A7	8368	cattatcgtttcAG	a

Table 1

Splice Site Data from Supplemental Table
3 in Reference 2 (Ocwieja).

As we identify the sequences that potentially makeup the mRNA for each of the proteins, we need to assess, for each protein, three characteristics in addition to how well the splice site sequence from the reference matches the one found in the HXB2 strain. First, we need to identify the start codon for the protein and be sure that no start codon occurs before it. Second, we need to locate the stop codon. Third, we need to make sure that sequence can generate the correct protein. We will use the first and last 6 or 7 amino acids generated as a validation of that. Further, given that the DNA code prior to the 743 cut contains the initial binding site for the reader for the gag group, we will assume that the reader for all of the spliced mRNAs use that site as well. Further, as noted above, it contains no start or stop codons.

a. mRNA2 – Vif Protein

Using the data in Supplementary Table 3 for the Vif protein we find the same Splice Site Sequence for A1 located in the HXB2 strain with the G of the intron to be spliced out located at position 4912. Thus, this mRNA results from the splicing of the 'g' at 743 to the 'g' at 4913. The first start codon (atg) after the splice appears at location 5041-43 and it is the start of the Vif protein. The protein ends with the stop codon (tag) at positions 5617-19. The sequence has (5620-5041 =) 193 codons and starts with amino acid sequence MENRWQV and

---

[4] Position of first base in exon being spliced to in HIV89.6 strain.

ends with amino acid sequence HTMNGH which agrees with those shown in Reference 3 (NCBI).

b. mRNA3 – Vpr Protein

Using the data in Supplementary Table 3 for the Vpr protein we find nearly the same Splice Site Sequence for A2 located in the HXB2 strain with the G of the intron to be spliced out located at position 5389. The only exception being that the HXB2 strain has a 'c' instead of a 't' in position 5379. Thus, this mRNA results from the splicing of the 'g' at 743 to the 'a' at 5390. The first start codon (atg) after the splice appears at location 5559-61 and it is the start of the Vpr protein. The protein ends with the stop codon (tag) at positions 5793-95. The sequence has (5796-5559 =) 79 codons and starts with amino acid sequence MEQAPED and ends with amino acid sequence QNWVST which agrees with those shown in reference 3 (NCBI).

c. mRNA4 – Tat Protein

Using the data in Supplementary Table 3 for the Tat protein we find nearly the same Splice Site Sequence for A3 located in the HXB2 strain with the G of the intron to be spliced out located at position 5777. The only exceptions being that HXB2 has a 'c' instead of a 't' in position 5768 and an added 't' in position 5774.Thus, this mRNA partially results from the splicing of the 'g' at 743 to the 'a' at 5778. The first start codon (atg) after the splice appears at location 5831-33 and it is the start of the Tat protein.

Reference 2 (Ocwieja) specifies that the mRNA for Tat undergoes additional splicing to remove a second intron. Using the Slice Site Sequence of ca|GTaagt for cut D4 as given in the reference, the second intron is found to start with the G in positions 6046. The end of the intron is defined by the G in the Splice Site Sequence cattatcgtttcAG|a for A7, which is found at position 8378 in the HXB2 strain. Thus, in this mRNA, the 'a' at 6045 is attached to the 'a' at 8379.

The protein ends with the stop codon (tag) at positions 8422-24. Since these values agree with those shown in Reference 3 (NCBI) for the coding sequence (CDS) that produces the Tat protein, i.e., join (5831..6045,8379..8424) no further verification of the amino acid sequence generated by the code is needed.

d. mRNA5 – Rev Protein

Using the data in Supplementary Table 3 for the Rev protein we find nearly the same Splice Site Sequence for A4b located in the HXB2 strain with the G of the intron to be spliced out located at position 5960. The only exception is that HXB2 has a 'c' instead of a 'g' in position 5955. Thus, this mRNA partially results from the splicing of the 'g' at 743 to the 'g' at 5961. The first start codon (atg) after the splice appears at location 5970-72 and it is the start of the Rev protein.

Reference 2 (Ocwieja) specifies that the mRNA for Rev undergoes additional splicing to remove a second intron. However, it is the same intron as was spliced out for Tat above. Thus, in both mRNAs, the 'a' at 6045 is attached to the 'a' at 8379.

The protein ends with the stop codon (tag) at positions 8651-53. Since these values agree with those shown in Reference 3 (NCBI) for the CDS that produces the Rev (trs/art) protein, i.e., join (5790..6045,8379..8653) no further verification of the amino acid sequence generated by the code is needed.

e. mRNA6 – Vpu Protein

Using the data in Supplementary Table 3 for the Vpu protein we find the same Splice Site Sequence for A5 located in the HXB2 strain with the 'G' of the intron to be spliced out located at position 5976. Thus, this mRNA would appear to results from the splicing of the 'g' at 743 to the 'g' at 5977. However, there are some issues. First, as the reader proceeds from the 5977 position, the first start codon (atg) it finds is at 6057-59. However, the next codon is the stop codon 'taa'. Further, Reference 4 (Excel) reports that the start codon is in positions 6062-64, but that the 't' has been replaced by a 'c' in the HXB2 strain. Reference 5 (Genomic) also reports that the Vpu CDS starts in position 6062 and ends at position 6310.

An analysis of the amino acids string generated by the sequence from 6062-6310 shows that they agree with the amino acid sequence shown in Reference 6 (Bioafrica). See data entered at the initial and final locations for the Vpu protein in the appendix.

What may be disconcerting about this is how the reader actually gets to the identified start codon at 6062-64. When it reads the 'taa' stop codon at 6060-6062 the data indicates that it does not actually stop and disassemble, but reads on. This is a unique function of the taa stop codon. See Post Script One for details. There does not seem to be any other way for the reader to reach the identified start codon. Further, the reader must shift one nucleotide at a time otherwise it would miss the fact that the second 'a' in the 'taa' stop codon is the leading 'a' in the start codon acg (atg). On the other hand, starting at 6062 and ending at 6310 does give the correct amino acid sequence for the Vpu protein. How the reader actually gets to the correct start position is beyond the scope of this effort.

f. mRNA7 – Env Protein

References 1 (Landmarks), 3 (NCBI), 4 (Excel) and 5 (Genomic), all specify that the coding for the Env protein is contained in positions 6225-8795 and indeed we find a start codon in positions 6225-27 and a 'taa' stop codon in positions 8793-95. However, it is unclear where the second exon, which contains this code, attaches to the first exon at the 743 position.

It is clear that the start of the second exon must be after the Vpu start codon at 6062. If it did not, the reader would be translating the Vpu protein. Further, it is obvious that the start of the second exon must be before the Env start codon at 6225. What might not be obvious is that there is at least one start codon, at 6177-79, and numerous stop codons in the code between positions 6062 and 6225. There is insufficient data to tell us the start location of the second exon for the Env protein.

g. mRNA8 – Nef Protein

While we do find the A7 Splice Site Sequence shown in Supplementary Table 3 for Nef, with the G at 8378, there are some issues with starting the second exon for the Nef protein at 8379. As the reader crosses this position in search of the Nef start codon it would first find 'tag' stop sites at 8422-24 and 8651-53 and an 'atg' start site at 8671-73. If it did happen to reach the 'atg' start codon at 8671, it would find a 'tag' stop codon just 4 codons later which should cause the reader to release the protein it was transcribing and disassemble. Thus, from the data available, it is not clear where Nef's second exon attaches to its first exon.

References 1 (Landmarks), 4 (Excel) and 5 (Genomic), all specify that the coding for the Nef protein is contained in positions 8797-9417 and indeed we find a start codon in positions 8797-99 and a 'tga' stop codon in positions 9415-17. It is interesting to note that this is the first use of the 'tga' stop codon we have observed in the virus.

We also note that the start of the Nef's start codon at 8797 is just two nucleotides from the end of the Env's stop codon, a 'taa', at 8795. Given the observation on the 'taa' stop codon in the discussion of the Vpu protein, it seems possible that the reader might end the Env protein at this point and continue to read until coming to the Nef start codon at the 8797-99 positions. That would mean that every time a Env protein is produced a Nef protein is produced as well.

Summary and Conclusions

Figure 9 shows that all seven of the mRNAs start with the 'g' in position 456 and end with the 'a' in position 9719. That is, they all have the same initial set of code and the same tail. All but the first mRNA undergo significant splicing. For mRNAs two through seven, the initial set of code ends at the 'g' nucleotide in position 743. The code spliced out varies with the protein to be translated. Tat and Rev undergo additional splicing. While Nef could have been shown separately, it is more interesting from an analytical point of view, to show that the translation of Nef might follow that of Env in mRNA7.

```
1a  g--------------- Gag Group -------------------------------------------------a
1b  g----------------------------------- Pol Group -----------------------------a

2   g--------g    Spliced Out     ----------------- Vif --------------------------a

3   g--------g    Spliced Out     ----------------- Vpr --------------------------a

4   g--------g    Spliced Out        ----------------- Tat 1 ------- Tat2 --------------a

5   g--------g    Spliced Out        ----------------- Rev1 -------- Rev2 ----------a

6   g--------g    Spliced Out        ----------------- Vpu ------------------a

7   g--------g    Spliced Out        ----------------- Env -------Nef----a

    ↑456   ↑743              |<  Various  >|                    9719↑
```

Figure 9 Overview of HIV-1 HXB2 mRNAs

As a researcher maybe one should not be surprised at the capabilities of Nature. However, the difference between Figures 8 and 9 seems astounding. Figure 8 can be looked as a storage media. It looks like a jumble of data packed away for use at an appropriate time. However, when it comes time to use the information, Nature has provided a means to transform this stored jumble into an exceedingly elegant set of mRNAs which the host can use to generate the required proteins. One must admire the beauty of Nature. On the other hand, maybe there is beauty in the arrangement shown in Figure 8 that we have not yet learned to appreciate.

APPENDIX

Selected HIV-1 HXB2 Sequences from
GenBank K03455.1 Annotated

1 tggaagggct aattcactcc caacgaagac aagatatcct tgatctgtgg atctaccaca ≠[5]

421 cctgca**tata agcagctgct** ttttgcctgt actg**ggtc**tc tctggttaga ccagatctga

    TATA ▶--◀ ▶-- 25 bp ID -------------◀▶-- 456 Start Unspliced mRNA[6]

481 gcctgggagc tctctggcta actagggaac ccactgctta agcctcaata aagcttgcct

≠

721 caagaggcga ggggcggcga ct**ggtgag**ta cgccaaaaat tttgactagc ggaggctaga

      D1[7] Splice Site Seq tg|GTgagt

    Retained for mRNAs 2-7 --◀▶≠≠ D1 Intron cut our starting at 744

781 aggagagaga t**g**ggtgcgag agcgtcagta ttaagcgggg gagaattaga tcgatgggaa

        ▶--790 Start of gag ----------------------------------

≠

2281 tcgtcacaa**t aa**aga**tag**ggg gggcaactaa aggaagctct attagataca ggagcagatg

    --------[ ]   [ ] Stop codons for gag

2341 atacagtatt agaagaa**atg** agtttgccag gaagatggaa accaaaaatg ataggggggaa

         [2358 Start of pol ---------------------------

≠

4861 aagaattaca aaaacaaatt acaaaaattc aaaatttt**cg ggttt**attac a**gg**gacagca

                A1 Slice Site Sequence cg ggtttattac AG|g

                     A1 starts at 4913 ▶.......

≠ _M__E__N__ R__W__Q__V _

5041 **atg**gaaaaca gatggcaggt gatgattgtg tggcaagtag acaggatgag gat**tag**aaca

  ▶ 5041 Start Vif ....

  -------------------------------------- 5096 pol Stop Codon◀

≠

5341 gaactagcag accaactaat tcatctgtat tacttt**gact** g**tttttcaga** ctctgctata

             Splice Site Sequence tgatt gtttttcAG|a

             A2 Starts at 5390 ▶ **********

                ≠_M __E__Q__A__ _P__E__D_

5521 ccacctttgc ctagtgttac gaaactgaca gaggatag**at g**gaacaagcc ccagaagacc

    A2******** ********** ********** ********▶ Vpr Starts at 5559 ***

        _H __T__M__N_ _G__H_

5581 aagggccaca gagggagcca cacaatgaat ggacac**tag**a gctttttagag gagcttaaga

             Vif....... ...... Vif Stop Codon at 5619 ◀

≠

        _Q__N_ _W__V__S__ T_

---

[5] ≠ indicates rows not included or sequence deletion.

[6]. Reference 3 (NCBI) has TSS starting at 455, but Reference 4 (Excel) indicates mRNA starts at 456.

[7] The D and A information is from Reference 2 (Ocwieja).

5761 tgtttatcca ttttcagaat tgggtgtcga catagcagaa taggcgttac tcgacagagg
tttattca ttt_cAGIa A3 Splice Site Sequence
▶ A3 Starts at 5778 ΦΦΦΦΦ ΦΦΦΦΦΦΦΦΦ ΦΦΦΦΦΦΦΦΦ
Vpr******* ********** ********** ****◀ Vpr Stops at 5795

5821 agagcaagaa atggagccag tagatcctag actagagccc tggaagcatc caggaagtca
A3ΦΦΦΦΦΦΦ ▶ Start Tat Part 1 ΦΦ ΦΦΦΦΦΦΦΦΦ ΦΦΦΦΦΦΦΦΦ
ΦΦΦΦΦΦΦΦΦ

≠

5941 tttcataaca aaagccttag gcatctccta tggcaggaag aagcggagac agcgacgaag
aaca aaaggcttAGIg A4b Splice Site Sequence
A4b Starts at 5961 ▶•••••••••▶ 5970 Start Rev Part 1 •••••••••
A5 Splice Site Sequence atctccta tggcAGIg
A5 Starts at 5977 ▶ooo ooooooooooo ooooooooooo

6001 agctcatcag aacagtcaga ctcatcaagc ttctctatca aagcagtaag tagtacatgt
D4 Cut Starts at 6046 calGTaag_t
Tat1ΦΦΦΦΦΦ Tat Part 1 Ends at 6045 ΦΦΦΦΦΦΦΦ ΦΦΦΦ◀D4 cut ########
Rev1••••••• Rev Part 1 Ends at 6045 ••••••••• ••••◀D4 cut ########
_M__Q__P_ _I__P__I__ V_

6061 aacgcaacct ataccaatag tagcaatagt agcattagta gtagcaataa taatagcaat
o▶ Vpu Starts at 6062 Note: code error[8] ooo ooooooooooo ooooooooooo

6121 agttgtgtgg tccatagtaa tcatagaata taggaaaata ttaagacaaa gaaaaataga

6181 caggttaatt gatagactaa tagaaagagc agaagacagt ggcaatgaga gtgaaggaga
Env Starts at 6225 ▶+++++ ++++++++++
_ W__D__V__D

6241 aatatcagca cttgtggaga tgggggtgga gatggggcac catgctcctt gggatgttga
__D__L_

6301 tgatctgtag tgctacagaa aaattgtggg tcacagtcta ttatggggta cctgtgtgga
ooooooooooo◀ Vpu Ends at 6310

≠

8341 atagagttag gcagggatat tcaccattat cgtttcagac ccacctccca accccgaggg
A7 Splice Site Sequence cattat cgtttcAGIa vvvvvvvvvv vvvvvvvvvv
8379 Start Tat 2nd part ######▶Φ ΦΦΦΦΦΦΦΦΦ ΦΦΦΦΦΦΦΦΦ
8379 Start Rev 2nd part ######▶• ••••••••••• •••••••••••

8401 gacccgacag gcccgaagga atagaagaag aaggtggaga gagagacaga gacagatcca
Tat2ΦΦΦΦΦ ΦΦΦΦΦΦΦΦΦ ΦΦΦ◀ 8424 End Tat 2nd Part

≠

8641 aactaaagaa tagtgctgtt agcttgctca atgccacagc catagcagta gctgagggga
Rev2••••••• ••◀ 8653 End Rev 2nd Part

≠

8761 gaataagaca gggcttggaa aggattttgc tataagatgg gtggcaagtg gtcaaaaagt
Env ++++++ ++++++++ Env Ends at 8795 ◀ ▶ Nef Starts at 8797 ^^^^^

8821 agtgtgattg gatggcctac tgtaagggaa agaatgagac gagctgagcc agcagcagat

≠

---

[8] Landmark Excel reports an error in the code: the 'c' should be a 't'.

9361 ctagcatttc atcacgtggc ccgagagctg catccggagt acttcaagaa ctgc**tga**cat
    Nef ^^^^^^ ^^^^^^^^^^ ^^^^^^^^^^ ^^^^^^^^^^ ^^^ 9417 End Nef ◄
≠
9661 tgactctggt aactagagat ccctcagacc cttttagtca gtgtggaaaa tctctagca//

References

1. Landmarks of the HIV-1 genome, HXB2 strain which can be found at http://www.hiv.lanl.gov/content/sequence/HIV/MAP/landmark.html

2. Ocwieja, et al, Dynamic regulation of HIV-1 mRNA populations analyzed by single-molecule..., NAR, Aug 25, 2012.

3. NCBI DNA Sequence for HIV-1 HXB2 Genome at http://www.ncbi.nlm.nih.gov/nuccore/1906382.

4. Excel - Reference Sequence for HXB2 Strain of HIV-1 (updated 6/27/2013) in MS Excel at http://www.hiv.lanl.gov/content/sequence/HIV/MAP/hxb2.xls

5. Genomic Regions in the HIV sequence database at http://www.hiv.lanl.gov/components/sequence/HIV/search/help.html#region

6. Gioafrica VPU - Viral Protein U at http://www.bioafrica.net/proteomics/VPUprot.html

CHAPTER 5

HUMAN AND VIRAL GENES
WITH UNIQUE IDENTIFIERS

The search for a functional unique identifier related to a quantum gene is an exercise in identifying how the transcription complex actually assembles in the 5' Upstream region of a segment of transcribable nuclear DNA. The element that makes initial contact with the nuclear DNA in the 5' Upstream region most likely is interacting with the unique identifier of the quantum gene. When the portion of the nuclear DNA in the 5' Upstream region where the initial contact is made becomes a recognizable known quantity to science, the unique identifier for a specific quantum gene will become a recognized entity. The exact science of how the transcription complex assembles at a particular location along the nuclear DNA is currently on the cutting edge of medical research.

Examining the HIV genome may provide an important clue to the unique identifier of a quantum gene. The HIV virion inserts RNA into the host T-Helper cell. The HIV genome is two strands of vRNA (viral RNA) each approximately 9600 nucleotides in length. The HIV RNA genome then undergoes reverse transcription to become DNA. The resultant viral DNA is approximately the same length as the original vRNA and becomes inserted into the T-Helper cell's nuclear DNA. Later, the cell transcribes HIV's viral DNA to produce a viral RNA that resembles the original HIV RNA, except that it is 600 nucleotides shorter in length.

The HIV genome is read from the 5' region to the 3' region. The HIV DNA genome is approximately 9719 base pairs in length. There does exist variation in the HIV genome. The following therefore is intended to act as an illustration rather than to be regarded as a set standard for the design and function of the HIV genome. HIV's genome is divided into several regions including: 5' LTR (1-634), gag (790-2292), pol (2085-5096), vif (5041-5619), vpr (5559-5850), env

(6225-8795), nef (8797-9417) and 3' LTR (9086-9719). Please see Chapter 4 for additional details.

The initial portion of the HIV DNA genome is termed the Long Terminal Repeat (LTR) located at the 5' region. The LTR is comprised of the regions indentified as U3, R and U5. The LTR is comprised of the nucleotide base pairs (bp) from 1-634.

The TATA box is considered a means of signaling to the cell's transcription machinery that a segment of transcribable genetic information follows downstream from that point. At bp 427 in the 5' LTR is located the first nucleotide of a TATA box. At bp 456 starts the messenger RNA of the HIV genome. Between the TATA box and the location of the transcribable messenger RNA of the HIV genome is a space of 25 nucleotide base pairs. The nucleotides of this 25 base pair segment are 'agcagctgcttttttgcctgtactgg'. This segment of 25-nucleotide base pairs may contain the 'unique identifier' of HIV to the human genome transcription machinery. See Figure 10. HIV has shown that it often utilizes mechanisms already present in the human cell, thus the HIV DNA genome having a unique identifier would be consistent with the identification of unique identifiers for human quantum genes.

HIV GENOME

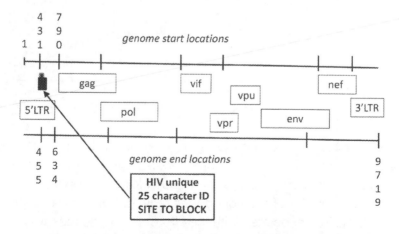

Figure 10 HIV genome with the 25-nucleotide unique identifier demonstratable between bp 430 and 456.

The actual HIV genome for HXB2 from nucleotide 0-1200 is provided in Figure 11. HIV may be mimicking a unique identifier that already exists in the human genome. When the human quantum gene is to be transcribed, the nuclear signaling protein or the control RNA that is used to identify the unique identifier is produced and seeks out the quantum gene. In some such cases, the nuclear signaling protein or control RNA locates the HIV genome and initiates the transcription process rather than locating the human quantum gene. The HIV replication process begins and takes over the normal process of the cell to produce copies of the HIV virion.

A search of the human genome of the nucleotides of HIV's 25 base pair unique identifier 5'-agcagctgcttttttgcctgtactgg-3' or some unique subset, if present in the human genome, may identify the identity of a quantum gene in the human genome. If genetic information were to be found downstream from this unique identifier in the human genome, a unique human quantum gene would be identified.

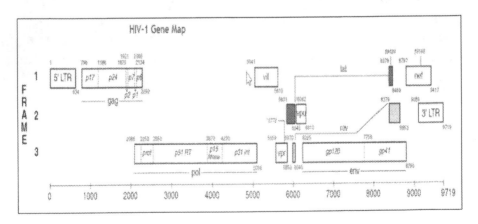

Figure 11 The genome for HIV HXB2

The HIV genome demonstrates the presence of both 'genes' and 'quantum genes'. If a gene is considered to be a segment of DNA that once transcribed produces a ribonucleic acid, then the genome of HIV is comprised of multiple genes. Given that there is only one unique identifier associated with the HIV genome dictates that some genes are bundled together under the assignment of only one unique identifier.

Bundling more than one gene to one unique identifier demonstrates nature's effort to conserve resources. If multiple unique genes are required to perform a specific task, such as construct the proteins necessary to produce HIV virions, then only the first gene in a particular series of genes needs to be locatable. Once the unique identifier associated with the first gene is located by a transcription complex all of the genes in the series will be transcribed, producing multiple ribonucleic acids products. Such bundling of genes represents a logical approach to increase efficiency in coding genetic instructions by compacting genetic information, represents a means to reduce errors in protein construction and cell structure production, and increases the proficiency of the transcription of certain proteins required to accomplish a specific outcome.

UNIQUE IDENTIFIERS IN HUMAN AND VIRAL GENOMES

The human genome consists of approximately 30,000 protein coding genes. We hypothesized there exists an organized means for transcription machinery to locate a specific gene. Transcription Binding Protein (TBP) is an initial transcription factor that binds to DNA to commence assembly of the transcription complex. TBP attaches to the DNA in the vicinity of the TATA box upstream from the transcription start site (TSS). Frequently there exists 25 nucleotides between the TATA box and the TSS. Twenty-five nucleotides would be sufficient to uniquely identify 200,000 differing genes for 5 billion species. It is estimated that 25% of human genes have a TATA box upstream from the TSS. We hypothesized there may be a unique numbering system associated with a subset of genes, and DNA may be divided into executable genes (locatable gene associated with a unique identifier) and follower genes (transcribed automatically following transcription of an executable gene). Eight human genes with a TATA box and four viral genomes which embed in human DNA are reported. The 25-nucleotide sequence downstream from the TATA box was converted to the numbering system a=0, g=1, c=2, t=3 as published in ESHG 2014 Abstract J16.03. NCBI BLAST analysis determined the complete TATA+25-nucleotide unique identifiers associated with the reported genes were not otherwise found intact in the human genome. More extensive study is forthcoming. The unique identifiers associated with embedded viral genomes may be utilized as inimitable targets for future anti-viral therapies and for use in future medical genetics therapies. See Table 2.

Gene Unique Identifiers				
Gene	25 Nucleotide Sequence Position	TATA-25 Unique Identifier	BLAST Closest Match 5'-3'	Numerical Conversion of Unique Identifier Using a=0, g=1, c=2, t=3
INS	2160-2184	TATA aagccagcgggggcccagcagccct	18/29	0012201211111222012012223
LEP	4975-4999	TATA agaggggcgggcaggcatggagccc	19/29	0101111211120112031101222
RMRP	134504-134528	TATA aaatactactctgtgaagctgagga	16/29	0003023023231310012310110
TPI1	573-597	TATA taagtgggcagtggccgcgactgcg	15/29	3001311120131122121023121
AGT	441-465	TATA aatagggcatcgtgacccggccggg	15/29	0030111203213102221122111
hGH	126-150	TATA aaaagggcccacaagagaccagctc	15/29	0000111222020010102201232
NOS2A	8271-8295	TATA aatacttcttggctgccagtgtgtt	15/29	0030233233112312201313133
TNF	1717-1741	TATA aaggcagttgttggcacacccagcc	16/29	0011201331331120202220122
HIV HXB2	431-455	TATA agcagctgcttttttgcctgtactgg	20/29	0120123123333312231302311
HSV-1 gC	96,145-96,169	TATA aattccggaaggggacacgggctac	18/29	0033221100111102021112302
VZV ORF21	30,734-30,758	TATA aagttaagtcagcgtagaatatacc	16/29	0013300132012130100303022
Smallpox	247-275	TATA cttttaattgaacaaaagagttaag	20/29	2333300331002000010133001

Table 2
Unique IDs for 8 human genes and 4 viral genes.

CHAPTER 6

THE WORK HORSE:
TRANSCRIPTION FACTOR IIIA

Ideally, a molecule could be developed to silence the HIV genome by modifying assets already in routine use by normal cells. Hormones direct cellular function and in some cases, such as the thyroid hormone, nuclear transcription. Nuclear signaling proteins generated in a cell's cytoplasm regulate nuclear function. These are examples of extranuclear proteins regulating nuclear function by engaging the DNA and either activating or blocking gene transcription.

Several nuclear and extranuclear ligands exist. These include hormones produced remotely outside the cell, intrinsic nuclear signaling proteins originating in the cytoplasm or smooth endoplasmic reticulum, and possibly control RNA molecules originating in the nucleus. Some hormones interact with nuclear receptors either combining with a nuclear receptor in the cytoplasm then migrating to the nucleus or combining with the nuclear receptor in the nucleus. Each of these modalities target a specific gene or grouping of genes once the molecule or molecular complex is in the nucleus. Some form of genetic identification must exist for the nuclear signaling protein complexes to activate or deactivate the proper genes as required. See Figure 12. Genes have unique identifiers.

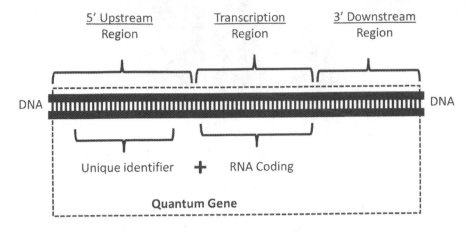

Figure 12 A gene's unique identifier

Taking advantage of the presence of a unique identifier associated with DNA embedded viruses, a nuclear binding protein could be fashioned to seek out the viral unique identifier. Therapeutic nuclear binding proteins would adhere to the DNA only in locations of the virus's unique identifier.

Several choices exist for therapeutic nuclear binding proteins. The Transcription Factor III A (TFIIIA) molecule has been shown to be generated in the cytoplasm of a cell and migrate to the nucleus of a cell. The TFIIIA molecule has been implicated in viral transcription. See Figure 13. Modifying the TFIIIA molecule to seek out HIV's unique identifier would cause the modified TFIIIA molecule to attach to the HIV genome when embedded in the human genome. The modified TFIIIA redesigned such that once it attaches to the embedded HIV genome, the configuration of the TFIIIA molecule prevents the formation of a transcription complex that would otherwise transcribe the HIV genome.

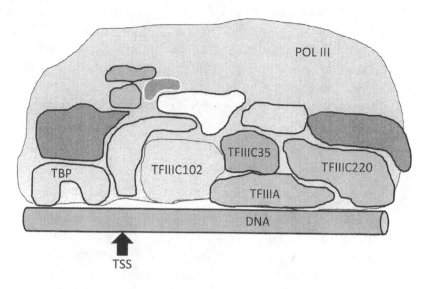

Figure 13 TFIIIA binds to DNA to assist initiation
of assembly of a transcription complex

The TFIIIA molecule is comprised of 365 amino acids. The generic
TFIIIA molecule is presented in Figure 14 in a concept drawing.

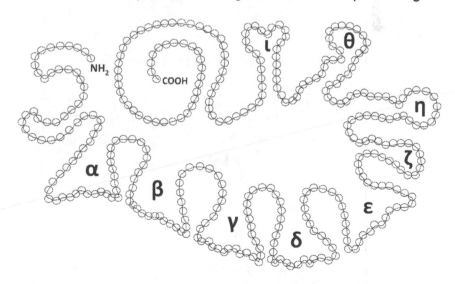

Figure 14 Concept drawing of the TFIIIA molecule

Combining the concept that HIV has a unique identifier and nuclear binding proteins travel from the cytoplasm to the nucleus, a transcription factor molecule can be modified to seek out and target HIV's unique identifier. A template for constructing a modified TFIIIA molecule is presented in Figure 15. The zinc fingers designated alpha, beta, gamma, delta and epsilon are the amino acid loops that bind to nuclear DNA. The zinc fingers designated zeta, eta, theta and iota are loops that bind with other transcription factors as the transcription complex becomes assembled.

Proper modification of zinc fingers: alpha, beta, gamma, delta, and epsilon causes the TFIIIA molecule to target the unique identifier of the HIV genome. Artful modification of the fingers designated zeta, eta, theta, and iota could prevent binding of transcription factors to the TFIIIA molecule when the TFIIIA molecule is bound to the DNA.

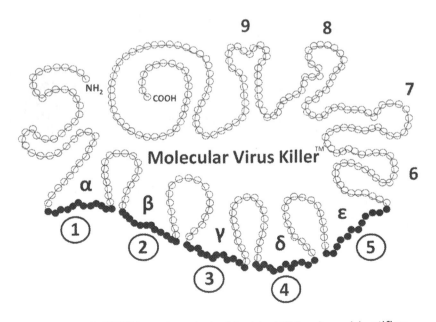

Figure 15 TFIIIA molecule to bind to HIV unique identifier

Figure 15 represents the generic molecule that may be termed a Molecular Virus Killer due to the concept whereby if a TFIIIA molecule is modified to target a specific virus, such a TFIIIA molecule would be capable of semi-permanently binding to a viral genome and preventing transcription of the virus's genetic material. If a virus's genome is prevented from being transcribed, then the virus is unable to generate copies of its virion and in effect the viral infection has been halted.

CHAPTER 7

STRUCTURE OF THE TFIIIA MOLECULE

There are twenty amino acids. Amino acids act as the building blocks to generate protein molecules. Figure 16 provides an illustration of the twenty amino acids.

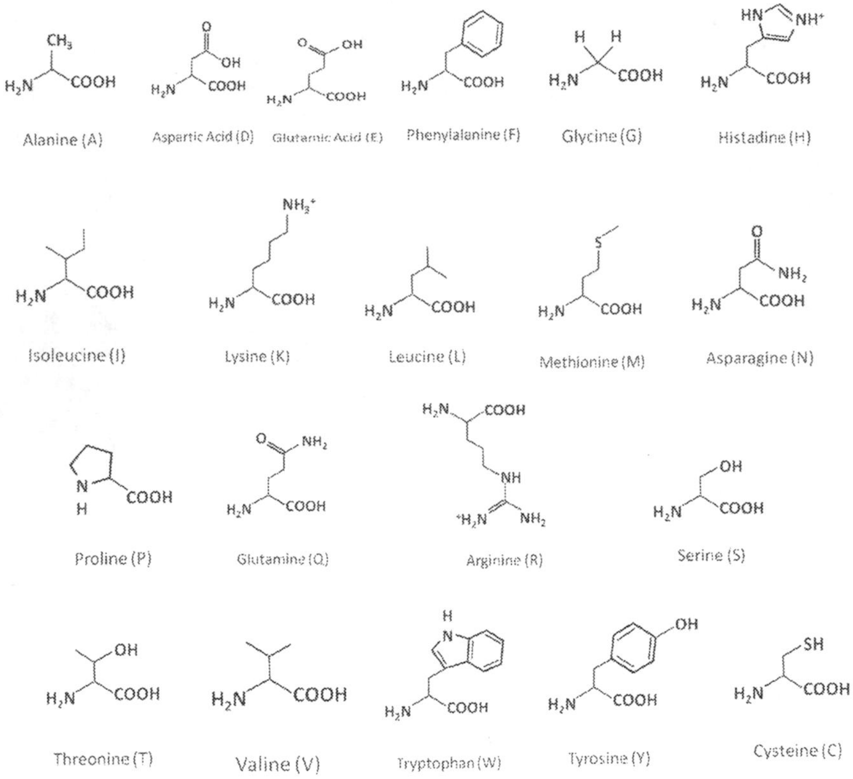

Figure 16 Amino Acids

The following three hundred sixty five amino acid sequence comprises the Transcription Factor III A molecule, Taxonomic identifier 9606 [NCBI]:

```
  1        10        20         30         40         50         60
MDPPAVVAES VSSLTIADAF IAAGESSAPT PPRPALPRRF ICSFPDCSAN YSKAWKLDAH
          70         80         90        100        110        120
LCKHTGERPF VCDYEGCGKA FIRDYHLSRH ILTHTGEKPF VCAANGCDQK FNTKSNLKKH
         130        140        150        160        170        180
FERKHENQQK QYICSFEDCK KTFKKHQQLK IHQCQHTNEP LFKCTQEGCG KHFASPSKLK
         190        200        210        220        230        240
RHAKAHEGYV CQKGCSFVAK TWTELLKHVR ETHKEEILCE VCRKTFKRKD YLKQHMKTHA
         250        260        270        280        290        300
PERDVCRCPR EGCGRTYTTV FNLQSHILSF HEESRPFVCE HAGCGKTFAM KQSLTRHAVV
         310        320        330        340        350        360
HDPDKKKMKL KVKKSREKRS LASHLSGYIP PKRKQGQGLS LCQNGESPNC VEDKMLSTVA
         365
VLTLG
```

The TFIIIA9606 is utilized naturally by a human cell to assist in the transcription of 5S RNA molecules.

The TFIIIA protein is comprised of nine zinc fingers. All nine zinc fingers may attach to the DNA in some situation. The fourth, fifth, sixth and seventh finger from 5- to the 3' end of the molecule may attach to an RNA molecule. The eight zinc finger may attach at times to a TFIIIC molecule. The ninth zinc finger may attach at times to TFIIID molecule.

The TFIIIA9606 is utilized naturally by a human cell to assist in the transcription of 5S RNA molecules. The TFIIIA molecule also assists in transcribing some viral DNA genomes

The following is taken from the NCBI website and represents how the gene which is responsible for the construct of the Transcription Factor III A molecule (Taxonomic identifier 9606 [NCBI]) is described:

```
FEATURES            Location/Qualifiers
     source         1..11166
                    /organism="Homo sapiens"
                    /mol _type="genomic DNA"
                    /db _xref="taxon:9606"
                    /chromosome="13"
     gene           1..11166
                    /gene="GTF3A"
                    /gene _synonym="AP2; TFIIIA"
                    /note="general transcription factor IIIA;
                    Derived by
                    automated computational analysis using gene
                    prediction
```

mRNA

```
method: BestRefSeq."
/db __xref="GeneID:2971"
/db __xref="HGNC:HGNC:4662"
/db __xref="MIM:600860"
join(1..395,2549..2649,5327..5423,5990..6078,8188
..8261,
9596..9676,10262..10491,10590..10649,10890..11166)
/gene="GTF3A"
/gene __synonym="AP2; TFIIIA"
/product="general transcription factor IIIA"
/note="Derived by automated computational
analysis using
gene prediction method: BestRefSeq."
/transcript __id="NM__002097.2"
/db __xref="GI:166063994"
/db __xref="GeneID:2971"
/db __xref="HGNC:HGNC:4662"
/db __xref="MIM:600860"
CDS join(195..395,2549..2649,5327..5423,5990..6078,
8188..8261,9596..9676,10262..10491,10590..10649,
10890..11054)
/gene="GTF3A"
/gene __synonym="AP2; TFIIIA"
/note="non-AUG (CUG) translation initiation
codon; Derived
by automated computational analysis using gene
prediction
method: BestRefSeq."
/codon __start=1
/product="transcription factor IIIA"
/protein __id="NP__002088.2"
/db __xref="GI:166063995"
/db __xref="CCDS:CCDS45019.1"
/db __xref="GeneID:2971"
/db __xref="HGNC:HGNC:4662"
/db __xref="MIM:600860"
```

CDS:'Coding DNA Sequence'

The amino acid sequence for general TFIIIA molecule. The TFIIIA molecule is comprised of 365 amino acid molecules. The amino acid sequence for the TFIIIA molecule is as follows:

/translation="MDPPAVVAESVSSLTIADAFIAAGESSAPTPPRPALPRRFICSF

PDCSANYSKAWKLDAHLCKHTGERPFVCDYEGCGKAFIRDYHLSRHILTHTGEKPFVC

AANGCDQKFNTKSNLKKHFERKHENQQKQYICSFEDCKKTFKKHQQLKIHQCQHTNEP

LFKCTQEGCGKHFASPSKLKRHAKAHEGYVCQKGCSFVAKTWTELLKHVRETHKEEIL

CEVCRKTFKRKDYLKQHMKTHAPERDVCRCPREGCGRTYTTVFNLQSHILSFHEESRP

FVCEHAGCGKTFAMKQSLTRHAVVHDPDKKKMKLKVKKSREKRSLASHLSGYIPPKRK

QGQGLSLCQNGESPNCVEDKMLSTVAVLTLG"

The gene that when transcribed generates the mRNA to produce the general TFIIIA molecule. Gene comprised of 11,166 nucleotides. The underlined segments are the nucleotide strings that represent bonding sites of the TFIIIA molecule's zinc fingers. Note the bonding sites are twelve amino acids in length. Thirty-six nucleotides are required to code for twelve amino acids (using the codon code methodology). The nucleotides comprising the DNA, when being used to code for an amino acid, function by three consecutive nucleotides coding for a single amino acid. There are sixty-four three-nucleotide combinations. Sixty-one of the three-nucleotide combinations code for the twenty amino acids. Three nucleotide combinations (taa, tag, tga) code specifically as stop codes. One three amino acid combination 'atg' codes for the amino acid methionine and also, in the proper setting, is recognized as a start code.

ORIGIN

```
   1 atgcgcgatc tcccggagca tgcgcagcag cggcgccgac gcggggcggt gcctggtgac
  61 cgcgcgcgct cccggaagtg tgccggcgtc gcgcgaaggt tcagcaggga gccgtgggcc
 121 gggcgcgccg gttcccggca cgtgtctcgg cacgtggcag cgcgcctggc cctgggcttg
 181 gaggcgccgg cgccctggat ccgccggccg tggtcgccga gtcggtgtcg tccttgacca
 241 tcgccgacgc gttcattgca gccggcgaga gctcagctcc gaccccgccg cgccccgcgc
 301 ttcccaggag gttcatctgc tccttccctg actgcagcgc caattacagc aaagcctgga
 361 agcttgacgc gcacctgtgc aagcacacgg gggagtgag gggggcgagg ctgccaaccc
 421 tgggcctagg gatgcgcgt ggccccgggg tagccactgc agtcgtggcc agggccgcag
 481 gccccgctgt gcagcgcgtt cagctttgac atccaggact tggggaagga gctgaggaag
 541 tagacaggaa gttgtaggac cttcgttctg cgaccttgat atccatggca ggggctcggg
 601 atttactaag cagtcattga tcgtgagtct cggccagcca agtgcctccc gtaatctgca
 661 aataagtgtg aggtttgagg gggcccaccg ctactagaca cctgccaaac actggcccct
 721 ggagctggta cagaagatgg gttacatgta ccaggggtcg tgaaagcagc atgtgctcat
 781 ttcttcgtaa ctccacactg gagagagcag tgagcaaaac aggcaaaccc aaggtttctg
 841 ctgccatgga cctttgttcc tgggtcgagc cgaccacagg ataggtggga atgacatgca
 901 gtgttgtggt caggaaaggc ctctctgtgt gagccgtgta agaaggaagg atctagccat
 961 gcagacattt gtgctaggta gagagaacac aaagggagcc tgtgaccctt ggggtgggag
1021 gcaggtgggt gtgtttgggt gcggagatca ccatatgagg tctgagaagt aggcccatta
1081 ggagtttgga ttttattttg aggggcaggag aatgtcagat accatgatat gacgtggcag
1141 cccatgtcac acacaagtga ggaaaacgag ggtcatggag gtcaaggaat ctgcccagct
1201 tcccagtttt tggcagagct aggcttcaca ctgcctcagc ttaaagccct taatttctta
1261 aaccactggg ctgcagtcca tacctttgcc ccttgcacct cctctaattt atgggccacc
1321 ttctccaggt gtcctccggg gcctcattcc ttaacctctc cagcactgga aggccgaccg
1381 cttcttcctt gagaccttct ctggttcttt tcctcttcct cgtctgccct tttcgttgga
1441 tcctcttctg ccctctgcat gttccacccc gcccagctcc ctcttgcggt cttacatagc
1501 caccggcatg actcataaca tcctttatgc tttgcccctc tgccttcct cttgcccgtt
1561 ctagcctcta aattctgggc tctgtattac cagtagatcc acgtaagagc ttgcctttcc
1621 ttttagaccg gtgtgctgta ttttggatac tggcgctacc agtttcctta atacaggttg
```

```
1681 aaaaacttgg agtcatcttt gttgtcccag atctctcatg cagattaatt tgacaaatgt
1741 ttattgagcc tactccacgc ctgccgctgt gcaaggttct gtggctccgc ccctggtggt
1801 atgtagctca ctgtgttcct gtttgcttgt tttgctctca gtactctcat ggaggcctcg
1861 gtgcctccct cctggacgcc ttggtagtat gcttttcata gtttgatgca ccaaactggt
1921 tatttggtta tttggggtgt gtgtttggct tttactatag gttcaaaatg agtcaccccc
1981 tcccaactcc tgggttacaa aaggtggttg catttagggt gttgagctgt tttctttgct
2041 tcgccctggc acctgtgagc tttttcaggt gtgacacact ttcctatagc tgtgcttggc
2101 attatcctag cacagaccct gggcttgtct gggatgagac aggcctccct cgttcctctg
2161 ccctaggctt gcttttttac atgttaaatc atgcggtggt ggggatccat gcagacaagc
2221 catgctaaca gccagggcgt ctttaagagg gggttgctgt gaaagcctgc tgccgggttg
2281 ggagcaggtt aaaaatgcta tgcctgctta ttttaaatgc tgttcatgga acaaaaatct
2341 gtgtagtgac tttgtgagaa gttgtgatgt ttatgttgtg taactttgtg caggaacact
2401 gcgtcttgca gtgggtgcac agctctgagt agaaaccacc tcttcatagg aagcctgtgg
2461 ccttaacact aggcagttta agcttttaaa taataccaga gttactaact agtgcagaag
2521 tgacatgctt tttctttttt cctgctag**ag accatttgtt tgtgactatg aagggtgtgg**
2581 **caaggccttc atcagggact accatctgag ccgccacatt ctgactcaca caggagaaaa**
2641 **gccgtttgt**g taagtagaga cctgtttta ggcttttgaa gtgggttgtg ttgggcatat
2701 agacccagta agaagattga tgttaactca cgagatcagg aatgtgaagc ctggcagggc
2761 tcggtggctc atgcctgtaa tcccagcact ttgggaggcg gagatgggca gatcacttga
2821 acccaggagt ttgagacaaa cctgggcaac atggtgaaac cccgtatgta caaaaataca
2881 aaaattagtc agggatggtg gtttgtgcct gtaatcctag ctacccagga ggctgagcta
2941 acataaaatg ctcatgggtg gggacaagct aaagtatatc aacacaatgg gataccctac
3001 agccaggaaa atgaatgcag atgctctctg caaagccatg agaaaatcac cagggcactt
3061 taattgaaaa accaaggtgc agaagagtcc tctttatgt gtgtaaaaaa
3121 gctaggggt aggggggagg gtgagtagtg ggtgtttggg aggcaggaag caactatatt
3181 tgtatttgtt cctatttgta aagaagtctt aaaagttaca taacaaaact aaaaatgtca
3241 tctgtttttgg gagcagtggg ggatcctggc caagtagggg gtggggatgg taggaaatgc
3301 catgcaacca ggaactactg gacatgactc ttccagctca tgatctaacc cagaccctgc
3361 ccctctttag ctgtagttcc ccgtttccca ctgctcgctg gacagtgcta cttggctatc
3421 tctgtgtctt cttaaattcc atgtggtagg ctgggtgtgg tggctcatgc ctgtaatccc
3481 agcactttga gaggctgagg tgggaggatt gctttgaggc caggagttca ggctgggcaa
3541 gatggtcagg tccatctcta ttaaagaaat aaataaataa aaaattccac atggcccaaa
3601 tttgtcacag tcaaactgag ctcacttttc tgtttgatct tctctcatgt tcttgtctgg
3661 agaggtggcc tcgctgtctg tccagtgacc catagcaaag ataaggcagc tccctggact
3721 ctccattctt tctcccatcc cttgcaacag gtgggttgcc agatcctgta actgacccat
3781 cagatccagc agccactgtc ttatctcggt cccttcctct ggctggaatg acagtttgca
3841 ggccagccct ctcccccagt gccctcccgt gtgcttccct taaagctgtg cagtgctttc
3901 aagcacggcc tacatgtgaa atccaggttt caagtgtgtc ctacaatgac ctgcgtgatt
3961 tagccctttt ctgcttatct tgccccattt gcttgacttg caggcatgaa gctgtggtcc
4021 agctgtgcta actaaccagc cccctctcca agtgtgccgg ggtctctcac gcccacttgg
4081 gtcttgtcag gactcttcct ggcctgtcct cctatcccat acccggttgg gttagatgcc
4141 tgtgtcaggt ttagagtgaa gaatggcagg aaccccagca caagagatgc ttaaacaaga
4201 tgggctcttt gtcttgtgcg actgaaatac agaaatacag aggcaggagc tctggagcct
4261 cttctgactg gtctctgcca tcctcatctt gggctttaac ctcactgtga tgcctgtttg
4321 ggcccatctg tcacataagc atgccactgg caggaaggag gaaagggcat aagaggcatg
4381 cccccttatt tagagacttt gtgggggttg agcaggatgg gctggactca gccatgagcc
4441 gccctaattg caggggaggc cggagagtgc actttctgtc ggccacctgc ccagctaaca
4501 ctcagcattc tgtccctgca gttagggggg cttctagggt ctctgccaca gcgcccctcc
4561 catttgtggg cctctgtgct gtgcctccca tggtcactgc tggcttgttt gtctctgctt
4621 ggccctagga atgggacagt gcctgcctca gggttatcag tgagtgatgg ctaagattga
4681 gcctgggaaa ggaagtcctg cttcatccct caagcttacg aaggctcatc acaagaggca
4741 caaattttct tttgggaaaa aaaaaaaaa aaaaggaaaa ggctttgcag aggatttaga
4801 tcattcaaag ccaagatgcc aagataaggg gaaccagaat ggcttggtaa gccagagaac
4861 ataatggtta tggttctgct ctaagtatct gttttacctc taatgataag ccaagacaag
4921 ttttatggag gcctttctgg aaatccagtt cataatgaca tctcaagcag cattaaggtt
4981 gtcagattct aagctgagaa taatttgtct taagcatgat ttaggcctag tgtaggcttt
5041 tgggactagt gtatttcacc ttcccatctg cccagtgtgt ataaaagatg actgatgtag
5101 tgtgtataat ttcagaagcc taatatgaaa aagcattttg ttacatgata gtcatcaggt
5161 tgagagtcta tgtggtatgg cttaacactc tggaattcgc taagactatt ttatagtatt
5221 actattcttt ggaagaatta gcttctataa agtaggaaga tatatgtgtc ttaaaacttc
5281 ttctcccttg gtttattaat attttggttt atataacttc ttacagt**tgt gcagccaatg**
5341 **gctgtgatc**a **aaaattcaac acaaaatcaa acttgaagaa acattttgaa cgcaaacatg**
5401 **aaaatcaaca aaaacaatat ata**gtaagta tgattttata tgcttaaatt ttttgagtat
5461 ttttacactt actgcctatg tttctgacat tttcagccag gtgcggtggc tcaagcctat
```

— 52 —

```
5521 aatcgtagct  tgaggccagg  aatttgagac  cagcctggga  aacatagtga  aatgctgtct
5581 ctgaaaaaaa  aaaacaaaaa  cagaaaacaa  aacaaaaaat  tttggggtaa  cagagaccct
5641 gtctctaaaa  aataaaagtg  aaaaataaag  ttttcgtcaa  ccaaattttg  tctgccaaat
5701 gtctgaattt  acttaatgcc  atcataatga  taaaggtttt  aatttggaag  cagacattgt
5761 gcaaattagt  gtattgggag  actattccaa  ctgaaacagt  tttgcttttt  caaatgttat
5821 atgattcttc  aaaccttttt  gagataaagc  agaattttac  agtaacaaaa  tgggtgaaag
5881 cagaaatttt  atacagtctc  caaaattgtt  ttatcttgag  gattctgtta  cgaactgttc
5941 attttgtttt  gactttccat  aagactaacg  agcctttaca  atttaacagt  gcagttttga
6001 agactgtaag  aagacccttta agaaacatca  gcagctgaaa  atccatcagt  gccagcatac
6061 caatgaacct  ctattcaagt  aggtacttca  tgtggctgaa  aatgcctgga  ttctaggtgt
6121 gaataagatt  ggaaatgcaa  gggtggtgtt  gagcattgtt  tcatgttttt  tggccatttg
6181 tatatcttct  gagaaatgtc  tgttcatatc  ctttgcccac  ttttcgatgg  attgtttttt
6241 tcttgctgat  ctgagttccc  tgtagatcct  ggatatacat  tctttattgg  atgcataatg
6301 tgccagtatt  ttctcccact  ctctgggttg  tctgtttact  ctgctgatta  tttctttttgc
6361 tgtgcagaag  cttttttagtt  taattaggtc  ccatttattt  atttctattt  ttgttgcatt
6421 tgctttcagg  gccttagtaa  gaattctttg  cctaggctga  tgtccagaag  tttttccaat
6481 gtttttcattt  tgaattttta  gtttcaggtc  ataaacttaa  tttgagttga  tttttgtata
6541 aggtgagaga  tagggatcca  gttttttccag  caccatttat  tgaatagga  gtcctttccc
6601 cagtttacgt  ttttatatgc  tttgttgaag  atcgggtggc  tgtaagtatt  tggctttatt
6661 tctgtttttgt  tccattggtc  taagtgccta  tttttaaacc  agtgccaccc  tgttttggta
6721 actgtagcct  cgtagtataa  tctgaagtct  ggtcaaagga  aaagaagtca  ctatatgaaa
6781 aagacacatg  cacacacgtt  tacagcagca  cagttcacaa  ttgcaaatac  atggagccaa
6841 tttaagtgcc  catcgaccaa  tgagtagata  aagaaaacgt  gatgtatata  caccatggaa
6901 tactacacag  ccataaaagg  gaacaaaatg  atgtcttttg  cagcagcttg  gatggagctg
6961 gaggccatta  ttctcagtga  agtaactcag  gaatggaaaa  ccaaatacca  tagttttcac
7021 taagtgggca  ctaaactatg  aggacaaaaa  gacacagtga  tttcataaac  tttggggact
7081 tggggtgggg  agtttgggga  ggggggtgag  ggatgaaaga  ctacatattg  ggtacagtgt
7141 atgctgcttg  agtgatggtg  cgctaaaatc  tcagcaccac  tataggattc  atccacgtaa
7201 cgaaaaaaca  cttgcaaccc  caaaagccat  tgaaatttaa  agcaacggtg  ggacaaatct
7261 tctgaaagct  tcctaatcaa  catttttctg  ttaaaatgta  ctgcatatgc  acatttatat
7321 attgggagca  ttttaaaggt  ttactttgct  ctgaaagaaa  tatttaatgt  gtttcaaaat
7381 aatttttgag  attattctag  ttgtggttaa  gcttaaaggc  tgagaaatta  cttaactatt
7441 caaatagagc  ctgtgcaact  atatgaaatg  tcattatgga  gacactcatt  atgcttttcc
7501 tgtagaacaa  aacaagtagt  tgggtttatc  tgcaattagg  gttttttgag  gaacgtgagg
7561 gtggctggac  aagttgggta  gacctgcaaa  agggccagcg  gctctctgca  tggctctggc
7621 catccggcac  tttccctttga  cttgcacagg  ctgccctgtg  ccttggagtt  gctgcagtga
7681 ccttgcctgt  ccttgcttgt  gggtctgctg  ctgctgcttt  gctgctgatg  gctttagcac
7741 agaggggggcc  cgtgcttttt  attgctcacc  agaggcagat  gcatctactg  ctgtgctgtc
7801 tcgcacaccc  cctatgcagc  atcattagga  aagctagaca  caagtgattc  agaatggctt
7861 aggggtttat  ctaagccaag  tcagataacc  tcttgaacta  tcttttttgta  gccatgaaag
7921 cagagtatat  ttccagaggt  ataaagatga  aaactgttta  aatgggtcaa  aaaaagtaac
7981 gtgactttttt  tctccaacag  tttgtttttgt  cctaaagctg  gtcaagtaac  ttgaatctca
8041 cctgtgatga  gagctacatt  ttaacatggg  tttggttatg  ggaagaggca  agactttggt
8101 gggagaaaca  ggacaaagtg  ccattgacct  tgagcggagt  tctctgtgaa  aatggattgg
8161 ctaatacctc  atgtgttgcc  aatgcaggtg  tacccaggaa  ggatgtggga  aacactttgc
8221 atcacccagc  aagctgaaac  gacatgccaa  ggcccacgag  ggtgtgtacg  gatagcctgg
8281 gtgtgctccg  aggggatgc  caaatcctgg  gcgccttttga  atctgttctg  tgatcacgct
8341 gaaaagatgg  gaaccctgtg  aacaggggac  accatcctgc  ttatttgggt  cttacactct
8401 tgtccaaaga  ggcactgtat  atgtctgttt  ttccactacc  gtatcattgc  tgttcacatg
8461 taatgtgttg  tttgttcaca  acaagcgcct  ggttacacat  tacactgacg  aatgtgctga
8521 tgctccagcc  atggctttga  tgcttctgtc  attttttaacc  tcttctatta  atatttactg
8581 cctgtgccat  tcttttcctt  gttggccatt  cacaaggctt  ggataatcgt  gtgacatttt
8641 gagagccatc  agatgttacg  tttctcaaaa  aaaaaaaaaa  aagacttgat  tatattaact
8701 atttgaatct  atgatctgtt  tccttgaggg  atttttgcta  atctgtattt  caatttccca
8761 ggtcctagaa  tttatgattt  tttttttttt  aagaggttag  tagctaacag  tgagaggcag
8821 cctcattgtt  tttagtttct  agttgggtgg  aactcagccc  tagtgttgta  tacttattaa
8881 tcccatttta  gtgctttgca  catatccatt  gttattcagt  gtttttctct  gggtccttcc
8941 agtttattttt  cttccttagc  tgtactcttt  taaaaaaaaa  aaacaaaaaa  aaactttttt
9001 tttttttttt  gtgataaagt  taaaatataa  tgtaccctac  tttttttgtg  cagtatgaca
9061 cttacaagat  ggccagacta  gaggaagcca  gaggtgggca  tggtaacact  actgaaaagt
9121 tggtggtgtg  ccatgacaa  gggaccgact  gcagagtatg  tttgctgagg  aaaatagagg
9181 cgaggataga  gcaggcaggg  gaagggaaat  aagacatgga  gataggaggt  taaagcagtt
9241 gggagtccat  acacagccta  cccaacttcc  tgagaactct  tagagaggaa  aaggcatcct
9301 taggcatcct  tcctgtgaag  tttgcctatt  ccgtgatcac  gctgagaaga  tgggaactct
```

```
  9361 gaagtttgct tcacaggaag gtaaaatcct taaagggagg caccttgctg tgccactgtt
  9421 cagttttact ataacatcaa tctttttttta gtttttattc ccacctcaag aggctgagtt
  9481 gaatactatt aggcggggaa tggaaaatta tataggcacc taagtttcct ttctagttat
  9541 ggtcagtgtt tacactgagt attcatgaca gacaatgcac caattttttt aatag gctat
  9601 gtatgtcaaa aaggatgttc ctttgtggca aaaacatgga cggaacttct gaaacatgtg
  9661 agagaaaccc ataaag gtaa ggcaggcatg aatggcaggc atggtgtaaa tgtttgtccc
  9721 cacagaactg atttagtgct tttcaagagt gaaatgctgt gtgctttaaa gtaaaagggt
  9781 ttctctatga tattttgtga agtgctgggt atgatgttgt tggaaaggtg agcagagctg
  9841 tgccaggtct ctgagccacc ccaccatgca caattagcat gctgaaggcg gtggcaggtc
  9901 tgtagtgaag aatttcggga ggcactgctg ttctgtggga ccgcctggga aacagtaccc
  9961 tgcatactgg gggacaagga aggacactgg tctgcttcat ttctgtacc tccccacagt
 10021 caccttcctg agagccctgc ctcttggcaa gtgaacaatg actgtgtggc atttaagaac
 10081 ttcagagaat tgagacaaac ttcctaggtg ataaaaactg gggttgtttc cttgggaatt
 10141 tctgatttgt atatagtgat caggtttcag gcactgaatg ttacttatat attaggtatt
 10201 aattttttct aaatggtaat atctggggaa atttgtgaaa tttgtctgtc tgtcccacca
 10261 gaggaaatac tatgtgaagt atgccggaaa acatttaaac gcaaagatta ccttaagcaa
 10321 cacatgaaaa ctcatgcccc agaaagggat gtatgtcgct gtccaagaga aggctgtgga
 10381 agaacctata caactgtgtt taatctccaa agccatatcc tctccttcca tgaggaaagc
 10441 cgcccttttg tgtgtgaaca tgctggctgt ggcaaaacat ttgcaatgaa agtaagcact
 10501 caccctcata ctcatggtcc tatagtctat gctttcacaa catggtttc atattaatat
 10561 ttcattaata actttctctt tcattgtag c aaagtctcac taggcatgct gttgtacatg
 10621 atcctgacaa gaagaaaatg aagctcaaa g taagttgaaa ctacttaggc aagcttagtt
 10681 ttcaagtgga aattgtttaa ggccagaagg agtctgtttg gaattctttt cacctgcttt
 10741 actgtttgag tctgcactac tgttgaagac tttacttcct cataaagcaa tgttgtacac
 10801 tatatctgct ggtacatatg actatcgtaa aattaactca gacagttttg attttgaatt
 10861 ctaatcgtgt gtcttcctta ttcccaaag g tcaaaaaatc tcgtgaaaaa cggagtttgg
 10921 cctctcatct cagtggatat atccctccca aaaggaaaca agggcaaggc ttatctttgt
 10981 gtcaaaacgg agagtcaccc aactgtgtgg aagacaagat gctctcgaca gttgcagtac
 11041 ttacccttgg ctaagaactg cactgctttg tttaaaggac tgcagaccaa ggagcgagct
 11101 ttctctcaga gcatgctttt ctttattaaa attactgatg cagaacattt gattccttat
 11161 catttc
```

Details of how the general TFIIIA molecule is constructed per coding instructions from the genetic code:

```
CDS          join(195..395,2549..2649,5327..5423,5990..6078,8188..8261,
                 9596..9676,10262..10491,10590..10649,10890..11054)
ORIGIN
TFIIIA GENE EXON ONE:


TFIIIA mRNA 5' UPSTREAM UNTRANSLATABLE SEGMENT:

         1 atg cgcgatc tcccggagca tgcgcagcag cggcgccgac gcggggcggt gcctggtgac
        61 cgcgcgcgct cccggaagtg tgccggcgtc gcgcgaaggt tcagcaggga gccgtgggcc
       121 gggcgcgccg gttcccggca cgtgtctcgg cacgtggcag cgcgcctggc cctgggcttg
       181 gaggcgccgg cgcc

*LOOP ALPHA BINDING TO DNA

TFIIIA MOLECULE AMINO ACIDS 1-47:
```

```
        L    D    P    P    A    V    V    A    E    S    V    S    S    L    T
195    ctg  gat  ccg  ccg  gcc  gtg  gtc  gcc  gag  tcg  gtg  tcg  tcc  ttg  acc


        I    A    D    A    F    I    A    A    G    E    S    S    A    P    T
240    atc  gcc  gac  gcg  ttc  att  gca  gcc  ggc  gag  agc  tca  gct  ccg  acc


        P    P    R    P    A    L    P    R    R    F    I    C    S    F    P
286    ccg  ccg  cgc  ccc  gcg  ctt  ccc  agg  agg  ttc  atc  tgc  tcc  ttc  cot


        D    C
330    gac  tgc
```

TFIIIA MOLECULE ZINC FINGER 'ONE' DNA BONDING SITES, AMINO ACIDS 48-59:

```
        S    A    N    Y    S    K    A    W    K    L    D    A
336    agc  gcc  aat  tac  agc  aaa  gcc  tgg  aag  ctt  gac  gcg
```

TFIIIA MOLECULE AMINO ACIDS 60-67:

```
        H    L    C    K    H    T    G    E
372    cac  ctg  tgc  aag  cac  acg  ggg  gag
```

TFIIIA GENE INTRON ONE:

```
396gtgag      ggggcgagg  ctgccaaccc
421tgggcctagg gatggcgcgt ggccccgggg tagccactgc agtcgtggcc agggccgcag
481gccccgctgt gcagcgcgtt cagctttgac atccaggact tggggaagga gctgaggaag
541tagacaggaa gttgtaggac cttcgttctg cgaccttgat atccatggca ggggctcggg
601atttactaag cagtcattga tcgtgagtct cggccagcca agtgcctccc gtaatctgca
661aataagtgtg aggtttgagg gggcccaccg ctactagaca cctgccaaac actggcccct
721ggagctggta cagaagatgg gttacatgta ccaggggtcg tgaaagcagc atgtgctcat
781ttcttcgtaa ctccacactg gagagagcag tgagcaaaac aggcaaaccc aaggtttctg
841ctgccatgga cctttgttcc tgggtcgagc cgaccacagg ataggtggga atgacatgca
901gtgttgtggt caggaaaggc ctctctgtgt gagccgtgta agaaggaagg atctagccat
961gcagacattt gtgctaggta gagagaacac aaagggagcc tgtgaccctt ggggtgggag
1021gcaggtgggt gtgtttgggt gcggagatca ccatatgagg tctgagaagt aggcccatta
1081ggagtttgga ttttattttg agggcaggag aatgtcagat accatgatat gacgtggcag
1141cccatgtcac acacaagtga ggaaaacgag ggtcatggag gtcaaggaat ctgcccagct
1201tcccagtttt tggcagagct aggcttcaca ctgcctcagc ttaaagccct taatttctta
1261aaccactggg ctgcagtcca tacctttgcc ccttgcacct cctctaattt atgggccacc
1321ttctccaggt gtcctccaggt gcctcattcc ttaacctctc cagcactgga aggccgaccg
1381cttcttcctt gagaccttct ctggttcttt tcctcttcct cgtctgccct tttcgttgga
1441tcctcttctg ccctctgcat gttccacccc gcccagctcc ctcttgcggt cttacatagc
1501caccggcatg actcataaca tcctttatgc tttgcccctc tgcccttcct cttgcccgtt
1561ctagcctcta aattctgggc tctgttattac cagtagatcc acgtaagagc ttgcctttcc
1621ttttagaccg gtgtgctgta ttttggatac tggcgctacc agtttcctta atacaggttg
1681aaaaacttgg agtcatcttt gttgtcccag atctctcatg cagattaatt tgacaaatgt
1741ttattgagcc tactccacgc ctgccgctgt gcaaggttct gtggctccgc ccctggtggt
1801atgtagctca ctgtgttcct gtttgcttgt tttgctccta gtactctcat ggaggcctcg
1861gtgcctccct cctggacgcc ttggtagtat gcttttcata gtttgatgca ccaaactggt
1921tatttggtta tttggggtgt gtgtttggct tttactatag gttcaaaatg agtcacccccc
1981tcccaactcc tgggttacaa aaggtggttg catttagggt gttgagctgt tttctttgct
2041tcgccctggc acctgtgagc ttttttcaggt gtgacacact ttcctatagc tgtgcttggc
2101attatcctag cacagaccct gggcttgtct gggatgaagc aggcctccct cgttcctctg
2161ccctaggctt gctttttttac atgttaaatc atgcggtggt ggggatccat gcagacaagc
2221catgctaaca gccagggcgt ctttaagagg gggttgctgt gaaagcctgc tgccgggttg
2281ggagcaggtt aaaaatgcta tgcctgctta ttttaaatgc tgttcatgga acaaaaatct
2341gtgtagtgac tttgtgagaa gttgtgatgt ttatgttgtg taactttgtg caggaacact
2401gcgtcttgca gtgggtgcac agctctgagt agaaaccacc tcttcatagg aagcctgtgg
2461ccttaacact aggcagttta agcttttaaa taataccaga gttactaact agtgcagaag
2521tgacatgctt tttctttttt cctgctag
```

TFIIIA GENE EXON TWO:

*LOOP BETA BINDING TO DNA

TFIIIA MOLECULE AMINO ACIDS 68-77:

```
         R    P    F    V    C    D    Y    E    G    C
   2549 aga  cca  ttt  gtt  tgt  gac  tat  gaa  ggg  tgt
```

TFIIIA MOLECULE ZINC FINGER 'TWO' DNA BONDING SITES, AMINO
ACIDS 78-89

```
         G    K    A    F    I    R    D    Y    H    L    S    R
   2579 ggc  aag  gcc  ttc  atc  agg  gac  tac  cat  ctg  agc  cgc
```

TFIIIA MOLECULE AMINO ACIDS 90-101:

```
         H    I    L    T    H    T    G    E    K    P    F    V
   2615 cac  att  ctg  act  cac  aca  gga  gaa  aag  ccg  ttt  gtg
```

TFIIIA GENE INTRON TWO:

2651 taa (STOP)

```
   2654 gtagaga    cctgttttta  ggcttttgaa  gtgggttgtg  ttgggcatat
   2701 agacccagta  agaagattga  tgttaactca  cgagatcagg  aatgtgaagc  ctggcagggc
   2761 tcggtggctc  atgcctgtaa  tcccagcact  ttgggaggcg  gagatgggca  gatcacttga
   2821 acccaggagt  ttgagacaaa  cctgggcaac  atggtgaaac  cccgtatgta  caaaaataca
   2881 aaaattagtc  agggatggtg  gtttgtgcct  gtaatcctag  ctacccagga  ggctgagcta
   2941 acataaaatg  ctcatggggtg  gggacaagct  aaagtatatc  aacacaatgg  gataccctac
   3001 agccaggaaa  atgaatgcag  atgctctctg  caaagccatg  agaaaatcac  cagggcactt
   3061 taattgaaaa  accaaggtgc  agaagagtcc  tctttaggct  acttttatgt  gtgtaaaaaa
   3121 gctaggggggt  aggggggaggg  gtgagtagtg  ggtgttgggt  aggcaggaag  caactatatt
   3181 tgtatttgtt  cctatttgta  aagaagtctt  aaaagttaca  taacaaaact  aaaaatgtca
   3241 tctgtttttgg  gagcagtggg  ggatcctggc  caagtagggg  gtggggatgg  taggaaatgc
   3301 catgcaacca  ggaactactg  gacatgactc  ttccagctca  tgatctaacc  cagaccctgc
   3361 ccctctttag  ctgtagttcc  ccgtttcccca  ctgctcgctg  gacagtgcta  cttggctatc
   3421 tctgtgtctt  cttaaattcc  atgtggtagg  ctgggtgtgg  tggctcatgc  ctgtaatccc
   3481 agcacttttga  gaggctgagg  tgggggaggatt  gctttgaggc  caggagttca  ggctgggcaa
   3541 gatggtcagg  tccatctcta  ttaaagaaat  aaataaataa  aaaattccac  atggcccaaa
   3601 tttgtcacag  tcaaactgag  ctcacttttc  tgtttgatct  tctctcatgt  tcttgtctgg
   3661 agaggtggcc  tcgctgtctg  tccagtgacc  catagcaaag  ataaggcagc  tccctggact
   3721 ctccattctt  tctcccatcc  cttgcaacag  gtgggttgcc  agatcctgta  actgacccat
   3781 cagatccagc  agccactgtc  ttatctcggt  ccettcctct  ggctggaatg  acagtttgca
   3841 ggccagccct  ctcccccagt  gccctcccgt  gtgcttccct  taaagctgtg  cagtgctttc
   3901 aagcacggcc  tacatgtgaa  atccaggttt  caagtgtgtc  ctacaatgac  ctgcgtgatt
   3961 tagccctttt  ctgcttatct  tgccccattt  gcttgacttg  caggcatgaa  gctgtggtcc
   4021 agctgtgcta  actaaccagc  cccctctcca  agtgtgccgg  ggtctctcac  gcccacttgg
   4081 gtcttgtcag  gactcttcct  ggcctgtcct  cctatcccat  acccggttgg  gttagatgcc
   4141 tgtgtcaggt  ttagagtgaa  gaatggcagg  aaccccagca  caagagatgc  ttaaacaaga
   4201 tgggctcttt  gtcttgtgcg  actgaaatac  agaaatacag  aggcaggagc  tctggagcct
   4261 cttctgactg  gtctctgcca  tcctcatctt  gggctttaac  ctcactgtga  tgcctgtttg
   4321 ggcccatctg  tcacataagc  atgccactgg  caggaaggag  gaaagggcat  aagaggcatg
   4381 ccccccttatt  tagagacttt  gtgggggttg  agcaggatgg  gctggactca  gccatgagcc
   4441 gccctaattg  cagggggaggc  cggagagtgc  actttctgtc  ggccacctgc  ccagctaaca
```

```
4501 ctcagcattc tgtccctgca gttaggggggg cttctagggt ctctgccaca gcgcccctcc
4561 catttgtggg cctctgtgct gtgcctccca tggtcactgc tggcttgttt gtctctgctt
4621 ggccctagga atgggacagt gcctgcctca gggttatcag tgagtgatgg ctaagattga
4681 gcctgggaaa ggaagtcctg cttcatccct caagcttacg aaggctcatc acaagaggca
4741 caaattttct tttgggaaaa aaaaaaaaaa aaaaggaaaa ggctttgcag aggatttaga
4801 tcattcaaag ccaagatgcc aagataaggg gaaccagaat ggcttggtaa gccagagaac
4861 ataatggtta tggttctgct ctaagtatct gttttacctc taatgataag ccaagacaag
4921 ttttatggag gcctttctgg aaatccagtt cataatgaca tctcaagcag cattaaggtt
4981 gtcagattct aagctgagaa taatttgtct taagcatgat ttaggcctag tgtaggcttt
5041 tgggactagt gtatttcacc ttcccatctg cccagtgtgt ataaagatg actgatgtag
5101 tgtgtataat ttcagaagcc taatatgaaa aagcattttg ttacatgata gtcatcaggt
5161 tgagagtcta tgtggtatgg cttadcactc tggaattcgc taagactatt ttatagtatt
5221 actattctt gg dagaatta gcttctataa agtaggaaga tatatgtgtc ttaaaacttc
5281 ttctcccttg gtttattaat attttggttt atataacttc ttacagt
```

TFIIIA GENE EXON THREE:

*LOOP GAMMA BINDING TO DNA

TFIIIA MOLECULE AMINO ACIDS 102-107:

	C	A	A	N	G	C
5328	tgt	gca	gcc	aat	ggc	tgt

TFIIIA MOLECULE ZINC FINGER 'THREE' DNA BONDING SITES, AMINO ACIDS 108-119

	D	Q	K	F	N	T	K	S	N	L	K	K
5349	gat	caa	aaa	ttc	aac	aca	aaa	tca	aac	ttg	aag	aaa

TFIIIA MOLECULE AMINO ACIDS 120-133:

	H	F	E	R	K	H	E	N	Q	Q	K	Q	Y	I
5381	cat	ttt	gaa	cgc	aaa	cat	gaa	aat	caa	caa	aaa	caa	tat	ata

TFIIIA GENE INTRON THREE:

```
5424 gtaagta    tgattttata tgcttaaatt ttttgagtat
5461 ttttacactt actgcctatg tttctgacat tttcagccag gtgcggtggc tcaagcctat
5521 aatcgtagct tgaggccagg aatttgagac cagcctggga aacatagtga aatgctgtct
5581 ctgaaaaaaa aaaacaaaaa cagaaaacaa aacaaaaaat tttgggggtaa cagagaccct
5641 gtctctaaaa aataaaagtg aaaaataaag ttttcgtcaa ccaaattttg tctgccaaat
5701 gtctgaattt acttaatgcc atcataatga taaaggtttt aatttggaag cagacattgt
5761 gcaaattagt gtattgggag actattccaa ctgaaacagt tttgcttttt caaatgttat
5821 atgattcttc aaaccttttt gagataaagc agaattttac agtaacaaaa tgggtgaaag
5881 cagaaatttt atacagtctc caaaattgtt ttatcttgag gattctgtta cgaactgttc
5941 attttgtttt gactttccat aagactaacg agcctttaca atttaacag
```

TFIIIA GENE EXON FOUR:

*LOOP DELTA BINDING TO DNA

TFIIIA MOLECULE AMINO ACIDS 134-139:

```
         C     S     F     E     D     C
 5990   tgc   agt   ttt   gaa   gac   tgt
```

TFIIIA MOLECULE ZINC FINGER 'FOUR' DNA BONDING SITES, AMINO ACIDS 140-151

```
        K     K     T     F     K     K     H     Q     Q     L     K     I
 6008  aag   aag   acc   ttt   aag   aaa   cat   cag   cag   ctg   aaa   atc
```

TFIIIA MOLECULE AMINO ACIDS 152-164:

```
        H     Q     C     Q     H     T     N     E     P     L     F     K
 6044  cat   cag   tgc   cag   cat   acc   aat   gaa   cct   cta   ttc   aag
```

TFIIIA GENE INTRON FOUR:

6080 tag (STOP)

```
6083 gtacttca    tgtggctgaa aatgcctgga ttctaggtgt
6121 gaataagatt  ggaaatgcaa gggtggtgtt gagcattgtt tcatgttttt tggccatttg
6181 tatatcttct  gagaaatgtc tgttcatatc ctttgcccac ttttcgatgg attgtttttt
6241 tcttgctgat  ctgagttccc tgtagatcct ggatatacat tctttattgg atgcataatg
6301 tgccagtatt  ttctcccact ctctgggttg tctgtttact ctgctgatta tttctttgc
6361 tgtgcagaag  ctttttagtt taattaggtc ccatttattt atttctattt ttgttgcatt
6421 tgctttcagg  gccttagtaa gaattctttg cctaggctga tgtccagaag tttttccaat
6481 gttttcattt  tgaattttta gtttcaggtc ataaacttaa tttgagttga tttttgtata
6541 aggtgagaga  tagggatcca gttttttccag caccatttat tgaatagggga gtcctttccc
6601 cagtttacgt  ttttatatgc tttgttgaag atcgggtggc tgtaagtatt tggctttatt
6661 tctgtttgt   tccattggtc taagtgccta tttttaaacc agtgccaccc tgtttggta
6721 actgtagcct  cgtagtataa tctgaagtct ggtcaaagga aaagaagtca ctatatgaaa
6781 aagacacatg  cacacacgtt tacagcagca cagttcacaa ttgcaaatac atggagccaa
6841 tttaagtgcc  catcgaccaa tgagtagata aagaaaacgt gatgtatata caccatggaa
6901 tactacacag  ccataaaagg gaacaaaatg atgtcttttg cagcagcttg gatggagctg
6961 gaggccatta  ttctcagtga agtaactcag gaatggaaaa ccaaatacca tagtttttcac
7021 taagtgggca  ctaaactatg aggacaaaaa gacacagtga tttcataaac tttggggact
7081 tggggtgggg  agtttgggga gggggtgag ggatgaaaga ctacatattg ggtacagtgt
7141 atgctgcttg  agtgatggtg cgctaaaatc tcagcaccac tataggattc atccacgtaa
7201 cgaaaaaaca  cttgcaaccc caaaagccat tgaaatttaa agcaacggtg ggacaaatct
7261 tctgaaagct  tcctaatcaa cattttctg ttaaaatgta ctgcatatgc acatttatat
7321 attgggagca  ttttaaaggt ttactttgct ctgaaagaaa tatttaatgt gtttcaaaat
7381 aatttttgag  attattctag ttgtggttaa gcttaaaggc tgagaaatta cttaactatt
7441 caaatagagc  ctgtgcaact atatgaaatg tcattatgga gacactcatt atgcttttcc
7501 tgtagaacaa  aacaagtagt tgggtttatc tgcaattagg gttttttgag gaacgtgagg
7561 gtggctggaa  aagttggtga gacctgcaaa agggccagcg gctctctgca tggctctggc
7621 catccggcac  tttcccttga cttgcacagg ctgccctgtg ccttggagtt gctgcagtga
7681 ccttgcctgt  ccttgcttgt gggtctgctg ctgctgcttt gctgctgatg gctttagcac
7741 agaggggggcc cgtgctttt attgctcaac agaggcagat gcatctactg ctgtgctgtc
7801 tcgcacaccc  cctatgcagc atcattagga aagctagaca caagtgattc agaatggctt
7861 aggggtttat  ctaagccaag tcagataacc tcttgaacta tctttttgta gccatgaaag
7921 cagagtatat  ttccagaggt ataaagatga aaactgtttta aatgggtcaa aaaaagtaac
7981 gtgacttttt  tctccaacag tttgtttttgt cctaaagctg gtcaagtaac ttgaatctca
8041 cctgtgatga  gagctacatt ttaacatggg tttggttatg ggaagaggca agactttggt
8101 gggagaaaca  ggacaaagtg ccattgacct tgagcggagt tctctgtgaa aatggattgg
8161 ctaataccctc atgtgttgcc aatgcagg
```

TFIIIA GENE EXON FIVE:

*LOOP EPSILON BINDING TO DNA

TFIIIA MOLECULE AMINO ACIDS 164-169:

```
        C      T      Q      E      G      C
8189   tgt    acc    cag    gaa    gga    tgt
```

TFIIIA MOLECULE BONDING TO DNA AMINO ACIDS 170-181:

```
        G    K    H    F    A    S    P    S    K    L    K    R
8207   ggg  aaa  cac  ttt  gca  tca  ccc  agc  aag  ctg  aaa  cga
```

TFIIIA MOLECULE AMINO ACIDS 182-187:

```
        H      A      K      A      H      E
8243   cat    gcc    aag    gcc    cac    gag
```

TFIIIA GENE EXON FIVE:

G
8261 ggt

```
8264 gtgtacg     gatagcctgg
8281 gtgtgctccg aggggatgc caaatcctgg gcgcctttga atctgttctg tgatcacgct
8341 gaaaagatgg gaaccctgtg aacaggggac accatcctgc ttatttgggt cttacactct
8401 tgtccaaaga ggcactgtat atgtctgttt ttccactacc gtatcattgc tgttcacatg
8461 taatgtgttg tttgttcaca acaagcgcct ggttacacat tacactgacg aatgtgctga
8521 tgctccagcc atggctttga tgcttctgtc atttttaacc tcttctatta atatttactg
8581 cctgtgccat tctttttcctt gttggccatt cacaaggctt ggataatcgt gtgacatttt
8641 gagagccatc agatgttacg tttctcaaaa aaaaaaaaaa aagacttgat tatattaact
8701 atttgaatct atgatctgtt tccttgaggg atttttgcta atctgtattt caatttccca
8761 ggtcctagaa tttatgattt tttttttttt aagaggttag tagctaacag tgagaggcag
8821 cctcattgtt tttagtttct agttgggtgg aactcagccc tagtgttgta tacttattaa
8881 tcccatttta gtgctttgca catatccatt gttattcagt gttttctct gggtccttcc
8941 agtttatttt cttccttagc tgtactcttt taaaaaaaaa aaacaaaaaa aaacttttt
9001 ttttttttt gtgataaagt taaaatataa tgtaccctac ttttttgtg cagtatgaca
9061 cttacaagat ggccagacta gaggaagcca gaggtgggca tggtaacact actgaaaagt
9121 tggtggtgtg ccatggacaa gggaccgact gcagagtatg tttgtgagg aaaatagagg
9181 cgaggataga gcaggcaggg gaagggaaat aagacatgga gataggaggt taaagcagtt
9241 gggagtccat acacagccta cccaacttcc tgagaactct tagagaggaa aaggcatcct
9301 taggcatcct tcctgtgaag tttgcctatt ccgtgatcac gctgagaaga tgggaactct
9361 gaagtttgct tcacaggaag gtaaaatcct taaagggagg caccttgctg tgccactgtt
9421 cagttttact ataacatcaa tctttttta gttttttattc ccacctcaag aggctgagtt
9481 gaatactatt aggcggggaa tggaaaatta tataggcacc taagtttcct ttctagttat
9541 ggtcagtgtt tacactgagt attcatgacca gacaatgcac caattttttt aata
```

TFIIIA GENE EXON SIX:

*LOOP ZETA BINDING TO TRANSCRIPTION FACTORS

TFIIIA MOLECULE AMINO ACIDS 188-195:

```
         G         Y
9595    ggc       tat

         V      C      Q      K      G      C
9601    gta    tgt    caa    aaa    gga    tgt
```

TFIIIA MOLECULE BIND TO TRANSCRIPTION FACTOR AMINO ACIDS 196-207:

```
       S     F     V     A     K     T     W     T     E     L     L     K
9619  tcc   ttt   gtg   gca   aaa   aca   tgg   acg   gaa   ctt   ctg   aaa
```

TFIIIA MOLECULE AMINO ACIDS 208-214:

```
       H     V     R     E     T     H     K
9655  cat   gtg   aga   gaa   acc   cat   aaa
```

GENE INTRON SIX

```
 9676 ggtaa        ggcaggcatg aatggcaggc atggtgtaaa tgtttgtccc
 9721 cacagaactg atttagtgct tttcaagagt gaaatgctgt gtgctttaaa gtaaaagggt
 9781 ttctctatga tattttgtga agtgctgggt atgatgttgt tggaaaggtg agcagagctg
 9841 tgccaggtct ctgagccacc ccaccatgca caattagcat gctgaaggcg gtggcaggtc
 9901 tgtagtgaag aatttcggga ggcactgctg ttctgtggga ccgcctggga aacagtaccc
 9961 tgcatactgg gggacaagga aggacactgg tctgcttcat tttctgtacc tccccacagt
10021 caccttcctg agagccctgc ctcttggcaa gtgaacaatg actgtgtggc atttaagaac
10081 ttcagagaat tgagacaaac ttcctaggtg ataaaaactg gggttgtttc cttgggaatt
10141 tctgatttgt atatagtgat caggtttcag gcactgaatg ttacttatat attaggtatt
10201 aatttttct aaatggtaat atctggggaa atttgtgaaa tttgtctgtc tgtcccacca
```

TFIIIA GENE EXON SEVEN:

*LOOP ETA BINDING TO TRANSCRIPTION FACTORS

TFIIIA MOLECULE AMINO ACIDS 215-222:

```
        E     E     I     L     C     E     Y     C
10261  gag   gaa   ata   cta   tgt   gaa   gta   tgc
```

TFIIIA MOLECULE AMINO ACIDS 223-234:

```
        R     K     T     F     K     R     K     D     Y     L     K     Q
10285  cgg   aaa   aca   ttt   aaa   cgc   aaa   gat   tac   ctt   aag   caa
```

TFIIIA MOLECULE AMINO ACIDS 235-253:

```
        H     M     K     T     H     A     P     E     R     D     V     C     R     C
10321  cac   atg   aaa   act   cat   gcc   cca   gaa   agg   gat   gta   tgt   cgc   tgt
```

```
        p           R           E           G           C
10363  cca         aga         gaa         ggc         tgt
```

*LOOP THETA BINDING TO TRANSCRIPTION FACTORS

TFIIIA MOLECULE AMINO ACIDS 254-265:

	G	R	T	Y	T	T	V	F	N	L	Q	S
10378	gga	aga	acc	tat	aca	act	gtg	ttt	aat	ctc	caa	agc

TFIIIA MOLECULE AMINO ACIDS 266-284:

	H	I	L	S	F	H	E	E	S	R	P	F
10414	cat	atc	ctc	tcc	ttc	cat	gag	gaa	agc	cgc	cct	ttt

	V	C	E	H	A	G	C
10450	gtg	tgt	gaa	cat	gct	ggc	tgt

*LOOP IOTA BINDING TO TRANSCRIPTION FACTORS

TFIIIA MOLECULE AMINO ACIDS 285-291:

	G	K	T	F	A	M	K
10471	ggc	aaa	aca	ttt	gca	atg	aaa

GENE INTRON SEVEN

```
10492 gtaagcact
10501 caccctcata ctcatggtcc tatagtctat gctttcacaa catggttttc atattaatat
10561 ttcattaata actttctctt tcattgtag
```

*LOOP IOTA (CONTINUED) BINDING TO TRANSCRIPTION FACTORS

TFIIIA MOLECULE AMINO ACIDS 292-296:

	Q	S	L	T	R
10590	caa	agt	ctc	act	agg

TFIIIA MOLECULE AMINO ACIDS 297-311:

	H	A	V	V	H	D	P	D	K	K	K	M	K
10605	cat	gct	gtt	gta	cat	gat	cct	gac	aag	aag	aaa	atg	aag

	L	K
10644	ctc	aaa

GENE INTRON EIGHT

```
10650 gtaagttgaa actacttagg caagcttagt t
10681 ttcaagtgga aattgtttaa ggccagaagg agtctgtttg gaattctttt cacctgcttt
10741 actgtttgag tctgcactac tgttgaagac tttacttcct cataaagcaa tgttgtacac
10801 tatatctgct ggtacatatg actatcgtaa aattaactca gacagttttg attttgaatt
10861 ctaatcgtgt gtcttcctta ttcccaaag
```

3′ END OF THE TFIIIA MOLECULE

TFIIIA MOLECULE AMINO ACIDS 312-365:

```
           V    K    K    S    R    E    K    R    S    L    A    S    H
    10890 gtc  aaa  aaa  tct  cgt  gaa  aaa  cgg  agt  ttg  gcc  tct  cat

           L    S    G    Y    I    P    P    K    R    K    Q    G    Q
    10929 ctc  agt  gga  tat  atc  cct  ccc  aaa  agg  aaa  caa  ggg  caa

           G    L    S    L    C    Q    N    G    E    S    P    N    C
    10968 ggc  tta  tct  ttg  tgt  caa  aac  gga  gag  tca  ccc  aac  tgt

           V    E    D    K    M    L    S    T    V    A    V    L    T
    11007 gtg  gaa  gac  aag  atg  ctc  tcg  aca  gtt  gca  gta  ctt  acc

    11046 L    G
          ctt  ggc
```

11052 taa (STOP)

TFIIIA GENE 3′ DOWNSTREAM REGION

```
    11055 gaactg      cactgctttg tttaaaggac tgcagaccaa ggagcgagct
    11101 ttctctcaga gcatgctttt ctttattaaa attactgatg cagaacattt gattccttat
    11161 catttc
```

CHAPTER 8

RE-DESIGNING THE TFIIIA MOLECULE

As shown in the previous chapter, the following three hundred sixty five amino acid sequence comprises the Transcription Factor III A molecule, Taxonomic identifier 9606 [NCBI]:

```
1          10          20          30          40          50          60
MDPPAVVAES  VSSLTIADAF  IAAGESSAPT  PPRPALPRRF  ICSFPDCSAN  YSKAWKLDAH
           70          80          90         100         110         120
LCKHTGERPF  VCDYEGCGKA  FIRDYHLSRH  ILTHTGEKPF  VCAANGCDQK  FNTKSNLKKH
          130         140         150         160         170         180
FERKHENQQK  QYICSFEDCK  KTFKKHQQLK  IHQCQHTNEP  LFKCTQEGCG  KHFASPSKLK
          190         200         210         220         230         240
RHAKAHEGYV  CQKGCSFVAK  TWTELLKHVR  ETHKEEILCE  VCRKTFKRKD  YLKQHMKTHA
          250         260         270         280         290         300
PERDVCRCPR  EGCGRTYTTV  FNLQSHILSF  HEESRPFVCE  HAGCGKTFAM  KQSLTRHAVV
          310         320         330         340         350         360
HDPDKKKMKL  KVKKSREKRS  LASHLSGYIP  PKRKQGQGLS  LCQNGESPNC  VEDKMLSTVA
365
VLTLG
```

The TFIIIA protein is comprised of nine zinc fingers. Generally, during the construct of a Transcription Complex, from the 5' to 3' end of the TFIIIA molecule zinc fingers 1-5 attach to a DNA segment while the remainder of the zinc fingers attach to other transcription factors. All nine zinc fingers may attach to the DNA in some situations. The fourth, fifth, sixth and seventh finger from 5' to the 3' end of the molecule may attach to an RNA molecule. The eight zinc finger may attach at times to a TFIIIC molecule. The ninth zinc finger may attach at times to TFIIID molecule.

The TFIIIA9606 is utilized naturally by a human cell to assist in the transcription of 5S RNA molecules. The TFIIIA molecule also assists in transcribing some viral DNA genomes.

For reference, Table 3 provides an Inverse table using IUPAC notation.

Amino Acid	Three Letter Abbreviation	One Letter Abbreviation	RNA Nucleotide Codes	DNA Nucleotide Codes
Alanine	Ala	A	GCU, GCC, GCA, GCG	GCT, GCC, GCA, GCG
Arginine	Arg	R	CGU, CGC, CGA, CGG, AGA, AGG	CGT, CGC, CGA, CGG, AGA, AGG
Asparagine	Asn	N	AAU, AAC	AAT, AAC
Aspartic acid	Asp	D	GAU, GAC	GAT, GAC
Cysteine	Cys	C	UGU, UGC	TGT, TGC
Glutamine	Gln	Q	CAA, CAG	CAA, CAG
Glutamic acid	Glu	E	GAA, GAG	GAA, GAG
Glycine	Gly	G	GGU, GGC, GGA, GGG	GGT, GGC, GGA, GGG
Histidine	His	H	CAU, CAC	CAT, CAC
Isoleucine	Ile	I	AUU, AUC, AUA	ATT, ATC, ATA
Leucine	Leu	L	UUA, UUG, CUU, CUC, CUA, CUG	TTA, TTG, CTT, CTC, CTA, CTG
Lysine	Lys	K	AAA, AAG	AAA, AAG
Methionine	Met	M	AUG	ATG
Phenylalanine	Phe	F	UUU, UUC	TTT, TTC
Proline	Pro	P	CCU, CCC, CCA, CCG	CCT, CCC, CCA, CCG
Serine	Ser	S	UCU, UCC, UCA UCG, AGU, AGC	TCT, TCC, TCA TCG, AGT, AGC
Threonine	Thr	T	ACU, ACC, ACA, ACG	ACT, ACC, ACA, ACG
Tryptophan	Typ	W	UGG	TGG
Tyrosine	Tyr	Y	UAU, UAC	TAT, TAC
Valine	Val	V	GUU, GUC, GUA, GUG	GTT, GTC, GTA, GTG

START *already Met	Met	---	AUG	ATG
STOP	---	---	UAA, UGA, UAG	TAA, TGA, TAG

Table 3

Inverse table using IUPAC notation.

In modifying the TFIIIA molecule to bind to HIV's unique identifier, the following design modifies only the binding segments in the nine zinc finger loops. The overall structure of the molecule has not been changed. Alterations of the elements in the 5' and 3' noncoding untranslatable regions of the mRNA that control the construct of the overall standard architecture of the TFIIIA molecule have been avoided. The amino acid to nucleotide binding elements of zinc fingers 1-5 are modified to generate a semi-permanent binding of the modified TFIIIA molecule to HIV's unique identifier. The modifications include changing the DNA binding sites of zinc finger loops alpha, beta, gamma, delta and epsilon. The amino acid asparagine (N) is utilized to attach to the nucleotide adenine (a). The amino acid arginine (R) is utilized to bind to the nucleic acid guanine (g). The amino acid glutamic acid (E) is utilized to bind to the nucleotide cytosine (c). The amino acid lysine (K) is utilized to attach to the nucleotide thymine (t). Zinc fingers 6-9 are modified to prevent binding of other transcription factors to the modified TFIIIA molecule. Amino acids with short side chains replace amino acids with long side chains in zinc finger loops zeta, eta, theta, and iota. Nonpolar amino acids with short side chains, such as alanine, are not capable of binding to other molecules. Filling zinc loops 6-9 with nonpolar amino acids with short size chains prevents assembly of a transcription complex by preventing other transcription factors from bonding to the modified TFIIIA molecule.

As reported by NCBI, the TFIIIA molecule as it is joined together as reported as CDS:

```
CDS join(195..395,2549..2649,5327..5423,5990..6078,8188..8261,
9596..9676,10262..10491,10590..10649,10890..11054)
```

ORIGIN

TFIIIA GENE EXON ONE:

TFIIIA mRNA 5′ UPSTREAM UNTRANSLATABLE SEGMENT:

```
  1 atgcgcgatc tcccggagca tgcgcagcag cggcgccgac gcggggcggt gcctggtgac
 61 cgcgcgcgct cccggaagtg tgccggcgtc gcgcgaaggt tcagcaggga gccgtgggcc
121 gggcgcgccg gttcccggca cgtgtctcgg cacgtggcag cgcgcctggc cctgggcttg
181 gaggcgccgg cgcc
```

*LOOP ALPHA BINDING TO DNA

TFIIIA MOLECULE AMINO ACIDS 1-47:

```
        L   D   P   P   A   V   V   A   E   S   V   S   S   L   T
    195 ctg gat ccg ccg gcc gtg gtc gcc gag tcg gtg tcg tcc ttg acc

        I   A   D   A   F   I   A   A   G   E   S   S   A   P   T
    240 atc gcc gac gcg ttc att gca gcc ggc gag agc tca gct ccg acc

        P   P   R   P   A   L   P   R   R   F   I   C   S   F   P
    286 ccg ccg cgc ccc gcg ctt ccc agg agg ttc atc tgc tcc ttc cct

        D   C
    330 gac tgc
```

TFIIIA MOLECULE ALPHA ZINC FINGER DNA BONDING SITES, AMINO ACIDS 48-59:

```
        S   A   N   Y   S   K   A   W   K   L   D   A
    336 agc gcc aat tac agc aaa gcc tgg aag ctt gac gcg
```

TFIIIA MOLECULE AMINO ACIDS 60-67:

```
        H   L   C   K   H   T   G   E
    372 cac ctg tgc aag cac acg ggg gag
```

TFIIIA GENE EXON TWO:

*LOOP BETA BINDING TO DNA

TFIIIA MOLECULE AMINO ACIDS 68-77:

```
         R   P   F   V   C   D   Y   E   G   C
    2549 aga cca ttt gtt tgt gac tat gaa ggg tgt
```

TFIIIA MOLECULE BETA ZINC FINGER DNA BONDING SITES, AMINO ACIDS 78-89

```
        G    K    A    F    I    R    D    Y    H    L    S    R
 2579  ggc  aag  gcc  ttc  atc  agg  gac  tac  cat  ctg  agc  cgc
```

TFIIIA MOLECULE AMINO ACIDS 90-101:

```
        H    I    L    T    H    T    G    E    K    P    F    V
 2615  cac  att  ctg  act  cac  aca  gga  gaa  aag  ccg  ttt  gtg
```

TFIIIA GENE EXON THREE:

*LOOP GAMMA BINDING TO DNA

TFIIIA MOLECULE AMINO ACIDS 102-107:

```
        C    A    A    N    G    C
 5328  tgt  gca  gcc  aat  ggc  tgt
```

TFIIIA MOLECULE ZINC FINGER 'THREE' DNA BONDING SITES,
AMINO ACIDS 108-119

```
        D    Q    K    F    N    T    K    S    N    L    K    K
 5349  gat  caa  aaa  ttc  aac  aca  aaa  tca  aac  ttg  aag  aaa
```

TFIIIA MOLECULE AMINO ACIDS 120-133:

```
        H    F    E    R    K    H    E    N    Q    Q    K    Q    Y    I
 5381  cat  ttt  gaa  cgc  aaa  cat  gaa  aat  caa  caa  aaa  caa  tat  ata
```

TFIIIA GENE EXON FOUR:

*LOOP DELTA BINDING TO DNA

TFIIIA MOLECULE AMINO ACIDS 134-139:

```
        C    S    F    E    D    C
 5990  tgc  agt  ttt  gaa  gac  tgt
```

TFIIIA MOLECULE DELTA ZINC FINGER DNA BONDING SITES, AMINO
ACIDS 140-151

```
        K    K    T    F    K    K    H    Q    Q    L    K    I
 6008  aag  aag  acc  ttt  aag  aaa  cat  cag  cag  ctg  aaa  atc
```

TFIIIA MOLECULE AMINO ACIDS 152-164:

```
       H    Q    C    Q    H    T    N    E    P    L    F    K
  6044 cat  cag  tgc  cag  cat  acc  aat  gaa  cct  cta  ttc  aag
```

TFIIIA GENE EXON FIVE:

*LOOP EPSILON BINDING TO DNA

TFIIIA MOLECULE AMINO ACIDS 164-169:

```
       C    T    Q    E    G    C
  8189 tgt  acc  cag  gaa  gga  tgt
```

TFIIIA MOLECULE EPSILON ZINC FINGER BONDING SITES, AMINO ACIDS 170-181:

```
       G    K    H    F    A    S    P    S    K    L    K    R
  8207 ggg  aaa  cac  ttt  gca  tca  ccc  agc  aag  ctg  aaa  cga
```

TFIIIA MOLECULE AMINO ACIDS 182-187:

```
  H  A  K  A  H  E
  8243 cat gcc aag gcc cac gag
```

TFIIIA GENE EXON SIX:

*LOOP ZETA BINDING TO TRANSCRIPTION FACTORS

TFIIIA MOLECULE AMINO ACIDS 188-195:

```
       G    Y
  9595 ggc  tat

       V    C    Q    K    G    C
  9601 gta  tgt  caa  aaa  gga  tgt
```

TFIIIA MOLECULE ZETA LOOP BIND TO TF, AMINO ACIDS 196-207:

```
       S    F    V    A    K    T    W    T    E    L    L    K
  9619 tcc  ttt  gtg  gca  aaa  aca  tgg  acg  gaa  ctt  ctg  aaa
```

TFIIIA MOLECULE AMINO ACIDS 208-214:

```
       H    V    R    E    T    H    K
  9655 cat  gtg  aga  gaa  acc  cat  aaa
```

TFIIIA GENE EXON SEVEN:

*LOOP ETA BINDING TO TRANSCRIPTION FACTORS

TFIIIA MOLECULE AMINO ACIDS 215-222:

```
          E    E    I    L    C    E    Y    C
    10261 gag  gaa  ata  cta  tgt  gaa  gta  tgc
```

TFIIIA MOLECULE ETA LOOP BINDING TO TF, AMINO ACIDS 223-234:

```
          R    K    T    F    K    R    K    D    Y    L    K    Q
    10285 cgg  aaa  aca  ttt  aaa  cgc  aaa  gat  tac  ctt  aag  caa
```

TFIIIA MOLECULE AMINO ACIDS 235-253:

```
          H    M    K    T    H    A    P    E    R    D    V    C    R    C
    10321 cac  atg  aaa  act  cat  gcc  cca  gaa  agg  gat  gta  tgt  cgc  tgt
```

```
          P    R    E    G    C
    10363 cca  aga  gaa  ggc  tgt
```

*LOOP THETA BINDING TO TRANSCRIPTION FACTORS

TFIIIA MOLECULE THETA LOOP BINDING TO TF, AMINO ACIDS 254-265:

```
          G    R    T    Y    T    T    V    F    N    L    Q    S
    10378 gga  aga  acc  tat  aca  act  gtg  ttt  aat  ctc  caa  agc
```

TFIIIA MOLECULE AMINO ACIDS 266-284:

```
          H    I    L    S    F    H    E    E    S    R    P    F
    10414 cat  atc  ctc  tcc  ttc  cat  gag  gaa  agc  cgc  cct  ttt
```

```
          V    C    E    H    A    G    C
    10450 gtg  tgt  gaa  cat  gct  ggc  tgt
```

*LOOP IOTA BINDING TO TRANSCRIPTION FACTORS

TFIIIA MOLECULE IOTA LOOP BIND TO TF, AMINO ACIDS 285-291:

```
          G    K    T    F    A    M    K
    10471 ggc  aaa  aca  ttt  gca  atg  aaa
```

*LOOP IOTA (CONTINUED) BINDING TO TRANSCRIPTION FACTORS

TFIIIA MOLECULE IOTA LOOP (continued), AMINO ACIDS 292-296:

```
       Q    S    L    T    R
10590 caa  agt  ctc  act  agg
```

TFIIIA MOLECULE AMINO ACIDS 297-311:

```
       H    A    V    V    H    D    P    D    K    K    K    M    K
10605 cat  gct  gtt  gta  cat  gat  cct  gac  aag  aag  aaa  atg  aag
```

```
       L    K
10644 ctc  aaa
```

3' END OF THE TFIIIA MOLECULE

TFIIIA MOLECULE AMINO ACIDS 312-365:

```
       V    K    K    S    R    E    K    R    S    L    A    S    H
10890 gtc  aaa  aaa  tct  cgt  gaa  aaa  cgg  agt  ttg  gcc  tct  cat
       L    S    G    Y    I    P    P    K    R    K    Q    G    Q
10929 ctc  agt  gga  tat  atc  cct  ccc  aaa  agg  aaa  caa  ggg  caa
```

```
       G    L    S    L    C    Q    N    G    E    S    P    N    C
10968 ggc  tta  tct  ttg  tgt  caa  aac  gga  gag  tca  ccc  aac  tgt
```

```
       V    E    D    K    M    L    S    T    V    A    V    L    T
11007 gtg  gaa  gac  aag  atg  ctc  tcg  aca  gtt  gca  gta  ctt  acc
```

```
11046 L    G
      ctt  ggc
```

```
11052 taa (STOP)
```

TFIIIA GENE 3' DOWNSTREAM REGION

```
11055 gaactg      cactgctttg tttaaaggac tgcagaccaa ggagcgagct
11101 ttctctcaga gcatgctttt ctttattaaa attactgatg cagaacattt gattccttat
11161 catttc
```

The binding sites of the TFIIIA molecule:

TFIIIA MOLECULE ALPHA ZINC FINGER DNA BONDING SITES, AMINO ACIDS 48-59:

```
      S    A    N    Y    S    K    A    W    K    L    D    A
336  agc  gcc  aat  tac  agc  aaa  gcc  tgg  aag  ctt  gac  gcg
```

TFIIIA MOLECULE BETA ZINC FINGER DNA BONDING SITES, AMINO ACIDS 78-89

```
       G    K    A    F    I    R    D    Y    H    L    S    R
2579  ggc  aag  gcc  ttc  atc  agg  gac  tac  cat  ctg  agc  cgc
```

— 70 —

TFIIIA MOLECULE GAMMA ZINC FINGER DNA BONDING SITES, AMINO ACIDS 108–119

```
         D   Q   K   F   N   T   K   S   N   L   K   K
    5349 gat caa aaa ttc aac aca aaa tca aac ttg aag aaa
```

TFIIIA MOLECULE DELTA ZINC FINGER DNA BONDING SITES, AMINO ACIDS 140–151

```
         K   K   T   F   K   K   H   Q   Q   L   K   I
    6008 aag aag acc ttt aag aaa cat cag cag ctg aaa atc
```

TFIIIA MOLECULE EPSILON ZINC FINGER BONDING SITES, AMINO ACIDS 170–181:

```
         G   K   H   F   A   S   P   S   K   L   K   R
    8207 ggg aaa cac ttt gca tca ccc agc aag ctg aaa cga
```

TFIIIA MOLECULE ZETA LOOP BIND TO TF, AMINO ACIDS 196–207:

```
         S   F   V   A   K   T   W   T   E   L   L   K
    9619 tcc ttt gtg gca aaa aca tgg acg gaa ctt ctg aaa
```

TFIIIA MOLECULE ETA LOOP BINDING TO TF, AMINO ACIDS 223–234:

```
          R   K   T   F   K   R   K   D   Y   L   K   Q
    10285 cgg aaa aca ttt aaa cgc aaa gat tac ctt aag caa
```

TFIIIA MOLECULE THETA LOOP BINDING TO TF, AMINO ACIDS 254–265:

```
          G   R   T   Y   T   T   V   F   N   L   Q   S
    10378 gga aga acc tat aca act gtg ttt aat ctc caa agc
```

TFIIIA MOLECULE IOTA LOOP BIND TO TF, AMINO ACIDS 285–291:

```
          G   K   T   F   A   M   K
    10471 ggc aaa aca ttt gca atg aaa
```

TFIIIA MOLECULE IOTA LOOP (continued), AMINO ACIDS 292–296:

```
          Q   S   L   T   R
    10590 caa agt ctc act agg
```

HIV's Unique Identifier: 25 character bp string:
'agcagctgcttttttgcctgtactgg'.

Human immunodeficiency virus 1 (HXB2), complete genome; HIV1/ HTLV-III/LAV reference genome, GenBank K03455.1. (Accessed October 20, 2013 at http://www.ncbi.nlm.nih.gov/nuccore/1906382.) The human immunodeficiency virus (HIV) type 1 HXB2 DNA genome at position 431 to 455 has the twenty-five nucleotide sequence 5'-agcagctgcttttgcctgtactgg-3' as a unique sequence located between HIV's TATA box and the TSS and is referred to as the unique identifier of HIV. This twenty-five nucleotide sequence does not appear intact in the naturally in the uninfected human genome. BLAST query of the human genome identifies 20/20 at 100% (agcagctgcttttgcctgt) of the 25 nucleotides comprising the unique identifier. BLAST is Basic Local Alignment Search Tool finds regions of proteins or nucleotide sequences in the database and calculates statistical significance of the matches; located ncbi.nlm.nih.gov/ BLAST/. NCBI: National Center for Biotechnology Information.

Building a transcription factor that would seek out and attach to these specific 25 nucleotides when the viral genome is embedded in the human DNA, could block transcription of the HIV genome. The TFIIIA molecule is a molecule occurring in nature that is incorporated in the transcription complex. The TFIIIA molecule binds to the DNA, as one of the first actions of the transcription complex, as the transcription complex begins to form at a site along the DNA where a gene is intended to be transcribed. The TFIIIA molecule is generated in the cytoplasm of the cell and is transported into the nucleus of the cell. Therefore, a synthetic therapeutic transcription factor molecule that is able to be delivered into the cytoplasm of the cell should migrate into the nucleus of the cell and take action in the nucleus of the cell as would a naturally occurring TFIIIA molecule.

An artistic two-dimensional rendering of a TFIIIA molecule was presented in Figure 15. There exists a 5' end to the molecule and a 3' end to the molecule. Between the 5' end of TFIIIA and the 3' end, there are nine loops, sometimes referred to as zinc fingers due to the manner by which they are constructed. Going from the 5' end of the molecule downstream to the 3' end of the molecule the first five loops designated alpha, beta, gamma, delta and epsilon are functional projections that cause the molecule to attach to the DNA at a certain binding site. The alpha loop is loop 1, the beta loop is loop 2, the gamma loop is loop 3, the delta loop is loop 4 and the epsilon loop is loop 5. The remaining four loops are functional projections that are meant to interact with other molecules. Molecular configuration distal in the molecule identifies the molecule as that is capable of migrating from the cytoplasm to the nucleus. A transcription complex is a macromolecule that is comprised of approximately forty differing protein molecules. One of the forty transcription factor molecules which congregate to form the transcription complex may include a TFIIIA molecule.

Figure 17 illustrates the atoms that comprise the four DNA nucleotides adenine, cytosine, guanine, and thymine.

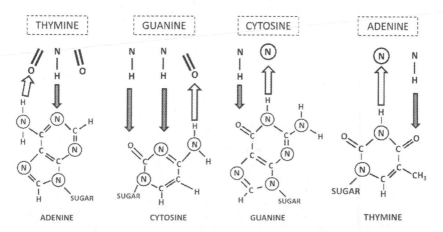

ADENINE   CYTOSINE   GUANINE   THYMINE

Figure 17 Construct of the four DNA nucleotides

Figure 18 illustrates the binding of adenine to thymine and guanine to cytosine when the nucleotides are arranged in DNA.

NUCLEOTIDE BINDING

THYMINE   GUANINE   CYTOSINE   ADENINE

ADENINE   CYTOSINE   GUANINE   THYMINE

Figure 18 Binding of the four DNA nucleotides
to respective nucleotides.

Figure 19 illustrates four amino acids that would semi-permanently bind to the DNA nucleotides. Illustrated is the binding of asparagine to adenine, binding of glutamic acid to cytosine, binding of arginine to guanine, and lysine to thymine.

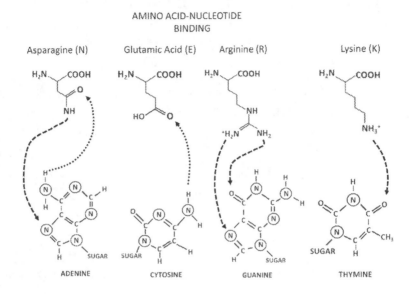

Figure 19 Binding of amino acids to nucleotides

Figure 20 illustrates the overall molecular design of the modified TFIIIA molecule designed to target the HIV genome when embedded in nuclear DNA.

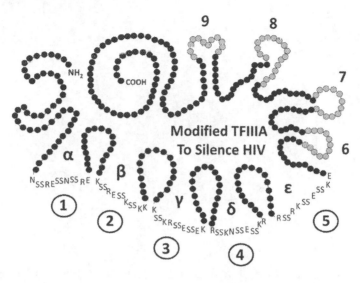

Figure 20 Modified TFIIIA molecule to target HIV genome

Figure 21 illustrates binding of amino acids to the nucleotides 431 to 436 of the HIV genome.

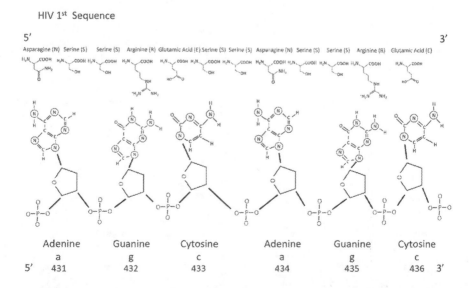

Figure 21 Binding of amino acids to the nucleotides 431 to 436

Figure 22 illustrates the bonds created by the amino acids to nucleotides 431 to 436 of the HIV genome.

HIV 1st Sequence (Zinc Finger: Alpha)

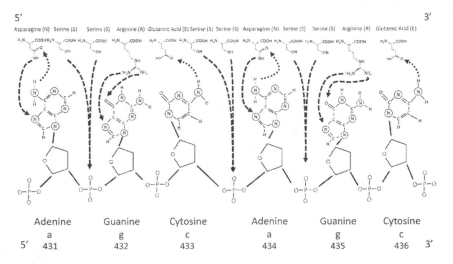

Figure 22 Binding of amino acids to nucleotides 431 to 436

Figure 23 illustrates the short hand notation of the letters assigned to the amino acids and the binding of amino acids to the nucleotides 431 to 436 of the HIV genome.

HIV 1st Sequence (Zinc Finger: Alpha)

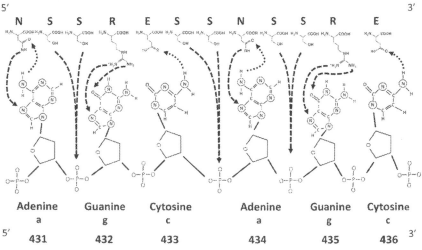

Figure 23 Binding of amino acids to the nucleotides 431 to 436

Figure 24 illustrates binding of amino acids to the nucleotides 437 to 442 of the HIV genome.

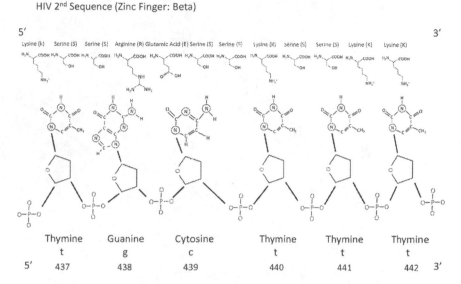

Figure 24 Binding of amino acids to the nucleotides 437 to 442

Figure 25 illustrates the bonds created by the amino acids to nucleotides 437 to 442 of the HIV genome.

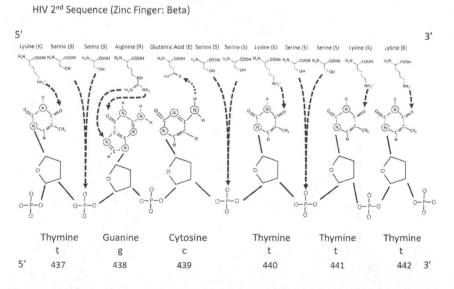

Figure 25 Bonds created by the amino acids to nucleotides 437 to 442

Figure 26 illustrates binding of amino acids to the nucleotides 443 to 448 of the HIV genome.

HIV 3rd Sequence (Zinc Finger: Gamma)

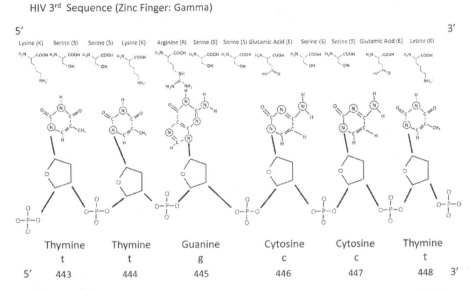

Figure 26 Binding of amino acids to the nucleotides 443 to 448

Figure 27 illustrates the bonds created by the amino acids to nucleotides 443 to 448 of the HIV genome.

HIV 3rd Sequence (Zinc Finger: Gamma)

Figure 27 Bonds created by the amino acids to nucleotides 443 to 448

Figure 28 illustrates binding of amino acids to the nucleotides 449 to 454 of the HIV genome.

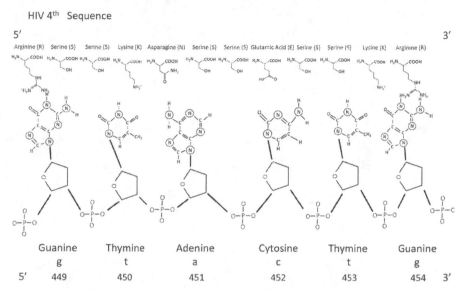

Figure 28 Binding of amino acids to the nucleotides 449 to 454

Figure 29 illustrates the bonds created by the amino acids to nucleotides 449 to 454 of the HIV genome.

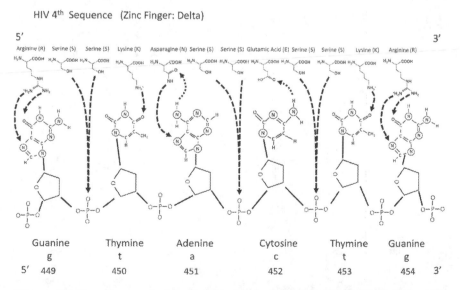

Figure 29 Bonds created by the amino acids to nucleotides 449 to 454

Figure 30 illustrates binding of amino acids to the nucleotides 455 to 460 of the HIV genome.

HIV 5th Sequence(Zinc Finger: Delta)

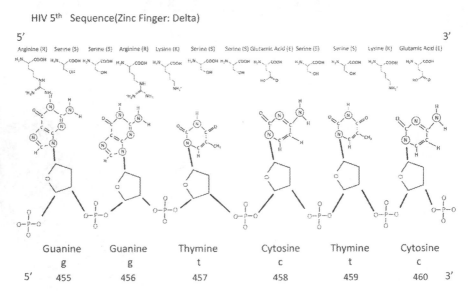

Figure 30 Binding of amino acids to the nucleotides 455 to 460

Figure 31 illustrates the bonds created by the amino acids to nucleotides 455 to 460 of the HIV genome.

HIV 5th Sequence (Zinc Finger: Epsilon)

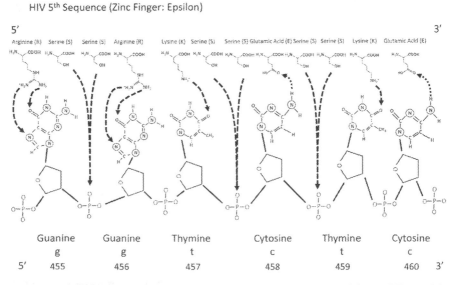

Figure 31 Bonds created by the amino acids to nucleotides 455 to 460

Figure 32 illustrates the modifications made to the Alpha Zinc Finger of the TFIIIA molecule.

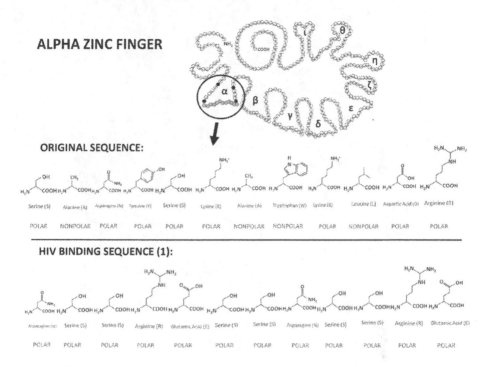

Figure 32 Modifications made to the Alpha Zinc Finger

Figure 33 illustrates the modifications made to the Beta Zinc Finger of the TFIIIA molecule.

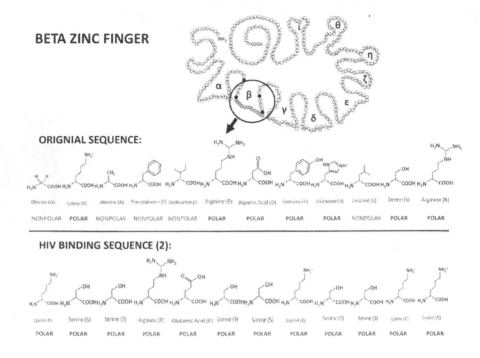

Figure 33 Modifications made to the Beta Zinc Finger

Figure 34 illustrates the modifications made to the Gamma Zinc Finger of the TFIIIA molecule.

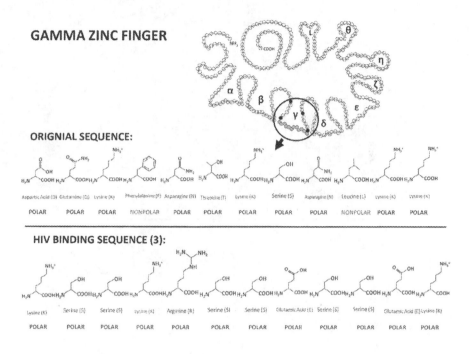

Figure 34 Modifications made to the Gamma Zinc Finger

Figure 35 illustrates the modifications made to the Delta Zinc Finger of the TFIIIA molecule.

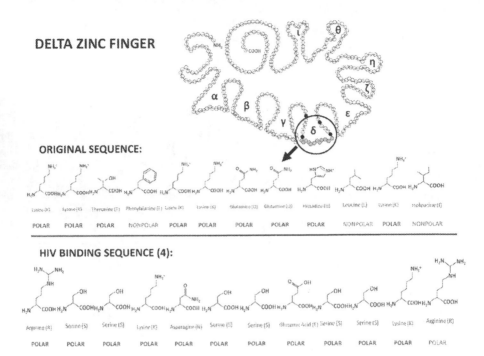

Figure 35 Modifications made to the Delta Zinc Finger

Figure 36 illustrates the modifications made to the Epsilon Zinc Finger of the TFIIIA molecule.

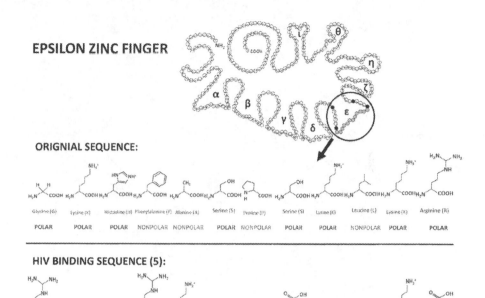

Figure 36 Modifications made to the Epsilon Zinc Finger

Figure 37 illustrates the modifications made to the Zeta Zinc Finger of the TFIIIA molecule.

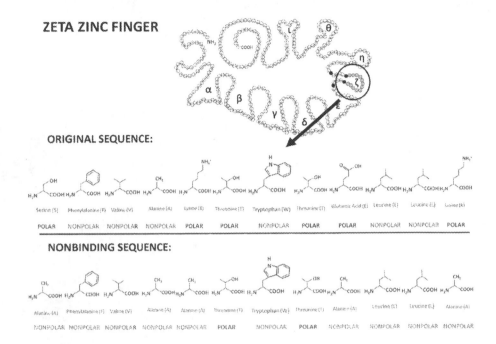

Figure 37 Modifications made to the Zeta Zinc Finger

Figure 38 illustrates the modifications made to the Eta Zinc Finger of the TFIIIA molecule.

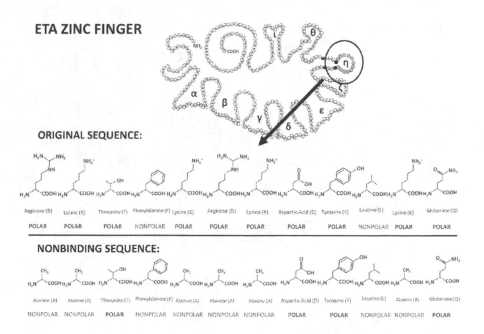

Figure 38 Modifications made to the Eta Zinc Finger

Figure 39 illustrates the modifications made to the Theta Zinc Finger of the TFIIIA molecule.

THETA ZINC FINGER

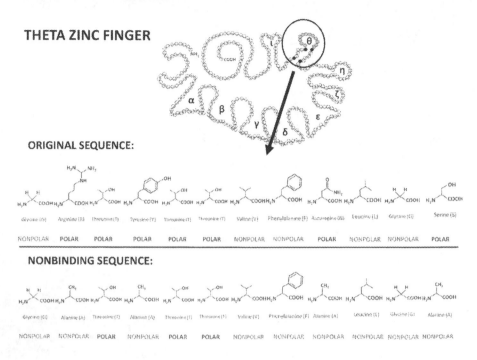

ORIGINAL SEQUENCE:

Glycine (G)	Arginine (R)	Threonine (T)	Tyrosine (Y)	Threonine (T)	Threonine (T)	Valine (V)	Phenylalanine (F)	Asparagine (N)	Leucine (L)	Glycine (G)	Serine (S)
NONPOLAR	POLAR	POLAR	POLAR	POLAR	POLAR	NONPOLAR	NONPOLAR	POLAR	NONPOLAR	NONPOLAR	POLAR

NONBINDING SEQUENCE:

Glycine (G)	Alanine (A)	Threonine (T)	Alanine (A)	Threonine (T)	Threonine (T)	Valine (V)	Phenylalanine (F)	Alanine (A)	Leucine (L)	Glycine (G)	Alanine (A)
NONPOLAR	NONPOLAR	POLAR	NONPOLAR	POLAR	POLAR	NONPOLAR	NONPOLAR	NONPOLAR	NONPOLAR	NONPOLAR	NONPOLAR

Figure 39 Modifications made to the Theta Zinc Finger

Figure 40 illustrates the modifications made to the Iota Zinc Finger of the TFIIIA molecule.

IOTA ZINC FINGER

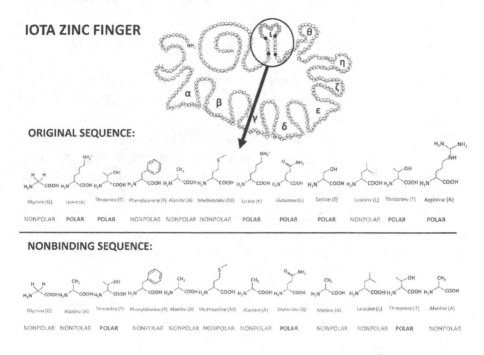

ORIGINAL SEQUENCE:

NONBINDING SEQUENCE:

Figure 40 Modifications made to the Iota Zinc Finger

To effect the binding of a therapeutic TFIIIA molecule to HIV's unique identifier, the first five loops of the TFIIIA molecule were modified. The naturally occurring as well as the modified amino acid sequence of loops 1-5, where the loops attach to the DNA are altered are presented in Table 4.

Number	Loop	Original Amino Acid Sequence	Modified Amino Acid Sequence
1	Alpha	SANYSKAWKLDA	NSSRESSNSSRE
2	Beta	GKAFIRDYHLSR	KSSRESSKSSKK
3	Gamma	DQKFNTKSNLKK	KSSKRSSESSEK
4	Delta	KKTFKKHQQLKI	RSSKNSSESSKR
5	Epsilon	GKHFASPSKLKR	RSSRKSSESSKE
6	Zeta	SFVAKTWTELLK	AFVAATWTALLA
7	Eta	RKTFKRKDYLKQ	AATFAAADYLAQ

| 8 | Theta | GRTYTTVFNLGS | GATATTVFALGA |
| 9 | Iota | GKTFAMKQSLTR | GATFAMAQALTA |

Table 4
Modification of amino acids for binding to HIV genome.

The modified HIV TFIIIA molecule may appear in the cytoplasm of a T-Helper cell by various delivery mechanisms. A form of TFIIIA molecule or pre-TFIIIA molecule might be delivered in the blood stream to the cell, and be absorbed through the cell membrane. A delivery vehicle, such as a modified virus virion might be employed to deliver the intact TFIIIA molecule to the target cell. As modeled by the life-cycle of the RNA virus Hepatitis C, a delivery vehicle such as a modified virus virion might be employed to deliver mRNA to a target cell, and once the mRNA has reached the target cell's cytoplasm the mRNA is translated to produce the therapeutic TFIIIA molecule.

Once the modified therapeutic TFIIIA molecule is in the cytoplasm of the T-Helper cell, then it should migrate to the nucleus similar to a naturally occurring TFIIIA molecule. Upon the modified therapeutic TFIIIA molecule reaching the nucleus and binding to the DNA at the site of the virus's unique identifier to silence the HIV genome, the modified TFIIIA becomes a Molecular Virus Killer.

The Molecular Virus Killer for HIV binds the alpha, beta, gamma, delta and epsilon loops (surfaces of loops 1-5) to the unique identifier at nucleotide position 431 to 455 along the HIV DNA genome. The binding of the modified TFIIIA molecule to the specific nucleotides comprising the unique identifier of HIV is as follows below:

NSSRESSNSSREKSSRESSKSSKKKSSKRSSESSEKRSSKNSSESSKRR
a   gc   a   gct   gc   t   ttt   tg   c   ctg   ta   c   tgg

In Figure 41, the modified TFIIIA molecule is illustrated to bind to the twenty-five nucleotides comprising HIV's unique identifier.

MOLECULAR VIRUS KILLER TO SILENCE HIV GENOME

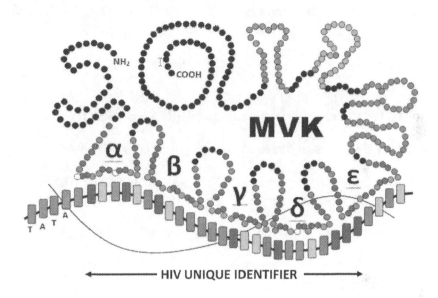

Figure 41 Modified TFIIIA binding to the HIV unique identifier

The naturally occurring Transcription Factor III A molecule, Taxonomic identifier 9606 [NCBI] (TFIIIA9606) may be found at http://www.uniprot.org/uniprot/Q92664. The TFIIIA9606 protein is 365 amino acids in length.

The TFIII A molecule is 365 amino acids in length. There are nine zinc fingers in the structure moving from the 5' (NH2) to 3' (COOH) end of the molecule designated as zinc finger 1, zinc finger 2, zinc finger 3, zinc finger 4, zinc finger 5, zinc finger 6, zinc finger 7, zinc finger 8, and zinc finger 9.

Zinc finger 1 is considered to include amino acids 40 to 64.

Within zinc finger 1, the amino acids 48 to 59 'SANYSKAWKLDA' are changed to the amino acid sequence 'NSSRESSNSSRE'.

Zinc finger 2 is considered to include amino acids 70 to 94.

Within zinc finger 2, amino acids 78 to 89 'GKAFIRDYHLSR' are changed to the amino acid sequence 'KSSRESSKSSKK'.

Zinc finer 3 is considered to include amino acids 100 to 125.

Within zinc finger 3, amino acids 108 to 119 'DQKFNTKSNLKK' are changed to the amino acid sequence 'KSSKRSSESSEK'.

Zinc finger 4 is considered to include amino acids 132 to 154.

Within zinc finger 4, amino acids 140 to 151 'KKTFKKHQQLKI' are changed to the amino acid sequence 'RSSKNSSESSKR'.

Zinc finger 5 is considered to include amino acids 162 to 186.

Within zinc finger 5, amino acids 170 to 181 'GKHFASPSKLKR' are changed to the amino acid sequence 'RSSRKSSESSKE'.

Zinc finger 6 is considered to include amino acids 189 to 213.

Zinc finger 6, amino acids 196 to 207 'SFVAKTWTELLK' are changed to the amino acid sequence 'AFVAATWTALLA'.

Zinc finger 7 is considered to include amino acids 217 to 239.

Within zinc finger 7, amino acids 223 TO 234 'RKTFKRKDYLKQ' are changed to the amino acid sequence 'AATFAAADYLAQ'.

Zinc finger 8 is considered to include amino acids 246 to 271.

Within zinc finger 8, amino acids 249 to 265 'PREGCGRTYTTVFNLQS' are changed to the amino acid sequence 'PAAGCGATYTTVFALQA'.

Zinc finger 9 is considered to include the amino acids 277 to 301.

Within zinc finger 9, amino acids 285 TO 296 'GKTFAMKQSLTR' are changed to the amino acid sequence 'GATFAMAQALTA'.

The modified form of the TFIIIA molecule is as follows with the original amino acid sequence comprising the molecule modified as mentioned above and the new amino acid sequences appearing in their defined position and underlined for clarity.

```
1         10          20          30          40          50          60
MDPPAVVAES VSSLTIADAF IAAGESSAPT PPRPALPRRF ICSFPDCNSS RESSNSSRESH
          70          80          90         100         110         120
LCKHTGERPF VCDYEGCKSS RESSKSSKKH ILTHTGEKPF VCAANGCKSS KRSSESSEKH
         130         140         150         160         170         180
FERKHENQQK QYICSFEDCR SSKNSSESSK RHQCQHTNEP LFKCTQEGCR SSRKSSESSK
         190         200         210         220         230         240
EHAKAHEGYV CQKGCAFVAA TWTALLAHVR ETHKEEILCE VCAATFAAAD YLAQHMKTHA
         250         260         270         280         290         300
PERDVCRCPA AGCGATATTV FALGAHILFS HEESRPFVCE HAGCGATFAM AQALTAHAVV
         310         320         330         340         350         360
HDPDKKKMKL KVKKSREKRS LASHLSGYIP PKRKQGQGLS LCQNGESPNC VEDKMLSTVA
         365
VLTLG
```

Table 5 shows the optional DNA codons for amino acids.

Amino Acid Used in Modification	Three Nucleotide Code	Three Nucleotide Code Used in DNA
S	TCT, TCC, TCA, TCG, AGT, AGC	TCT, TCC, TCA, TCG, AGT, AGC
N	AAT, AAC	AAT, AAC
R	CGU, CGC, CGA, CGG, AGA, AGG	CGC, CGA, CGG, AGA, AGG
E	GAA, GAG	GAA, GAG
K	AAA, AAG	AAA, AAG

Table 5

Sequence for the modified TFIIIA protein and the mRNA sequence to produce it showing the Nine Fingers

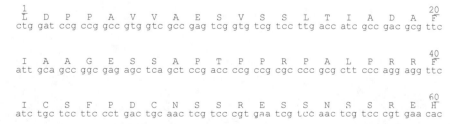

```
1                                                            20
L   D   P   P   A   V   V   A   E   S   V   S   S   L   T   I   A   D   A   F
ctg gat ccg ccg gcc gtg gtc gcc gag tcg gtg tcg tcc ttg acc atc gcc gac gcg ttc

                                                             40
I   A   A   G   E   S   S   A   P   T   P   P   R   P   A   L   P   R   R   F
att gca gcc ggc gag agc tca gct ccg acc ccg ccg cgc ccc gcg ctt ccc agg agg ttc

                                                             60
I   C   S   F   P   D   C   N   S   S   R   E   S   S   N   S   S   R   E   H
atc tgc tcc ttc cct gac tgc aac tcg tcc cgt gaa tcg tcc aac tcg tcc cgt gaa cac
```

```
       L   C   K   H   T   G   E   R   P   F   V   C   D   Y   E   G   C   K   S   S 80
      ctg tgc aag cac acg ggg gag aga cca ttt gtt tgt gac tat gaa ggg tgt aag tct tcc


       R   E   S   S   K   S   S   K   K   H   I   L   T   H   T   G   E   K   P   F 100
      cgt gaa tcg tcc aaa tct tcc aaa aag cac att ctg act cac aca gga gaa aag ccg ttt


       V   C   A   A   N   G   C   K   S   S   K   R   S   S   E   S   S   E   K   H 120
      gtt tgt gca gcc aat ggc tgt aag tct tcc aaa agg tca tcc gag tcg tcc gag aag cat


       F   E   R   K   H   E   N   Q   Q   K   Q   Y   I   C   S   F   E   D   C   R 140
      ttt gaa cgc aaa cat gaa aat caa caa aaa caa tat ata tgc agt ttt gaa gac tgt cgc


       S   S   K   N   S   S   E   S   S   K   R   H   Q   C   Q   H   T   N   E   P 160
      tcc tcc aaa aac tcg tcc gag tcg tcc aaa agg cat cag tgc cag cat acc aat gaa cct


       L   F   K   C   T   Q   E   G   C   R   S   S   R   K   S   S   E   S   S   K 180
      cta ttc aag tgt acc cag gaa gga tgt cgc agc tcc cgt aaa tct tcc gag tcg tcc aaa


       E   H   A   K   A   H   E   G   Y   V   C   Q   K   G   C   A   F   V   A   A 200
      gag cat gcc aag gcc cac gag ggc tat gta tgt caa aaa gga tgt gca ttc gtg gcc gcc


       T   W   T   A   L   L   A   H   V   R   E   T   H   K   E   E   I   L   C   E 220
      acc tgg acc gca ctc ctg gcc cat gtg aga gaa acc cat aaa gag gaa ata cta tgt gaa


       Y   C   A   A   T   F   A   A   A   D   Y   L   A   Q   H   M   K   T   H   A 240
      gta tgc gca gcc acc ttt gcc gca gcc gac tat ctc gcc cag cac atg aaa act cat gcc


       P   E   R   D   V   C   R   C   P   R   E   G   C   G   A   T   A   T   T   V 260
      cca gaa agg gat gta tgt cgc tgt cca aga gaa ggc tgt ggc gcc acc gca aca act gtg


       F   A   L   G   A   H   I   L   S   F   H   E   E   S   R   P   F   V   C   E 280
      ttt gcc ctc ggc gcg cat atc ctc tcc ttc cat gag gaa agc cgc cct ttt gtg tgt gaa


       H   A   G   C   G   A   T   F   A   M   A   Q   A   L   T   A   H   A   V   V 300
      cat gct ggc tgt ggc gcc acc ttt gcc atg gcc cag gcg ctg acc gca cat gct gtt gta


       H   D   P   D   K   K   K   M   K   L   K   V   K   K   S   R   E   K   R   S 320
      cat gat cct gac aag aag aaa atg aag ctc aaa gtc aaa aaa tct cgt gaa aaa cgg agt


       L   A   S   H   L   S   G   Y   I   P   P   K   R   K   Q   G   Q   G   L   S 340
      ttg gcc tct cat ctc agt gga tat atc cct ccc aaa agg aaa caa ggg caa ggc tta tct


       L   C   Q   N   G   E   S   P   N   C   V   E   D   K   M   L   S   T   V   A 360
      ttg tgt caa aac gga gag tca ccc aac tgt gtg gaa gac aag atg ctc tcg aca gtt gca


       V   L   T   L   G 365  STOP
      gta ctt acc ctt ggc  taa
```

CHAPTER 9

REVERSE TRANSLATION: BUILDING A THERAPEUTIC mRNA

Once the therapeutic target is known and protein sequence is developed to generate a protein to engage the therapeutic target, an mRNA molecule can be designed to be translated to produce the desired protein. See Figure 42.

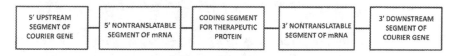

Figure 42 Design of an mRNA gene

Basics of Messenger RNA Molecules

Messenger RNA molecules are divided into three regions. The three regions include (1) the 5' untranslatable region, (2) the coding region, and (3) the 3' untranslatable region. An 'untranslatable region' represents a segment of a messenger RNA molecule that does not code for a protein and is not used to yield a protein and therefore 'translation' does not occur in such a region. The 'coding region' is the portion of the mRNA that is decoded by the ribosomes by the process known as translation to produce a particular protein molecule. A sequence of three nucleotides present in the coding region of a mRNA molecule represents a unit of information referred to as a codon. Codons code for all of the 20 amino acids used to construct protein molecules and also for START and STOP commands. The configuration of the 3' untranslatable region, in part, determines the half-life survival of the messenger RNA molecule.

In the process known as translation, a ribosome decodes the codons present in the coding region in the mRNA, initiating the protein manufacturing process at a START codon, then interfacing with charged transport RNAs (tRNA) carrying the amino acids that match the sequence of codons in the mRNA as the ribosome traverses the length of the coding region of the mRNA molecule. The ribosome functions as a protein factory by taking amino acids delivered by charged tRNAs and binding the amino acids together in the order dictated by the sequence of codon instructions coded into the mRNA template as directed by the manner of the nucleic acid arrangement in the mRNA molecule. Protein synthesis ceases when a ribosome encounters a STOP code. The protein molecule is then released by the ribosome. Ribosomes do not decode the nucleotide sequences to produce proteins in a mRNA's 5' untranslatable region or a mRNA's 3' untranslatable region.

Re-Designing a Messenger RNA's coding region

To redesign a messenger RNA molecule's coding region, involves leaving the existing mRNA molecule 5' and 3' untranslatable ends intact, but changes the translatable portion of the mRNA molecule. In this case, the mRNA molecule is designed similar to a normal mRNA molecule that would produce a TFIIIA molecule, but the translatable portion of newly designed mRNA molecule has been altered to produce a modified TFIIIA molecule to seek out and neutralize the HIV genome.

CHAPTER 10

REVERSE TRANSCRIPTION: BUILDING A THERAPEUTIC DNA SEQUENCE

Once the therapeutic target is known and protein sequence is developed to generate a protein to engage the therapeutic target, and an mRNA molecule is designed to be translated to produce the desired protein, then using reverse transcription, the desired DNA segment can be developed to produce the mRNA molecule that will generate the desired protein.

Basics of a Gene

A gene is comprised of a number of segments loosely strung together along a particular section of DNA. In general, there are at least three global segments associated with a gene which include: (1) the Upstream 5' flanking region, (2) the transcriptional unit and (3) the Downstream 3' flanking region. See Figure 5. The term 'upstream' refers to DNA sequencing that occurs prior to the transcription start site (TSS) if viewed from the 5' end to the 3' end of the DNA; while the term 'downstream' refers to DNA sequencing located after the TSS.

The Upstream 5' flanking region of a gene is comprised of the 'enhancer region', the 'promoter-proximal region', and 'promoter region'.

The 'transcriptional unit' begins at a location designated 'transcription start site', which is located in a site called the 'initiator region' (inR), which may be described in a general form as Py_2CAPy_5. The transcription unit is comprised of the combination of segments of DNA nucleotides to be transcribed into RNA and spacing units known as 'introns' that are not transcribed or if transcribed are later removed post transcription, such that they do not appear in the final RNA molecule. In the case of a gene coding for a mRNA molecule, the transcription unit will contain all three elements of the mRNA, which includes: (1) the 5' noncoding region, (2) the translational region and (3) the 3' noncoding region.

The Downstream 3' flanking region contains DNA nucleotides that are not transcribed and may contain what has been termed an 'enhancer region'. An enhancer region in the Downstream 3' flanking region may promote the gene previously transcribed to be transcribed again.

The 'enhancer region' may or may not be present in the Upstream 5' flanking region. If present in the Upstream 5' flanking region, the enhancer region helps facilitate the reading of the gene by encouraging formation of the transcription mechanism. An enhancer may be 50 to 1500 base pairs in length occupying a position upstream from the transcription start site.

On either side of the DNA sequencing comprising a gene and its flanking regions, may be inactive DNA that act as boundaries, which have been termed 'insulator elements'.

The 'transcription mechanism', also referred to as 'the transcription machinery' or the 'transcription complex' (TC) in humans, is reported to be comprised of over forty separate proteins that assemble together to ultimately function in a concerted effort to transcribe the nucleotide sequence of the DNA into RNA. The transcription mechanism includes elements such as 'general transcription factor Sp1', 'general transcription factor NF1', 'general transcription factor TATA-binding protein', 'TF$_{II}$D', 'basal transcription complex', and a 'RNA polymerase protein' to name only a few of the approximately seventy proposed elements that may combine to form a transcription complex. The elements of the transcription mechanism function as (1) a means to recognize the location of the start of a gene, (2) as proteins to bind the transcription mechanism to the DNA such that transcription may occur and (3) as means of transcribing the DNA nucleotide coding to produce a RNA molecule or a precursor RNA molecule.

There are at least three RNA polymerase proteins which include: RNA polymerase I, RNA polymerase II, and RNA polymerase III.

RNA polymerase I tends to be dedicated to transcribing genetic information that will result in the formation of rRNA molecules. RNA polymerase II tends to be dedicated to transcribing genetic information that will result in the formation of mRNA molecules. RNA polymerase III appears to be dedicated to transcribing genetic information that results in the formation of tRNAs, small cellular RNAs and viral RNAs.

The 'promoter proximal region' is located upstream from the TSS and upstream from the core promoter region. See Figure 6. The 'promoter proximal region' includes two sub-regions termed the GC box and the CAAT box. The 'GC box' appears to be a segment rich in guanine-cytosine nucleotide sequences. The GC box binds to the 'general transcription factor Sp1' of the transcription mechanism. The 'CAAT box' is a segment which contains the nucleotide sequence 'ggccaatct' located approximately 75 base pairs (bps) upstream from the transcription start site. The CAAT box binds to the 'general transcription factor NF1' of the transcription mechanism.

The 'core promoter' region is considered the shortest sequence within which RNA polymerase II can initiate transcription of a gene The core promoter may include the inR and either a TATA box or a 'downstream promoter element' (DPE). The inR is the region designated Py_2CAPy_5 that surrounds the transcription start site. The TATA box is located 25 base pairs (bps) upstream from the TSS. The TATA box acts as a site of attachment of the $TF_{II}D$, which is a promoter for binding of the RNA polymerase II molecule. The DPE may appear 28 bps to 32 bps downstream from the TSS. The DPE acts as an alternative site of attachment for the $TF_{II}D$ when the TATA box is not present.

Re-Designing a Nuclear Gene

To redesign a nuclear gene to generate a modified TNFIIIA molecule, the existing DNA sequence that produces a TNFIIIA molecule is altered to remove the 5' and 3' nontranscribable regions. The translatable region of the existing DNA sequence is then modified to generate the desired mRNA molecule to produce a modified TFIIIA molecule to seek out and neutralize the HIV genome.

A 5' and 3' nontranscribable regions are then inserted on the modified DNA sequence so that the gene can be properly transcribed like a naturally occurring nuclear gene.

CHAPTER 11

CONCEPT OF THE COURIER GENE

A courier gene is a composite gene. The concept of a courier gene is to take a known naturally occurring gene and insert a therapeutic segment of DNA into the transcription reading segment of this known gene. The composite courier gene is to be integrated into the native DNA of a cell. The concept of the courier gene is further expanded to theorize that the intent of the courier gene is that for a known naturally occurring stimulus which will trigger the reading of the courier gene, the resultant transcription of the synthetic courier gene will generate a mRNA that will migrate from the nucleus to be translated to produce therapeutic proteins to result in the medical management of a disease state.

A courier gene is constructed such that the 5' upstream segment and the 3' downstream segment of the composite gene are taken from one naturally occurring gene, while the transcription reading segment is taken from an entirely different gene. The transcription reading segment may be taken in its entirety from an existing naturally occurring gene, or the transcription reading segment may be a modified representation of a naturally occurring gene, or the transcription reading segment may be a fully synthetic segment of DNA. See Figure 43.

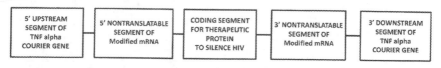

Figure 43 Concept of a Courier Gene to Combat HIV

In this text, the courier gene is comprised of a composite of a naturally occurring Tumor Necrosis Factor (TNF) alpha gene and the modified transcription reading segment from a Transcription Factor IIIA (TFIIIA) gene. It is theorized that in the event that the immune system of a cell is activated by the presence of Human

Immunodeficiency Virus (HIV), transcription of the TNF alpha gene would occur. In the event the synthetic courier TNF alpha gene is transcribed, an mRNA molecule would be produced and translation of this mRNA molecule would produce a modified TFIIIA molecule designed to seek out and neutralize the HIV genome. Excessive amounts of the modified TFIIIA molecule would be disposed of naturally by the cell. See Figure 44.

COURIER GENE TO TRANSPORT
EMBEDDED DNA VACCINE

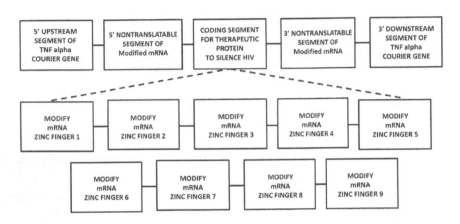

Figure 44 Courier Gene Concept to Target HIV

CHAPTER 12

THE TNF GENE

```
FEATURES     Location/Qualifiers
   source    1..7240
             /organism="Homo sapiens"
             /mol _type="genomic DNA"
             /db _xref="taxon:9606"

   gene      1750..4519
             /gene="TNF"
   mRNA      join(1750..2105,2718..2763,2951..2998,3300..4519)
             /gene="TNF"
             /product="tumor necrosis factor (TNF superfamily, member
             2)"
   CDS       join(1920..2105,2718..2763,2951..2998,3300..3721)
             /gene="TNF"
             /codon _start=1
             /product="tumor necrosis factor (TNF superfamily, member
             2)"
             /protein _id="AAO21132.1"
             /db _xref="GI:27802685"
```

/translation="MSTESMIRDVELAEEALPKKTGGPQGSRRCLFLSLFSFLIVAGA
TTLFCLLHFGVIGPQREEFPRDLSLISPLAQAVRSSSRTPSDKPVAHVVANPQAEGQL
QWLNRRANALLANGVELRDNQLVVPSEGLYLIYSQVLFKGQGCPSTHVLLTHTISRIA
VSYQTKVNLLSAIKSPCQRETPEGAEAKPWYEPIYLGGVFQLEKGDRLSAEINRPDYL
DFAESGQVYFGIIAL"

THE TNF GENE

```
   1 ctgctgatag  tcccggagct  ttcaagaagg  attctttcct  cccaggggac  cacacctccc
  61 tgaatatccc  tgatgtctgt  ctggctgagg  atttcaagcc  tgcctaggaa  ttcccagccc
 121 aaagctgttg  gtctgtccca  ccagctaggt  ggggcctaga  tccacacaca  gaggaagagc
 181 aggcacatgg  aggagcttgg  gggatgacta  gaggcaggga  ggggactatt  tatgaaggca
 241 aaaaaattaa  attatttatt  tatggaggat  ggagagaggg  gaataataga  agaacatcca
 301 aggagaaaca  gagacaggcc  caagagatga  agagtgagag  ggcatgcgca  caaggctgac
 361 caagagagaa  agaagtaggc  atgagggatc  acagggcccc  agaaggcagg  gaaaggctct
 421 gaaagccagc  tgccgaccag  agccccacac  ggaggcatct  gcaccctcga  tgaagcccaa
 481 taaacctctt  ttctctgaaa  tgctgtctgc  ttgtgtgtgt  gtgtctggga  gtgagaactt
 541 cccagtctat  ctaaggaatg  gagggaggga  cagagggctc  aaagggagca  agagctgtgg
 601 ggagaacaaa  aggataaggg  ctcagagagc  ttcagggata  tgtgatggac  tcaccaggtg
 661 aggccgccag  actgctgcag  gggaagcaaa  ggagaagctg  agaagatgaa  ggaaaagtca
 721 gggtctggag  gggcgggggt  cagggagctc  ctgggagata  tggccacatg  tagcggctct
 781 gaggaatggg  ttacaggaga  cctctgggca  gatgtgacca  cagcaatggg  taggagaatg
 841 tccaggggcta  tggaagtcga  gtatggggac  ccccccctta  acgaagacag  ggccatgtag
 901 agggccccag  ggagtgaaag  agcctccagg  acctccaggt  atggaataca  ggggacgttt
 961 aagaagatat  ggccacacac  tggggccctg  agaagtgaga  gcttcatgaa  aaaaatcagg
1021 gaccccagag  ttccttggaa  gccaagactg  aaaccagcat  tatgagtctc  cgggtcagaa
1081 tgaaagaaga  aggcctgccc  cagtggggtc  tgtgaattcc  cggggtgat  ttcactcccc
1141 ggggctgtcc  caggcttgtc  cctgctaccc  ccacccagcc  tttcctgagg  cctcaagcct
1201 gccaccaagc  ccccagctcc  ttctccccgc  agggacccaa  acacaggcct  caggactcaa
1261 cacagctttt  ccctccaacc  ccgtttttctc  tccctcaagg  actcagcttt  ctgaagcccc
1321 tcccagttct  agttctatct  ttttcctgca  tcctgtctgg  aagttagaag  gaaacagacc
1381 acagacctgg  tccccaaaag  aaatggaggc  aataggtttt  gaggggcatg  gggacggggt
1441 tcagcctcca  gggtcctaca  cacaaatcag  tcagtggccc  agaagacccc  cctcggaatc
1501 ggagcaggga  ggatgggag  tgtgaggggt  atccttgatg  cttgtgtgtc  cccaactttc
1561 caaatccccg  ccccgcgat  ggagaagaaa  ccgagacaga  aggtgcaggg  cccactaccg
1621 cttcctccag  atgagctcat  gggtttctcc  accaaggaag  ttttccgctg  gttgaatgat
1681 tctttccccg  ccctcctctc  gccccaggga  ca**tataaagg**  **cagttgttgg**  **cacacccagc**
1741 **c**agcagacg**c**  **tccctcagca**  **aggacagcag**  **aggaccagct**  **aagagggaga**  **gaagcaacta**
1801 **cagacccccc**  **cctgaaaaca**  **accctcagac**  **gccacatccc**  **ctgacaagct**  **gccaggcagg**
1861 **ttctcttcct**  **ctcacatact**  **gacccacggc**  **tccaccctct**  **ctcccctgga**  **aaggacacca**
1921 **tgagcactga**  **aagcatgatc**  **cgggacgtgg**  **agctggccga**  **ggaggcgctc**  **cccaagaaga**
1981 **caggggggcc**  **ccagggctcc**  **aggcggtgct**  **tgttcctcag**  **cctcttctcc**  **ttcctgatcg**
2041 **tggcaggcgc**  **caccacgctc**  **ttctgcctgc**  **tgcactttgg**  **agtgatcggc**  **ccccagaggg**
2101 **aagaggtgag**  **tgcctggcca**  **gccttcatcc**  **actctcccac**  **ccaagggaaa**  **atggagacgc**
2161 **aagagaggga**  **gagagatgga**  **atgggtgaaa**  **gatgtgcgct**  **gatagggagg**  **gatggagaga**
2221 **aaaaaacgtg**  **gagaaagacg**  **gggatgcaga**  **aagagatgtg**  **gcaagagatg**  **gggaagagag**
2281 **agagagaaag**  **atggagagac**  **aggatgtctg**  **gcacatggaa**  **ggtgctcact**  **aagtgtgtat**
2341 **ggagtgaatg**  **aatgaatgaa**  **tgaatgaatg**  **aacaagcaga**  **tatataaata**  **agatatgaag**
2401 **acagatgtgg**  **ggtgtgagaa**  **gagagatgaa**  **ggaagaaaca**  **agtgatatga**  **ataaagatgg**
2461 **tgagacagaa**  **agagagcggg**  **aaatatgaca**  **gctaaggaga**  **gagatggggg**  **agataaggag**
2521 **aaagaagat**  **agggtgtctg**  **gcacacagaa**  **gacactcagg**  **gaaagagctg**  **ttgaatgcct**
2581 **ggaaggtgaa**  **tacacagatg**  **aatggagaga**  **gaaaaccaga**  **cacctcaggg**  **ctaagagcgc**
2641 **aggccagaca**  **ggcagccagc**  **tgttcctcct**  **ttaagggtga**  **ctccctcgat**  **gttaaccatt**
2701 **ctccttctcc**  **ccaacagttc**  **cccagggacc**  **tctctctaat**  **cagccctctg**  **gcccaggcag**
2761 **tcagtaagtg**  **tctccaaacc**  **tctttcctaa**  **ttctggggttt**  **gggtttggg**  **gtagggttag**
2821 **taccggtatg**  **gaagcagtgg**  **gggaaattta**  **aagtttttggt**  **cttgggggag**  **gatggatgga**
2881 **ggtgaaagta**  **ggggggtatt**  **ttctaggaag**  **tttaagggtc**  **tcagcttttt**  **cttttctctc**
2941 **tcctcttcag**  **gatcatcttc**  **tcgaaccccg**  **agtgacaagc**  **ctgtagccca**  **tgtttgtaggt**
3001 **aagagctctg**  **aggatgtgtc**  **ttggaacttg**  **gagggctagg**  **atttgggggat**  **tgaagcccgg**
3061 **ctgatggtag**  **gcagaacttg**  **gagacaatgt**  **gagaaggact**  **cgctgagctc**  **aagggaaggg**
3121 **tggaggaaca**  **gcacaggcct**  **tagtgggata**  **ctcagaacgt**  **catggccagg**  **tgggatgtgg**
3181 **gatgacagac**  **agagaggaca**  **ggaaccggat**  **gtggggtggg**  **cagagctcga**  **gggccaggat**
3241 **gtggagagtg**  **aaccgacatg**  **gccacactga**  **ctctcctctc**  **cctctcctctc**  **tccctccagc**
3301 **aaacctcaa**  **gctgagggc**  **agctccagtg**  **gctgaaccgc**  **cgggccaatg**  **ccctcctggc**
3361 **caatggcgtg**  **gagctgagag**  **ataaccagct**  **ggtggtgcca**  **tcagagggcc**  **tgtacctcat**
3421 **ctactcccag**  **gtcctcttca**  **agggccaagg**  **ctgcccctcc**  **acccatgtgc**  **tcctcaccca**
3481 **caccatcagc**  **cgcatcgccg**  **tctcctacca**  **gaccaaggtc**  **aacctcctct**  **ctgccatcaa**
3541 **gagcccctgc**  **cagagggaga**  **ccccagaggg**  **ggctgaggcc**  **aagccctggt**  **atgagcccat**
3601 **ctatctggga**  **ggggtcttc**  **agctgggaga**  **gggtgaccga**  **ctcagcgctg**  **agatcaatcg**
3661 **gcccgactat**  **ctcgactttg**  **ccgagtctgg**  **gcaggtctac**  **tttgggatca**  **ttgccctgtg**
3721 **aggaggacga**  **acatccaacc**  **ttcccaaacg**  **cctccccctgc**  **cccaatccct**  **ttattacccc**
3781 **ctccttcaga**  **caccctcaac**  **ctcttctggc**  **tcaaaaagag**  **aattgggggc**  **ttagggtcgg**
3841 **aacccaagct**  **tagaacttta**  **agcaacaaga**  **ccaccacttc**  **gaaacctggg**  **attcaggaat**
3901 **gtgtggcctg**  **cacagtgaag**  **tgctggcaac**  **cactaagaat**  **tcaaactggg**  **gcctccagaa**
3961 **ctcactgggg**  **cctacagctt**  **tgatccctga**  **catctggaat**  **ctggagacca**  **gggagccttt**
4021 **ggttctggcc**  **agaatgctgc**  **aggacttgag**  **aagacctcac**  **ctagaaattg**  **acacaagtgg**
4081 **accttaggcc**  **ttcctctctc**  **cagatgtttc**  **cagacttcct**  **tgagacacgg**  **agcccagccc**
4141 **tccccatgga**  **gccagctccc**  **tctatttatg**  **tttgcacttg**  **tgattattta**  **ttatttattt**
4201 **attatttatt**  **tatttacaga**  **tgaatgtatt**  **tatttgggag**  **accggggtat**  **cctggggggac**
4261 **ccaatgtagg**  **agctgccttg**  **gctcagacat**  **gttttccgtg**  **aaaacggagc**  **tgaacaatag**
4321 **gctgttccca**  **tgtagccccc**  **tggcctctgt**  **gccttctttt**  **gattatgttt**  **tttaaaatat**
4381 **ttatctgatt**  **aagttgtcta**  **aacaatgctg**  **atttggtgac**  **caactgtcac**  **tcattgctga**
4441 **gcctctgctc**  **cccaggggag**  **ttgtgtctgt**  **aatcgcccta**  **ctattcagtg**  **gcgagaaata**
4501 **aagtttgctt**  **agaaaagaa** a  catggtctcc  ttcttggaat  taattctgca  tctgcctctt
4561 cttgtgggtg  ggaagaagct  ccctaagtcc  tctctccaca  ggctttaaga  tccctcggac
4621 ccagtcccat  ccttagactc  ctagggccct  ggagacccta  cataaacaaa  gcccaacaga
4681 atattccccca  tcccccagga  aacaagaccc  tgaacctaat  tacctctccc  tcagggcatg
4741 ggaatttcca  actctgcaac  ttcaatcct  tgctgggaaa  atcctgcagc  tcaggtgaga
4801 tttccggctg  ttgcagctgg  ccagcagtcc  ggagagagct  ggagaggagc  cgcattctca
4861 ggtacctgaa  tcacacagcc  aagggacttc  cagagattcg  ggtgtctagg  cttcaaatca
4921 ccctgtccta  actctgcaac  ctgaaccagc  cacttaacct  atctatccaa  tggggatagg
```

```
4981 aatgtccacc acacataggg catgtgagag aaggcctgac ctccatcaga ggacctcact
5041 cagcccttgg cacagtgggc acttagtgaa ttctggcttc cttcaaccag tttccagctg
5101 ttctatcccc ttccattctc tcagtgggtg aaatcgaaga gactgaggac aataaagaac
5161 aaggaaccga actgccggac gtggtggcat gcacctgtaa tcctaccact ttgcaaggcc
5221 aaggtgagag gatcgcttga acccaggagt tccagagcaa cctgggcaac atagtgagat
5281 cctgtctcta tttttaaaa aagaatgaaa catagggata agatgtgggt gaaggactca
5341 catgccggct tggtcccact ggtctttgtg gtgaaggagg ggagaggtga gaggtgggta
5401 atccggaaag agaaaagcac cccctccctg gatgaaggct cttctggaga gagtcaaaga
5461 caaataaggg tggggcgcag tggctcatgc ctgttatccc aacactttgg gaggctgagg
5521 tgggaggacc acttgagccc actagttcaa gaccagcctg tgcaacatag caagaccttg
5581 tttctagaaa aaaaattaaa gattagtcag gtgtagtggt gcatgcctgt aatcctagct
5641 cctcaggagg ctgaggcagg aggatcactc aagcccagga gtttgaggtt acagtaagct
5701 atgatcatgc cactgtaccc ccgtctgggt gacagaacga gaccctgtct caaaaaaata
5761 ataattccaa aaacaaatat ggagacggaa attgagcccc cctagactgg gagcccccac
5821 tgagttcgga aattaggctt tacctccagc cctggggtgc caggcaggag aaaaccatgt
5881 ggtaggctga gggggtaggg tgacccattg gggtgaccta gataggggcct tgggtcaccc
5941 tctgcctcct ccagcctgtg gctgaaagtc agccatgaag taatggggga cactgttact
6001 catcccagaa gcacccacac ttactcactt ttgggaaggg ggacctaaag tgtgaaaaaa
6061 aggtgaggat tttccgtctc accctaaatg ggacaccta agtggggcat cggttttttcc
6121 tcctccccag aacttcctgg tgttttcagg caccacaggc tccttcctgc catccccatc
6181 tctctctaat attctcccct tctttctcct tcagcctcct cccttcagac cccatgagcc
6241 ttgaattaag ctccttggag gagaagagtt gactgtcggg taggagacag agaggccttc
6301 aggcagctct aggggggagaa gtgcgggggcc cctccaggct tcattcctct gtcatgatag
6361 gggcttactc tgctgctggg cctttctgag tggtgcttgc tgggctctgt aatgacccct
6421 ctcactgttg gggggtaccc aagagaaaag agtatggtgc agagtctggt tgggaccatg
6481 tggccctgaa aatcaggatg cctagagaag cttcggagtt tgagaagtcc cccttcctcc
6541 caccctccaa ctgggctaat ggtggtgcct ggccattcag aggcagggag ggggtgggac
6601 aggcagacca tcatcccctag gagcaaaggc catacactgt gttgtgatga attgtttcaa
6661 gcaaccagaa gagtactgag aatatttaac ccgcacccgt gcacccaccc tgaattaaga
6721 cgtgtgtcgc aactcagcat ctttatcggc agcactgaag ctttccattc tttattttca
6781 tcaggttcaa aatcaatttc caaacagtct cctacatttt tcccactgcc atggggtcct
6841 gggcgtccgg gccccccaata ttcacgcact cgcaccacgc actcatattc cctcacccca
6901 ccatcacggc cccaaagaag gtcttccctc tcgcgaagtc caccatatcg gggtgactga
6961 tgttgacgta caccctctcg cccctccgga gctgcaccag gccgccgaac cccacgctcg
7021 tgtaccagag aggcccgtac ccttgtctcc tggccgggtc cagcactgga gtcaccgtct
7081 cggcgccctc gagcagcagc tcgggagtgc ccggcccgta ggcgcccccc gcccggtaca
7141 gagagctgcg cagcgtgacc gagcggccct ggggtccccc gccgccaggg ggcgcccggc
7201 cccggtagcc gacgagacag tagaggtaat agaggccgtc
```

Homo sapiens chromosome 6, GRCh38 Primary Assembly

TNF alpha GENE 5' UPSTREAM REGION:

```
   1 ctgctgatag tcccggagct ttcaagaagg attctttcct cccaggggac cacacctccc
  61 tgaatatccc tgatgtctgt ctggctgagg atttcaagcc tgcctaggaa ttcccagccc
 121 aaagctgttg gtctgtccca ccagctaggt ggggcctaga tccacacaca gaggaagagc
 181 aggcacatgg aggagcttgg gggatgacta gaggcaggga ggggactatt tatgaaggca
 241 aaaaaattaa attatttatt tatggaggat ggagagaggg gaataataga agaacatcca
 301 aggagaaaca gagacaggcc caagagatga agagtgagag ggcatgcgca caaggctgac
 361 caagagagaa agaagtaggc atgagggatc acagggcccc agaaggcagg gaaaggctct
 421 gaaagccagc tgccgaccag agccccacac ggaggcatct gcaccctcga tgaagcccaa
 481 taaacctctt ttctctgaaa tgctgtctgc ttgtgtgtgt gtgtctggga gtgagaactt
 541 cccagtctat ctaaggaatg gagggaggga cagagggctc aaagggagca agagctgtgg
 601 ggagaacaaa aggataaggg ctcagagagc ttcagggata tgtgatggac tcaccaggtg
 661 aggccgccag actgctgcag gggaagcaaa ggagaagctg agaagatgaa ggaaaagtca
 721 gggtctggag gggcgggggt cagggagctc ctgggagata tggccacatg tagcggctct
 781 gaggaatggg ttacaggaga cctctgggga gatgtgacca cagcaatggg taggagaatg
 841 tccagggcta tggaagtcga gtatggggac ccccccctta acgaagacag ggccatgtag
 901 agggccccag ggagtgaaag agcctccagg acctccaggt atggaataca ggggacgttt
 961 aagaagatat ggccacacac tggggccctg agaagtgaga gcttcatgaa aaaaatcagg
1021 gaccccagag ttccttggaa gccaagactg aaaccagcat tatgagtctc cgggtcagaa
1081 tgaaagaaga aggcctgccc cagtggggtc tgtgaattcc cggggggtgat ttcactcccc
1141 ggggctgtcc caggcttgtc cctgctaccc ccacccagcc tttcctgagg cctcaagcct
1201 gccaccaagc ccccagctcc ttctccccgc tggagcccaa acacaggcct caggactcaa
1261 cacagctttt ccctccaacc ccgttttctc tccctcaagg actcagcttt ctgaagcccc
1321 tcccagttct agttctatct ttttcctgca tcctgtctgg aagttagaag gaaacagacc
1381 acagacctgg tccccaaaag aaatggaggc aataggtttt gaggggcatg gggacg9gggt
1441 tcagcctcca gggtcctaca cacaaatcag tcagtggccc agaagacccc cctcggaatc
1501 ggagcaggga ggatggggag tgtgaggggt atccttgatg cttgttgtgtc cccaactttc
1561 caaatccccg ccccagcgat ggagaagaaa ccgagacaga aggtgcaggg cccactaccg
1621 cttcctccag atgagctcat gggtttctcc accaaggaag ttttccgctg gttgaatgat
1681 tctttccccg ccctcctctc gccccaggga ca
```

TATA BOX + TNF alpha 25-NUCLEOTIDE UNIQUE IDENTIFIER:

1713 **tataaagg cagttgttgg cacacccagcc**

RESIDUAL NUCLEOTIDES:

1742 agcagacg

TNF alpha mRNA:

```
1750 ctccctcagca aggacagcag aggaccagct aagagggaga gaagcaacta
1801 cagacccccc cctgaaaaca accctcagac gccacatccc ctgacaagct gccaggcagg
1861 ttctcttcct ctcacatact gacccacggc tccaccctct ctccctgga aaggacacca
1921 tgagcactga aagcatgatc cgggacgtgg agctggccga ggaggcgctc cccaagaaga
1981 caggggggcc ccagggctcc aggcggtgct tgttcctcag cctcttctcc ttcctgatcg
2041 tggcaggcgc caccacgctc ttctgcctgc tgcactttgg agtgatcggc ccccagaggg
2101 aagaggtgag tgcctggcca gccttcatcc actctcccac ccaaggggaa atggagacgc
2161 aagagaggga gagagatggg atgggtgaaa gatgtgcgct gataggagg gatggagaga
2221 aaaaaacgtg gagaaagacg gggatgcaga aagagatgtg gcaagagatg gggaagagag
2281 agagagaaag atggagagac aggatgtctg gcacatggaa ggtgctcact aagtgtgtat
2341 ggagtgaatg aatgaatgaa tgaatgaatg aacaagcaga tatataaata agatatggag
2401 acagatgtgg ggtgtgagaa gagagatggg ggaagaaaca agtgatatga ataaagatgg
2461 tgagacagaa agagagcggg aaatatgaca gctaaggaga gagatgggg agataaggag
2521 agaagaagat agggtgtctg gcacacagaa gacactcagg gaaagagctg ttgaatgcct
2581 ggaaggtgaa tacacagatg aatggagaga gaaaaccaag cacctcaggg ctaagagcgc
2641 aggccagaca ggcagccagc tgttcctcct ttaaggtga ctccctcgat gttaaccatt
2701 ctccttctcc ccaacagttc cccagggacc tctctctaat cagccctctg gcccaggcag
2761 tcagtaagtg tctccaaacc tctttcctaa ttctgggttt gggtttgggg gtaggttag
2821 taccggtatg gaagcagtgg gggaaattta aagttttggt cttggggag gatgggatgga
2881 ggtgaaagta ggggggtatt ttctaggaag tttaagggtc tcagcttttt cttttctctc
2941 tcctcttcag gatcatcttc tcgaacccg agtgacaagc ctgtagccca tgttgtaggt
3001 aagagctctg aggatgtgtc ttggaacttg gagggctagg atttggggat tgaagcccgg
3061 ctgatggtag gcagaacttg gagacaatgt gagaaggact cgctgagctc aagggaaggg
3121 tggaggaaca gcacaggcct tagtgggata ctcagaacgt catggccagg tgggatgtgt
3181 gatgacagac agagaggaca ggaaccggat gtggggtggg cagagctcga gggccaggat
3241 gtggagagtg aaccgacatg gccacactga ctctcctctc cctctctccc tccctccagc
3301 aaaccctcaa gctgaggggc agctccagtg gctgaaccgc cgggccaatg ccctcctggc
3361 caatggcgtg gagctgagag ataaccagct ggtggtgcca tcagagggcc tgtacctcat
3421 ctactcccag gtcctcttca agggccaagg ctgcccctcc acccatgtgc tcctcaccca
3481 caccatcagc cgcatcgccg tctcctacca gaccaaggtc aacctcctct ctgccatcaa
3541 gagcccctgc cagagggaga ccccagaggg ggctgaggcc aagccctggt atgagcccat
3601 ctatctggga ggggtcttcc agctggagaa gggtgaccga ctcagcgctg agatcaatcg
```

```
3661 gcccgactat  ctcgactttg  ccgagtctgg  gcaggtctac  tttgggatca  ttgccctgtg
3721 aggaggacga  acatccaacc  ttcccaaacg  cctcccctgc  cccaatccct  ttattacccc
3781 ctccttcaga  caccctcaac  ctcttctggc  tcaaaaagag  aattgggggc  ttagggtcgg
3841 aacccaagct  tagaacttta  agcaacaaga  ccaccacttc  gaaacctggg  attcaggaat
3901 gtgtggcctg  cacagtgaag  tgctggcaac  cactaagaat  tcaaactggg  gcctccagaa
3961 ctcactgggg  cctacagctt  tgatccctga  catctggaat  ctggagacca  gggagccttt
4021 ggttctggcc  agaatgctgc  aggacttgag  aagacctcac  ctagaaattg  acacaagtgg
4081 accttaggcc  ttcctctctc  cagatgtttc  cagacttcct  tgagacacgg  agcccagccc
4141 tccccatgga  gccagctccc  tctatttatg  tttgcacttg  tgattattta  ttatttattt
4201 attatttatt  tatttacaga  tgaatgtatt  tatttgggag  accggggtat  cctgggggac
4261 ccaatgtagg  agctgccttg  gctcagacat  gttttccgtg  aaaaoggagc  tgaacaatag
4321 gctgttccca  tgtagccccc  tggcctctgt  goottctttt  gattatgttt  tttaaaatat
4381 ttatctgatt  aagttgtcta  aacaatgctg  atttggtgac  caactgtcac  tcattgctga
4441 gcctctgcto  cccagggggg  ttgtgtctgt  aatcgcccta  ctattcagtg  gcgagaaata
4501 aagtttgctt  agaaaagaa
```

TNF alpha GENE 3′ DOWNSTREAM REGION:

```
4520 a catggtctcc              ttcttggaat taattctgca tctgcctctt
```

```
4561 cttgtgggtg  ggaagaagct  ccctaagtcc  tctctccaca  ggctttaaga  tccctcggac
4621 ccagtcccat  ccttagactc  ctagggccct  ggagacccta  cataaacaaa  gcccaacaga
4681 atattcccca  tcccccaagga aacaagagcc  tgaacctaat  tacctctccc  tcagggcatg
4741 ggaatttcca  actctgggaa  ttccaatcct  tgctgggaaa  atcctgcagc  tcaggtgaga
4801 tttccggctg  ttgcagctgg  ccagcagtcc  ggagagagct  ggagaggagc  cgcattctca
4861 ggtacctgaa  tcacacagcc  aagggacttc  cagagattcg  ggtgtctagg  cttcaaatca
4921 ccctgtccta  actctgcaac  ctgaaccagc  cacttaacct  atctatccaa  tggggatagg
4981 aatgtccacc  acacataggg  catgtgagag  aaggcctgac  ctccatcaga  ggacctcact
5041 cagcccttgg  cacagtgggc  acttagtgaa  ttctggcttc  cttcaaccag  tttccagctg
5101 ttctatcccc  ttccattctc  tcagtgggtg  aaatcgaaga  gactgaggac  aataaagaac
5161 aaggaaccga  actgccggac  gtggtggcat  gcacctgtaa  tcctaccact  ttgcaaggcc
5221 aaggtgagag  gatcgcttga  acccaggagt  tccagagcaa  cctgggcaac  atagtgagat
5281 cctgtctcta  tttttaaaa   aagaatgaaa  cataggaata  agatgtgggt  gaaggactca
5341 catgccggct  tggtcccact  ggtctttgtg  gtgaaggagg  ggagaggtga  gaggtgggta
5401 atccggaaag  agaaaagcac  cccctccctg  gatgaaggct  cttctggaga  gagtcaaaga
5461 caaataaggg  tggggcgcag  tggctcatgc  ctgttatccc  aacactttgg  gaggctgagg
5521 tgggaggacc  acttgagccc  actagttcaa  gaccagcctg  tgcaacatag  caagaccttg
5581 tttctagaaa  aaaaattaaa  gattagtcag  gtgtagtggt  gcatgcctgt  aatcctagct
5641 cctcaggagg  ctgaggcagg  aggatcactc  aagcccagga  gtttgaggtt  acagtaagct
5701 atgatcatgc  cactgtaccc  ccgtctgggt  gacagaacga  gaccctgtct  caaaaaaata
5761 ataattccaa  aaacaaatat  ggagacggaa  attgagcccc  cctagactgg  gagcccccac
5821 tgagttcgga  aattaggctt  tacctccagc  cctggggtgc  caggcaggag  aaaaccatgt
5881 ggtaggctga  gggggtaggg  tgacccattg  gggtgaccta  gatagggcct  tgggtcaccc
5941 tctgcctcct  ccagcctgtg  gctgaaagtc  agccatgaag  taatggggga  cactgttact
6001 catcccagaa  gcacccacac  ttactcactt  ttgggaaggg  ggacctaaag  tgtgaaaaaa
6061 aggtgaggat  tttccgtctc  accctaaatg  ggacacccta  agtggggcat  cggttttttcc
6121 tcctccccag  aacttcctgg  tgttttccagg  caccacaggc  tccttcctgc  catccccatc
6181 tctctctaat  attctcccct  tctttctcct  tcagcctcct  cccttcagac  cccatgagcc
6241 ttgaattaag  ctccttggag  gagaagagtt  gactgtcggg  taggagacag  agaggccttc
6301 aggcagctct  aggggggagaa gtgcggggcc  cctccaggct  tcattcctct  gtcatgatag
6361 gggcttactc  tgctgctggg  cctttctgag  tggtgcttgc  tgggctctgt  aatgacccct
6421 ctcactgttg  gggggtaccc  aagagaaaag  agtatggtgc  agagtctggt  tgggaccatg
6481 tggccctgaa  aatcaggatg  cctagagaag  cttcggagtt  tgagaagtcc  cccttcctcc
6541 caccctccaa  ctgggctaat  ggtggggcct  ggccattcag  aggcagggag  ggggtgggac
6601 aggcagacca  tcatccctag  gagcaaaggc  catacactgt  gttgtgatga  attgtttcaa
6661 gcaaccagaa  gagtactgag  aatatttaac  ccgcacccgt  gcacccaccc  tgaattaaga
6721 cgtgtgtcgc  aactcagcat  ctttatcggc  agcactgaag  ctttccattc  tttattttca
6781 tcaggttcaa  aatcaatttc  caaacagtct  cctacatttt  tcccactgcc  atggggtcct
6841 gggcgtccgg  gccccccaata ttcacgcact  cgcaccacgc  actcatattc  cctcacccca
6901 ccatcacggc  cccaaagaag  gtcttccctc  tcgcgaagtc  caccatatcg  gggtgactga
6961 tgttgacgta  caccctctcg  ccctccgga   gctgcaccag  gccgccgaac  cccacgctcg
7021 tgtaccagag  aggcccgtac  ccttgtctcc  tggccgggtc  cagcactgga  gtcaccgtct
7081 cggcgccctc  gagcagcagc  tcgggagtgc  ccggcccgta  ggcgcccccc  gcccggtaca
7141 gagagctgcg  cagcgtgacc  gagcggccct  ggggggtcccc  gccgccaggg  ggcgcccggc
7201 cccggtagcc  gacgagacag  tagaggtaat  agaggccgtc
```

CHAPTER 13

RE-DESIGNING THE TNF GENE

A DNA sequence has been designed to be embedded into the human genome (Table 6), when transcribed is intended to generate a mRNA, this mRNA when translated to produce a therapeutic Transcription Factor IIIA (TFIIIA) molecule to engage the HIV genome (GenBank K03455.1). We modified TFIIIA molecule (NC_000013), altering zinc fingers 1-5, to bond to HIV's unique identifier, 'agcagctgcttttgcctgtactgg', nucleotides 431-455, the 25 nucleotides located between the TATA box and transcription start site. We studied amino acid-nucleotide binding characteristics. Permanently binding a TFIIIA to HIV's unique identifier is intended to prevent transcription of the HIV genome. Using a reverse transcription process, we developed a transcribable segment of DNA. The Tumor Necrosis Factor alpha (TNF) gene (AY214167.1) is active in CD4+ lymphocytes, including the reservoir for HIV. The transcribable sequence of DNA coding for the therapeutic TFIIIA molecule replaces the TNF's original mRNA's protein coding sequence from nucleotides 1750-4519. The modified TNF gene utilizes TNF gene's original 5' upstream and 3' downstream signaling segments. The modified TNF gene acts as a courier to transport the embedded DNA vaccine sequence. Likened to the HIV genome, the modified TNF gene is inserted into the human genome and functions like an alternative copy of the TNF gene. The embedded DNA vaccine undergoes transcription, producing mRNAs which generate TFIIIAs designed to seek out and silence the HIV genome, creating a cell defensible against intracellular HIV infection.

Embedded DNA vaccine

	5' Upstream TNF alpha gene sequence AY214167.1	TFIIIA Zinc Fingers	Modified TFIIIA gene sequence (as Amino Acids) NC_000013	3' Downstream TNF alpha gene sequence AY214167.1
Original:	1-1749	---	1-11166	4520-7240
Modified:	1-1749	---	1750-12915	12916-15636
---	---	---	---	---
---	--------------------	1-Original:	336-371	--------------------
---	--------------------	Sequence:	SANYSKAWKLDA	--------------------
---	--------------------	1-Modified:	2085-2120	--------------------
---	--------------------	Coding:	NSSRESSNSSRE	--------------------
---	--------------------	2-Original:	2579-2614	--------------------
---	--------------------	Sequence:	GKAFIRDYHLSR	--------------------
---	--------------------	2-Modified:	4328-4363	--------------------
---	--------------------	Coding:	KSSRESSKSSKK	--------------------
---	--------------------	3-Original:	5346-5381	--------------------
---	--------------------	Sequence:	DQKFNTKSNLKK	--------------------
---	--------------------	3-Modified:	7095-7130	--------------------
---	--------------------	Coding:	KSSKRSSESSEK	--------------------
---	--------------------	4-Original:	6008-6043	--------------------
---	--------------------	Sequence:	KKTFKKHQQLKI	--------------------
---	--------------------	4-Modified:	7757-7792	--------------------
---	--------------------	Coding:	RSSKNSSESSKR	--------------------
---	--------------------	5-Original:	8207-8242	--------------------
---	--------------------	Sequence:	GKHFASPSKLKR	--------------------
---	--------------------	5-Modified:	9956-9991	--------------------
---	--------------------	Coding:	RSSRKSSESSKE	--------------------

Table 6

TNF alpha GENE 5' UPSTREAM REGION:

```
   1 ctgctgatag tcccggagct ttcaagaagg attctttcct cccaggggac cacacctccc
  61 tgaatatccc tgatgtctgt ctggctgagg atttcaagcc tgcctaggaa ttcccagccc
 121 aaagctgttg gtctgtccca ccagctaggt ggggcctaga tccacacaca gaggaagagc
 181 aggcacatgg aggagcttgg gggatgacta gaggcaggga ggggactatt tatgaaggca
 241 aaaaaattaa attatttatt tatggaggat ggagagaggg gaataataga agaacatcca
 301 aggagaaaca gagacaggcc caagagatga agagtgagag ggcatgcgca caaggctgac
 361 caagagagaa agaagtaggc atgagggatc acagggcccc agaaggcagg gaaaggctct
 421 gaaagccagc tgccgaccag agccccacac ggaggcatct gcaccctcga tgaagcccaa
 481 taaacctctt ttctctgaaa tgctgtctgc ttgtgtgtgt gtgtctggga gtgagaactt
 541 cccagtctat ctaaggaatg gagggaggga cagagggctc aaagggagca agagctgtgg
 601 ggagaacaaa aggataaggg ctcagagagc ttcagggata tgtgatgagc tcaccaggtg
 661 aggccgccag actgctgcag gggaagcaaa ggagaagctg agaagatgaa ggaaaagtca
 721 gggtctggag gggcggggt gggggagctc ctgggagata tggcccacatg tagcggctct
 781 gaggaatggg ttacaggaga cctctgggga gatgtgacca cagcaatggg taggagaatg
 841 tccagggcta tggaagtcga gtatggggac ccccccctta acgaagacag ggccatgtag
 901 agggccccag ggagtgaaag agcctccagg acctccaggt atggaataca ggggacgttt
 961 aagaagatat ggccacacac tggggccctg agaagtgaga gcttcatgaa aaaaatcagg
1021 gaccccagag ttccttggaa gccaagactg aaaccagcat tatgagtctc cgggtcagaa
1081 tgaaagaaga aggcctgccc cagtggggtc tgtgaattcc cggggggtgat ttcactcccc
1141 ggggctgtcc caggcttgtc cctgctaccc ccacccagcc tttcctgagg cctcaagcct
1201 gccaccaagc ccccagctcc ttctcccccgc agggacccaa acacaggcct caggactcaa
1261 cacagctttt ccctccaacc ccgttttctc tccctcaagg actcagcttt ctgaagcccc
1321 tcccagttct agttctatct ttttcctgca tcctgtctgg aagttagaag gaaacagacc
1381 acagacctgg tccccaaaag aaatggaggc aataggtttt gaggggcatg gggacggggt
1441 tcagcctcca gggtcctaca cacaaatcag tcagtggccc agaagacccc cctcggaatc
1501 ggagcaggga ggatggggag tgtgaggggt atccttgatg cttgtgtgtc ccaacttttc
1561 caaatccccg ccccgcgat ggagaagaaa ccgagacaga aggtgcaggg cccactaccg
1621 cttcctccag atgagctcat gggtttctcc accaaggaag ttttccgctg gttgaatgat
1681 tctttccccg ccctcctctc gccccaggga ca
```

TATA BOX + TNF alpha 25-NUCLEOTIDE UNIQUE IDENTIFIER:

1713 **tataaagg cagttgttgg cacacccagcc**

RESIDUAL NUCLEOTIDES:

1742 agcagacg

TNF alpha mRNA:

```
1750 ctccctcagca aggacagcag aggaccagct aagagggaga gaagcaacta
1801 cagacccccc cctgaaaaca accctcagac gccacatccc ctgacaagct gccaggcagg
1861 ttctcttcct ctcacatact gacccacggc tccacccctct ctccctgga aaggacacca
1921 tgagcactga aagcatgatc cgggacgtgg agctggccga ggaggcgctc cccaagaaga
1981 caggggggcc ccagggctcc aggccgtgct tgttcctcag cctcttctct ttcctgatcg
2041 tggcaggcgc caccacgctc ttctgcctgc tgcactttgg agtgatcggc ccccagaggg
2101 aagaggtgag tgcctggcca gccttcatcc actctcccac ccaaggggaa atggagacgc
2161 aagagggaga gagatgggg atgggtgaaa gatgtgcgct gataggagg gatggagaga
2221 aaaaaacgtg gagaaagacg gggatgcaga aagagatgtg gcaagagatg gggaagagag
2281 agagagaaag atggagagac aggatgtctg gcacatggaa ggtgctcact aagtgtgtat
2341 ggagtgaatg aatgaatgaa tgaatgaatg aacaagcaga tatataaata agatatggag
2401 acagatgtgg ggtgtgagaa gagagatggg ggaagaaaca agtgatatga ataaagatgg
2461 tgagacagaa agagacgggg aaatatgaca gctaaggaga gagatggggg agataaggag
2521 agaagaagat agggtgtctg gcacacagaa gacaactcagg gaaagagctg ttgaatgcct
2581 ggaaggtgaa tacacagatg aatggagaga gaaaaccaga cacctcaggg ctaagagcgc
2641 aaggccagaca ggcagccagc tgttcctcct ttaaggggtga ctccctcgat gttaaccatt
2701 ctccttctcc ccaacagttc cccaggggacc tctctctaat cagccctctg gcccaggcag
2761 tcagtaagtg tctccaaacc tctttcctaa ttctgggttt gggtttgggg gtagggttag
2821 taccggtatg gaagcagtgg gggaaattta aagttttggt cttgggggag gatggatgga
2881 ggtgaaagta gggggtatt ttctaggaag tttaagggtc tcagcttttt cttttctctc
2941 tcctcttcag gatcatcttc tcgaaccccg agtgacaagc ctgtagccca tgttgtaggt
3001 aagagctctg aggatgtgtc ttggaacttg gagggctagg atttgggggat tgaagcccgg
3061 ctgatggtag gcagaacttg gagacaatgt gagaaggact cgctgagctc aagggaaggg
3121 tggaggaaca gcacaggcct tagtggggata ctcagaacgt catggccagg tgggatgtgg
3181 gatgacagac agagaggaca ggaaccggat gtggggtggg cagagctcga gggccaggat
3241 gtggagagtg aaccgacatg gccacactga ctctcctctc cctctctccc tccctccagc
3301 aaacccctcaa gctgaggggc agctccagtg gctgaaccgc cgggccaatg ccctcctggg
3361 caatggcgtg gagctcgagag ataaccagct ggtggtgcca tcagagggcc tgtacctcat
3421 ctactccagg gtcctcttca agggccaagg ctgcccctcc acccatgtgc tcctcacccca
3481 caccatcagc cgcatcgccg tctcctacca gaccaaggtc aacctcctct ctgccatcaa
3541 gagccctgc cagaggggaga ccccagaggg ggctgaggcc aagccctggt atgagcccat
3601 ctatctgggg ggggtcttcc agctgggaga gggtgaccga ctcagcgctg agatcaatcg
3661 gcccgactat ctcgactttg ccgagtctgg gcaggtctac tttgggggatca ttgccctgtg
3721 aggaggacga acatccaacc ttcccaaacg cctcccctgc cccaatccct ttattaccc
```

— 110 —

```
3781 ctccttcaga  caccctcaac  ctcttctggc  tcaaaaagag  aattgggggc  ttagggtcgg
3841 aacccaagct  tagaacttta  agcaacaaga  ccaccacttc  gaaacctggg  attcaggaat
3901 gtgtggcctg  cacagtgaag  tgctggcaac  cactaagaat  tcaaactggg  gcctccagaa
3961 ctcactgggg  cctacagctt  tgatccctga  catctggaat  ctggagacca  gggagccttt
4021 ggttctggcc  agaatgctgc  aggacttgag  aagacctcac  ctagaaattg  acacaagtgg
4081 accttaggcc  ttcctctctc  cagatgtttc  cagacttcct  tgagacacgg  agcccagccc
4141 tccccatgga  gccagctccc  tctatttatg  tttgcacttg  tgattatttta ttatttattt
4201 attatttatt  tatttacaga  tgaatgtatt  tatttgggag  accggggtat  cctgggggag
4261 ccaatgtagg  agctgccttg  gctcagacat  gtttttccgtg aaaacggagc  tgaacaatag
4321 gctgttccca  tgtagcccccc tggcctctgt  gccttcttttt gattatgttt  tttaaaatat
4381 ttatctgatt  aagttgtcta  aacaatgctg  atttggtgac  caactgtcac  tcattgctga
4441 gcctctgctc  cccaggggag  ttgtgtctgt  aatcgcccta  ctattcagtg  gcgagaaata
4501 aagtttgctt  agaaaagaa
```

TNF alpha GENE 3' DOWNSTREAM REGION:

```
4520 a catggtctcc ttcttggaat taattctgca tctgcctctt
```

```
4561 cttgtgggtg  ggaagaagct  ccctaagtcc  tctctccaca  ggctttaaga  tccctcggac
4621 ccagtcccat  ccttagactc  ctagggccct  ggagaccta   cataaacaaa  gcccaacaga
4681 atattcccca  tccccccagga aacaagagcc  tgaacctaat  tacctctccc  tcagggcatg
4741 ggaatttcca  actctgggaa  ttccaatcct  tgctgggaaa  atcctgcagc  tcaggtgaga
4801 tttccggctg  ttgcagctgg  ccagcagtcc  ggagagagct  ggagaggagc  cgcattctca
4861 ggtacctgaa  tcacacagcc  aagggacttc  cagagattcg  ggtgtctagg  cttcaaatca
4921 ccctgtccta  actctgcaac  ctgaaccagc  cacttaacct  atctatccaa  tggggatagg
4981 aatgtccacc  acacatagg   catgtgagag  aaggcctgac  ctccatcaga  ggacctcact
5041 cagcccttgg  cacagtgggc  acttagtgaa  ttctggcttc  cttcaaccag  tttccagctg
5101 ttctatcccc  ttccattctc  tcagtgggtg  aaatcgaaga  gactgaggac  aataaagaac
5161 aaggaaccga  actgccggac  gtggtggcat  gcacctgtaa  tcctaccact  ttgcaaggcc
5221 aaggtgagag  gatcgcttga  acccaggagt  tccagagcaa  cctgggcaac  atagtgagat
5281 cctgtctcta  tttttttaaaa  aagaatgaaa  cataggaata  agatgtgggt  gaaggactca
5341 catgccggct  tggtcccact  ggtctttgtg  gtgaaggagg  gggagggtga  gaggtgggta
5401 atccggaaag  agaaaagcac  cccctccctg  gatgaaggct  cttctggaga  gagtcaaaga
5461 caaataaggg  tggggcgcag  tggctcatgc  ctgttatccc  aacactttgg  gaggctgagg
5521 tgggaggacc  acttgagccc  actagttcaa  gaccagcctg  tgcaacatag  caagaccttg
5581 tttctagaaa  aaaaattaaa  gattagtcag  gtgtagtggt  gcatgcctgt  aatcctagct
5641 cctcaggagg  ctgaggcagg  aggatcactc  aagcccagga  gtttgaggtt  acagtaagct
5701 atgatcatgc  cactgtaccc  ccgtctgggt  gacagaacga  gaccctgtct  caaaaaaata
5761 ataattccaa  aaacaaatat  gggagacggaa attgagcccc  cctagactgg  gagccccccac
5821 tgagttcgga  aattaggctt  tacctccagc  cctggggtgc  caggcaggag  aaaaccatgt
5881 ggtaggctga  ggggggtaggg tgacccattg  gggtgaccta  gatagggcct  tgggtcaccc
5941 tctgcctcct  ccagcctgtg  gctgaaagtc  agccatgaag  taatggggga  cactgttact
6001 catcccagaa  gcacccacac  ttactcactt  ttgggaaggg  ggacctaaag  tgtgaaaaaa
6061 aggtgaggat  tttccgtctc  accctaaatg  ggacacccta  agtggggcat  cggttttttcc
6121 tcctccccag  aacttcctgg  tgttttcagg  caccacaggc  tccttcctgc  catccccatc
6181 tctctctaat  attctcccct  tctttctcct  tcagcctcct  cccttcagac  cccatgagcc
6241 ttgaattaag  ctccttggag  gagaagagtt  gactgtcggg  taggagacag  agagggccttc
6301 aggcagctct  aggggggagaa gtgcggggcc  cctccaggct  tcattcctct  gtcatgatag
6361 gggcttactc  tgctgctggg  cctttctgag  tggtgcttgc  tgggctctgt  aatgacccct
6421 ctcactgttg  gggggtaccc  aagagaaaag  agtatggtgc  agagtctggt  tgggaccatg
6481 tggccctgaa  aatcaggatg  cctagagaag  cttcggagtt  tgagaagtcc  cccttcctcc
6541 caccctccaa  ctgggctaat  ggtggggcct  ggccattcag  aggcagggag  ggggtgggac
6601 aggcagacca  tcatccctag  gagcaaaggc  catacactgt  gttgtgatga  attgtttcaa
6661 gcaaccagaa  gagtactgag  aatatttaac  ccgcacccgt  gcacccaccc  tgaattaaga
6721 cgtgtcgc   aactcagcat  ctttatcggc  agcactgaag  ctttccattc  tttattttca
6781 tcaggttcaa  aatcaatttc  caaacagtct  cctacatttt  tcccactgcc  atgggtcct
6841 gggcgtccgg  gcccccaata  ttcacgcact  cgcaccacgc  actcatattc  cctcacccca
6901 ccatcacggc  cccaaagaag  gtcttccctc  tcgcgaagtc  caccatatcg  gggtgactga
6961 tgttgacgta  caccctctcg  ccctccggaa  gctgcaccag  gccgccgaac  cccacgctcg
7021 tgtaccagag  aggcccgtac  ccttgtctcc  tggccgggtc  cagcactgga  gtcaccgtct
7081 cggcgccctc  gagcagcgagc tcgggagtgc  ccggcccgta  ggcgccccc   gcccggtaca
7141 gagagctgcg  cagcgtgacc  gagcggccct  gggggtcccc  gccgccaggg  ggcgcccggc
7201 cccggtagcc  gacgagacag  tagaggtaat  agaggccgtc
```

TNF alpha GENE 5' UPSTREAM REGION:

```
   1 ctgctgatag  tcccggagct  ttcaagaagg  attctttcct  cccaggggac  cacacctccc
  61 tgaatatccc  tgatgtctgt  ctggctgagg  atttcaagcc  tgcctaggaa  ttcccagccc
 121 aaagctgttg  gtctgtccca  ccagctaggt  ggggcctaga  tccacacaca  gaggaaagagc
 181 aggcacatgg  aggagcttgg  gggatgacta  gaggcaggga  ggggactatt  tatgaaggca
 241 aaaaaattaa  attatttatt  tatggaggat  ggagagaggg  gaataataga  agaacatcca
 301 aggagaaaca  gagacaggcc  caagagatga  agagtgagag  ggcatgcgca  caaggctgac
 361 caagagagaa  agaagtaggc  atgagggatc  acagggcccc  agaaggcagg  gaaaggctct
 421 gaaagccagc  tgccgaccag  agccccacac  ggaggcatct  gcaccctcga  tgaagcccaa
 481 taaacctctt  ttctctgaaa  tgctgtctgc  ttgtgtgtgt  gtgtctggga  gtgagaactt
```

```
 541 cccagtctat ctaaggaatg gagggaggga cagagggctc aaagggagca agagctgtgg
 601 ggagaacaaa aggataaggg ctcagagagc ttcagggata tgtgatggac tcaccaggtg
 661 aggccgccag actgctgcag gggaagcaaa ggagaagctg agaagatgaa ggaaaagtca
 721 gggtctggag gggcgggggt cagggagctc ctgggagata tggccacatg tagcggctct
 781 gaggaatggg ttacaggaga cctctgggga gatgtgacca cagcaatggg taggagaatg
 841 tccagggcta tggaagtcga gtatggggac cccccccttta acgaagacag ggccatgtag
 901 agggccccag ggagtgaaag agcctccagg acctccaggt atggaataca ggggacgttt
 961 aagaagatat ggccacacac tggggccctg agaagtgaga gcttcatgaa aaaaatcagg
1021 gaccccagag ttccttggaa gccaagactg aaaccagcat tatgagtctc cgggtcagaa
1081 tgaaagaaga aggcctgccc cagtggggtc tgtgaattcc cggggtgat ttcactcccc
1141 ggggctgtcc caggcttgtc cctgctaccc ccacccagcc tttcctgagg cctcaagcct
1201 gccaccaagc ccccagctcc ttctccccgc agggacccaa acacaggcct caggactcaa
1261 cacagctttt ccctcaacc ccgtttttctc tccctcaagg actcagcttt ctgaagcccc
1321 tcccagttct agttctatct ttttcctgca tcctgtctgg aagttagaag gaaacagacc
1381 acagacctgg tccccaaaag aaatggaggc aataggtttt gaggggcatg gggacggggt
1441 tcagcctcca gggtcctaca cacaaatcag tcagtggccc agaagacccc cctcggaatc
1501 ggagcaggga ggatggggag tgtgaggggt atccttgatg cttgtgtgtc cccaactttc
1561 caaatccccg ccccccgcgat ggagaagaaa ccgagacaga aggtgcaggg cccactaccg
1621 cttcctccag atgagctcat gggtttctcc accaaggaag ttttccgctg gttgaatgat
1681 tctttccccg ccctcctctc gccccaggga ca
```

TATA BOX + TNF alpha 25-NUCLEOTIDE UNIQUE IDENTIFIER:

1713 **tataaagg   cagttgttgg   cacacccagcc**

RESIDUAL NUCLEOTIDES:

1742 agcagacg

Modified TFIIIA mRNA:

TFIIIA GENE EXON ONE:

TFIIIA mRNA 5' UPSTREAM UNTRANSLATABLE SEGMENT:

```
  1 atgcgcgatc tcccggagca tgcgcagcag cggcgccgac gcggggcggt gcctggtgac
 61 cgcgcgcgct cccggaagtg tgccggcgtc gcgcgaaggt tcagcaggga gccgtgggcc
121 gggcgcgccg gttcccggca cgtgtctcgg cacgtggcag cgcgcctggc cctgggcttg
181 gaggcgccgg cgcc
```


*LOOP ALPHA BINDING TO DNA

TFIIIA MOLECULE AMINO ACIDS 1-47:

```
      L   D   P   P   A   V   V   A   E   S   V   S   S   L   T
    195 ctg gat ccg ccg gcc gtg gtc gcc gag tcg gtg tcg tcc ttg acc


      I   A   D   A   F   I   A   A   G   E   S   S   A   P   T
    240 atc gcc gac gcg ttc att gca gcc ggc gag agc tca gct ccg acc


      P   P   R   P   A   L   P   R   R   F   I   C   S   F   P
    286 ccg ccg cgc ccc gcg ctt ccc agg agg ttc atc tgc tcc ttc cct


      D   C
    330 gac tgc
```

TFIIIA MOLECULE ZINC FINGER 'ONE' DNA BONDING SITES, AMINO ACIDS 48-59:

```
      N    S    S    R    E    S    S    N    S    S    R    E
336  aac  tcg  tcc  cgt  gaa  tcg  tcc  aac  tcg  tcc  cgt  gaa
```

TFIIIA MOLECULE AMINO ACIDS 60-67:

```
      H    L    C    K    H    T    G    E
372  cac  ctg  tgc  aag  cac  acg  ggg  gag
```

TFIIIA GENE INTRON ONE:

```
 396 gtgag      ggggcgagg ctgccaaccc
 421 tgggcctagg gatggcgcgt ggccccgggg tagccactgc agtcgtggcc agggccgcag
 481 gccccgctgt gcagcgcgtt cagctttgac atccaggact tggggaagga gctgaggaag
 541 tagacaggaa gttgtaggac cttcgttctg cgaccttgat atccatggca ggggctcggg
 601 atttactaag cagtcattga tcgtgagtct cggccagcca agtgcctccc gtaatctgca
 661 aataagtgtg aggtttgagg gggcccaccg ctactagaca cctgccaaac actggcccct
 721 ggagctggta cagaagatgg gttacatgta ccagggtcg tgaaagcagc atgtgctcat
 781 ttcttcgtaa ctccacactg gagagagcag tgagcaaaac aggcaaaccc aaggtttctg
 841 ctgccatgga cctttgttcc tgggtcgagc cgaccacagg ataggtggga atgacatgca
 901 gtgttgtggt caggaaaggc ctctctggt gagccgtgta agaaggaagg atctagccat
 961 gcagacattt gtgctaggta gagagaacac aaagggagcc tgtgaccctt ggggtgggag
1021 gcaggtgggt gtgtttgggt gcggagatca ccatatgagg tctgagaagt aggcccatta
1081 ggagtttgga ttttattttg agggcaggag aatgtcagat accatgatat gacgtggcag
1141 cccatgtcac acacaagtga ggaaaacgag ggtcatggag gtcaaggaat ctgcccagct
1201 tcccagtttt tggcagagct aggcttcaca ctgcctcagc ttaaagccct taatttctta
1261 aaccactggg ctgcagtcca taccttttgcc ccttgcacct cctctaattt atgggccacc
1321 ttctccaggt gtcctccggg gcctcattcc ttaacctctc cagcactgga aggccgaccg
1381 cttcttcctt gagacctct ctggttcttt tcctcttcct cgtctgccct tttcgttgga
1441 tcctcttctg ccctctgcat gttccacccc gcccagctcc ctcttgcggt cttacatagc
1501 caccggcatg actcataaca tcctttatgc tttgcccctc tgcccttcct cttgcccgtt
1561 ctagcctcta aattctgggc tctgtattac cagtagatcc acgtaagagc ttgcctttcc
1621 ttttagaccg gtgtgctgta ttttggatac tggcgctacc agtttccta atacaggttg
1681 aaaaacttgg agtcatcttt gttgtcccag atctctcatg cagattaatt tgacaaatgt
1741 ttattgagcc tactccacgc ctgccgctgt gcaaggttct gtggctccgc ccctggtggt
1801 atgtagctca ctgtgttcct gtttgcttgt tttgctccta gtactctcat ggaggcctcg
1861 gtgcctccct cctggacgcc ttggtagtat gcttttcata gtttgatgca ccaaactggt
1921 tatttggtta tttgggtgt gtgtttggct tttactatag gttcaaaatg agtcaccccc
1981 tcccaactcc tgggttacaa aaggtggttg catttagggt gttgagctgt tttctttgct
2041 tcgccctggc acctgtgagc tttttcaggt gtgacacact ttcctatagc tgtgcttggc
2101 attatcctag cacagaccct gggcttgtct gggatgagac aggcctccct cgttcctctg
2161 ccctaggctt gcttttttac atgttaaatc atgcggtggt ggggatccat gcagacaagc
2221 catgctaaca gccaggcgt ctttaagagg gggttgctgt gaaagcctgc tgccgggttg
2281 ggagcaggtt aaaaatgcta tgcctgctta ttttaaatgc tgtccatgga acaaaaatct
2341 gtgtagtgac tttgtgagaa gttgtgatgt ttatgttgtg taactttgtg caggaacact
2401 gcgtcttgca gtgggtgcac agctctgagt agaaaccacc tcttcatagg aagcctgtgg
2461 ccttaacact aggcagttta agctttttaaa taataccaga gttactaact agtgcagaag
2521 tgacatgctt tttcttttttt cctgctag
```

TFIIIA GENE EXON TWO:

*LOOP BETA BINDING TO DNA

TFIIIA MOLECULE AMINO ACIDS 68-77:

```
       R    P    F    V    C    D    Y    E    G    C
2549  aga  cca  ttt  gtt  tgt  gac  tat  gaa  ggg  tgt
```

TFIIIA MOLECULE ZINC FINGER 'TWO' DNA BONDING SITES, AMINO ACIDS 78-89

```
        K    S    S    R    E    S    S    K    S    S    K    K
  2579 aag  tct  tcc  cgt  gaa  tcg  tcc  aaa  tct  tcc  aaa  aag
```

TFIIIA MOLECULE AMINO ACIDS 90-101:

```
        H    I    L    T    H    T    G    E    K    P    F    V
  2615 cac  att  ctg  act  cac  aca  gga  gaa  aag  ccg  ttt  gtg
```

TFIIIA GENE INTRON TWO:

```
  2651 taa           (STOP)

  2654 gtagaga    cctgttttta ggcttttgaa gtgggttgtg ttgggcatat
  2701 agacccagta agaagattga tgttaactca cgagatcagg aatgtgaagc ctggcagggc
  2761 tcggtggctc atgcctgtaa tcccagcact ttgggaggcg gagatgggca gatcacttga
  2821 acccaggagt ttgagacaaa cctgggcaac atggtgaaac cccgtatgta caaaaataca
  2881 aaaattagtc agggatggtg gtttgtgcct gtaatcctag ctacccagga ggctgagcta
  2941 acataaaatg ctcatgggtg gggacaagct aaagtatatc aacacaatgg gataccctac
  3001 agccaggaaa atgaatgcag atgctctctg caaagccatg agaaaatcac cagggcactt
  3061 taattgaaaa accaaggtgc agaagagtcc tctttaggct acttttatgt gtgtaaaaaa
  3121 gctagggggt agggggaggg gtgagtagtg ggtgttgggt aggcaggaag caactatatt
  3181 tgtatttgtt cctatttgta aagaagtctt aaaagttaca taacaaaact aaaaatgtca
  3241 tctgttttgg gagcagtggg ggatcctggc caagtagggg gtggggatgg taggaaatgc
  3301 catgcaacca ggaactactg gacatgactc ttccagctca tgatctaacc cagaccctgc
  3361 ccctctttag ctgtagttcc ccgtttccca ctgctcgctg gacagtgcta cttggctatc
  3421 tctgtgtctt cttaaattcc atgtggtagg ctgggtgtgg tggctcatgc ctgtaatccc
  3481 agcactttga gaggctgagg tgggaggatt gctttgaggc caggagttca ggctgggcaa
  3541 gatggtcagg tccatctcta ttaaagaaat aaataaataa aaaattccac atggcccaaa
  3601 tttgtcacag tcaaactgag ctcacttttc tgtttgatct tctctcatgt tcttgtctgg
  3661 agaggtggcc tcgctgtctg tccagtgacc catagcaaag ataaggcagc tccctggact
  3721 ctccattctt tctcccatcc cttgcaacag gtggttgcc agatcctgta actgacccat
  3781 cagatccagc agccactgtc ttatctcggt cccttcctct ggctggaatg acagtttgca
  3841 ggccagccct ctcccccagt gccctcccgt gtgcttccct taaagctgtg cagtgctttc
  3901 aagcacggcc tacatgtgaa atccaggttt caagtgtgtc ctacaatgac ctgcgtgatt
  3961 tagccctttt ctgcttatct tgccccattt gcttgacttg caggcatgaa gctgtggtcc
  4021 agctgtgcta actaaccagc cccctctcca agtgtgccgg ggtctctcac gcccacttgg
  4081 gtcttgtcag gactcttcct ggcctgtcct cctatcccat acccggttgg gttagatgcc
  4141 tgtgtcaggt ttagagtgaa gaatggcagg aaccccagca caagagatgc ttaaacaaga
  4201 tgggctcttt gtcttgtgcg actgaaatac agaaatacag aggcaggagc tctggagcct
  4261 cttctgactg gtctctgcca tcctcatctt gggctttaac ctcactgtga tgcctgtttg
  4321 ggcccatctg tcacataagc atgccactgg caggaaggag gaaaggccat aagaggcatg
  4381 cccccttatt tagagacttt gtggggttg agcaggatgg gctggactca gccatgagcc
  4441 gccctaattg caggggaggc cggagagtgc actttctgtc ggccacctgc ccagctaaca
  4501 ctcagcattc tgtccctgca gttaggggg cttctagggt ctctgccaca gcgcccctcc
  4561 catttgtggg cctctgtgct gtgcctccca tggtcactgc tggcttgttt gtctctgctt
  4621 ggccctagga atgggacagt gcctgcctca gggttatcag tgagtgatgg ctaagattga
  4681 gcctgggaaa ggaagtcctg cttcatccct caagcttacg aaggctcatc acaagaggca
  4741 caaattttct tttgggaaaa aaaaaaaaaa aaaaggaaaa ggctttgcag aggatttaga
  4801 tcattcaaag ccaagatgcc aagataaggg gaaccagaat ggcttggtaa gccagagaac
  4861 ataatggtta tggttctgct ctaagtatct gttttacctc taatgataag ccaagacaag
  4921 ttttatggag gcctttctgg aaatccagtt cataatgaca tctcaagcag cattaaggtt
  4981 gtcagattct aagctgagaa taatttgtct taagcatgat ttaggcctag tgtaggcttt
  5041 tgggactagt gtatttcacc ttcccatctg cccagtgtgt ataaaagatg actgatgtag
  5101 tgtgtataat ttcagaagcc taatatgaaa aagcattttg ttacatgata ctcatcaggt
  5161 tgagagtcta tgtgtgtatgg cttaacactc tggaattcgc taagactatt ttatagtatt
  5221 actattcttt ggaagaatta gcttctataa agtaggaaga tatatgtgtc ttaaaacttc
  5281 ttctcccttg gtttattaat attttggttt atataacttc ttacagt
```

TFIIIA GENE EXON THREE:

*LOOP GAMMA BINDING TO DNA

TFIIIA MOLECULE AMINO ACIDS 102-107:

```
        C    A    A    N    G    C
  5328 tgt  gca  gcc  aat  ggc  tgt
```

TFIIIA MOLECULE ZINC FINGER 'THREE' DNA BONDING SITES,
AMINO ACIDS 108-119

```
       K   S   S   K   R   S   S   E   S   S   E   K
  5349 aag tct tcc aaa agg tca tcc gag tcg tcc gag aag
```

TFIIIA MOLECULE AMINO ACIDS 120-133:

```
       H   F   E   R   K   H   E   N   Q   Q   K   Q   Y   I
  5381 cat ttt gaa cgc aaa cat gaa aat caa caa aaa caa tat ata
```

TFIIIA GENE INTRON THREE:

```
  5424 gtaagta      tgattttata tgcttaaatt ttttgagtat
  5461 ttttacactt actgcctatg tttctgacat tttcagccag gtgcggtggc tcaagcctat
  5521 aatcgtagct tgaggccagg aatttgagac cagcctggga aacatagtga aatgctgtct
  5581 ctgaaaaaaa aaaacaaaaa cagaaaacaa aacaaaaaat tttgggtaa  cagagaccct
  5641 gtctctaaaa aataaaagtg aaaaataaag ttttcgtcaa ccaaattttg tctgccaaat
  5701 gtctgaattt acttaatgcc atcataatga taaaggtttt aatttggaag cagacattgt
  5761 gcaaattagt gtattgggag actattccaa ctgaaacagt tttgcttttt caaatgttat
  5821 atgattcttc aaaccttttt gagataaagc agaattttac agtaacaaaa tgggtgaaag
  5881 cagaaatttt atacagtctc caaaattgtt ttatcttgag gattctgtta cgaactgttc
  5941 attttgtttt gactttccat aagactaacg agcctttaca atttaacag
```

TFIIIA GENE EXON FOUR:

*LOOP DELTA BINDING TO DNA

TFIIIA MOLECULE AMINO ACIDS 134-139:

```
        C    S    F    E    D    C
  5990 tgc  agt  ttt  gaa  gac  tgt
```

TFIIIA MOLECULE ZINC FINGER 'FOUR' DNA BONDING SITES, AMINO
ACIDS 140-151

```
       R   S   S   K   N   S   S   E   S   S   K   R
  6008 cgc tcc tcc aaa aac tcg tcc gag tcg tcc aaa agg
```

TFIIIA MOLECULE AMINO ACIDS 152-164:

```
       H   Q   C   Q   H   T   N   E   P   L   F   K
  6044 cat cag tgc cag cat acc aat gaa cct cta ttc aag
```

TFIIIA GENE INTRON FOUR:

6080 tag (STOP)

```
6083 gtacttca   tgtggctgaa aatgcctgga ttctaggtgt
6121 gaataagatt ggaaatgcaa gggtggtgtt gagcattgtt tcatgttttt tggccatttg
6181 tatatcttct gagaaatgtc tgttcatatc ctttgcccac ttttcgatgg attgttttt
6241 tcttgctgat ctgagttccc tgtagatcct ggatatacat tctttattgg atgcataatg
6301 tgccagtatt ttctcccact ctctgggttg tctgtttact ctgctgatta tttcttttgc
6361 tgtgcagaag cttttttagtt taattaggtc ccatttattt atttctattt ttgttgcatt
6421 tgctttcagg gccttagtaa gaattctttg cctaggctga tgtccagaag tttttccaat
6481 gtttttcattt tgaattttta gtttcaggtc ataaacttaa tttgagttga tttttgtata
6541 aggtgagaga tagggatcca gtttttccag caccatttat tgaataggga gtcctttccc
6601 cagtttacgt ttttatatgc tttgttgaag atcgggtggc tgtaagtatt tggctttatt
6661 tctgtttttgt tccattggtc taagtgccta ttttaaacc agtgccaccc tgtttttggta
6721 actgtagcct cgtagtataa tctgaagtct ggtcaaagga aaagaagtca ctatatgaaa
6781 aagacacatg cacacacgtt tacagcagca cagttcacaa ttgcaaatac atggagccaa
6841 tttaagtgcc catcgaccaa tgagtagata aagaaaacgt gatgtatata caccatggaa
6901 tactacacag ccataaaagg gaacaaaatg atgtcttttg cagcagcttg gatggagctg
6961 gaggccatta ttctcagtga agtaactcag gaatggaaaa ccaaatacca tagtttttcac
7021 taagtgggca ctaaactatg aggacaaaaa gacacagtga tttcataaac tttggggact
7081 tggggtgggg agtttgggga ggggggtgag ggatgaaaga ctacatattg ggtacagtgt
7141 atgctgcttg agtgatggtg cgctcaaaatc tcagcaccac tataggattc atccacgtaa
7201 cgaaaaaaca cttgcaaccc caaaagccat tgaaatttaa agcaacggtg ggacaaatct
7261 tctgaaagct tcctaatcaa cattttttctg ttaaaatgta ctgcatatgc acatttatat
7321 attgggagca ttttaaaggt ttactttgct ctgaaagaaa tatttaatgt gtttcaaaat
7381 aatttttgag attattctag ttgtggttaa gcttaaaggc tgagaaatta cttaactatt
7441 caaatagagc ctgtgcaact atatgaaatg tcattatgga gacactcatt atgcttttcc
7501 tgtagaacaa aacaagtagt tgggtttatc tgcaattagg gtttttttgag gaacgtgagg
7561 gtggctggac aagttgggta gacctgcaaa agggccagcg gctctctgca tggctctggc
7621 catccggcac tttcccttga cttgcacagg ctgccctgtg ccttggagtt gctgcagtga
7681 ccttgcctgt ccttgcttgt gggtctgctg ctgctgcttt gctgctgatg gctttagcac
7741 agaggggggcc cgtgcttttt attgctcacc agaggcagat gcatctactg ctgtgctgtc
7801 tcgcacaccc cctatgcagc atcattagga aagctagaca caagtgattc agaatggctt
7861 aggggtttat ctaagccaag tcagataacc tcttgaacta tcttttttgta gccatgaaag
7921 cagagtatat ttccagaggt ataaagatga aaactgttta aatgggtcaa aaaaagtaac
7981 gtgacttttt tctccaacag tttgtttttgt cctaaagctg gtcaagtaac ttgaatctca
8041 cctgtgatga gagctacatt ttaacatggg tttggttatg ggaagaggca agactttggt
8101 gggagaaaca ggacaaagtg ccattgacct tgagcggagt tctctgtgaa aatggattgg
8161 ctaataccctc atgtgttgcc aatgcagg
```

TFIIIA GENE EXON FIVE:

*LOOP EPSILON BINDING TO DNA

TFIIIA MOLECULE AMINO ACIDS 164-169:

```
        C   T   Q   E   G   C
   8189 tgt acc cag gaa gga tgt
```

TFIIIA MOLECULE BONDING TO DNA AMINO ACIDS 170-181:

```
        R   S   S   R   K   S   S   E   S   S   K   E
   8207 cgc agc tcc cgt aaa tct tcc gag tcg tcc aaa gag
```

TFIIIA MOLECULE AMINO ACIDS 182-187:

```
        H   A   K   A   H   E
   8243 cat gcc aag gcc cac gag
```

TFIIIA GENE EXON FIVE:

```
        G
8261 ggt
```

```
8264 gtgtacg    gatagcctgg
8281 gtgtgctccg agggggatgc caaatcctgg gcgcctttga atctgttctg tgatcacgct
8341 gaaaagatgg gaaccctgtg aacagggga  accatcctgc ttatttgggt cttacactct
8401 tgtccaaaga ggcactgtat atgtctgttt ttccactacc gtatcattgc tgttcacatg
8461 taatgtgttg tttgttcaca acaagcgcct ggttacacat tacactgacg aatgtgctga
8521 tgctccagcc atggctttga tgcttctgtc atttttaacc tcttctatta atatttactg
8581 cctgtgccat tcttttcctt gttggccatt cacaaggctt ggataatcgt gtgacatttt
8641 gagagccatc agatgttacg tttctcaaaa aaaaaaaaaa aagacttgat tatattaact
8701 atttgaatct atgatctgtt tccttgaggg atttttgcta atctgtattt caatttccca
8761 ggtcctagaa tttatgattt tttttttttt aagaggttag tagctaacag tgagaggcag
8821 cctcattgtt tttagtttct agttgggtgg aactcagccc tagtgttgta tacttattaa
8881 tcccatttta gtgctttgca catatccatt gttattcagt gtttttctct gggtccttcc
8941 agtttatttt cttccttagc tgtactcttt taaaaaaaaa aaacaaaaaa aaactttttt
9001 tttttttttt gtgataaagt taaaatataa tgtaccctac ttttttttgtg cagtatgaca
9061 cttacaagat ggccagacta gaggaagcca gaggtgggca tggtaacact actgaaaagt
9121 tggtggtgtg ccatggacaa gggaccgact gcagagtatg tttgctgagg aaaatagagg
9181 cgaggataga gcaggcaggg gaagggaaat aagacatgga gataggaggt taaagcagtt
9241 gggagtccat acacagccta cccaacttcc tgagaactct tagagaggaa aaggcatcct
9301 taggcatcct tcctgtgaag tttgcctatt ccgtgatcac gctgagaaga tgggaactct
9361 gaagtttgct tcacaggaag gtaaaatcct taaagggagg caccttgctg tgccactgtt
9421 cagttttact ataacatcaa tcttttttta gttttttattc ccacctcaag aggctgagtt
9481 gaatactatt aggcgggga a tggaaaatta tataggcacc taagtttcct ttctagttat
9541 ggtcagtgtt tacactgagt attcatgaca gacaatgcac caattttttt aata
```

TFIIIA GENE EXON SIX:

*LOOP ZETA BINDING TO TRANSCRIPTION FACTORS

TFIIIA MOLECULE AMINO ACIDS 188-195:

```
        G   Y
9595 ggc tat
```

```
        V   C   Q   K   G   C
9601 gta tgt caa aaa gga tgt
```

TFIIIA MOLECULE BIND TO TRANSCRIPTION FACTOR AMINO ACIDS 196-207:

```
        A   F   V   A   A   T   W   T   A   L   L   A
9619 gca ttc gtg gcc gcc acc tgg acc gca ctc ctg gcc
```

TFIIIA MOLECULE AMINO ACIDS 208-214:

```
        H   V   R   E   T   H   K
9655 cat gtg aga gaa acc cat aaa
```

GENE INTRON SIX

```
 9676 ggtaa        ggcaggcatg aatggcaggc atggtgtaaa tgtttgtccc
 9721 cacagaactg atttagtgct tttcaagagt gaaatgctgt gtgctttaaa gtaaaagggt
 9781 ttctctatga tattttgtga agtgctgggt atgatgttgt tggaaaggtg agcagagctg
 9841 tgccaggtct ctgagccacc ccaccatgca caattagcat gctgaaggcg gtggcaggtc
 9901 tgtagtgaag aatttcggga ggcactgctg ttctgtggga ccgcctggga aacagtaccc
 9961 tgcatactgg gggacaagga aggacactgg tctgcttcat tttctgtacc tccccacagt
10021 caccttcctg agagccctgc ctcttggcaa gtgaacaatg actgtgtggc atttaagaac
10081 ttcagagaat tgagacaaac ttcctaggtg ataaaaactg gggttgtttc cttgggaatt
10141 tctgatttgt atatagtgat caggttttcag gcactgaatg ttacttatat attaggtatt
10201 aatttttttct aaatggtaat atctggggaa atttgtgaaa tttgtctgtc tgtcccacca
```

TFIIIA GENE EXON SEVEN:

*LOOP ETA BINDING TO TRANSCRIPTION FACTORS

TFIIIA MOLECULE AMINO ACIDS 215-222:

```
          E    E    I    L    C    E    Y    C
    10261 gag  gaa  ata  cta  tgt  gaa  gta  tgc
```

TFIIIA MOLECULE AMINO ACIDS 223-234:

```
          A    A    T    F    A    A    A    D    Y    L    A    Q
    10285 gca  gcc  acc  ttt  gcc  gca  gcc  gac  tat  ctc  gcc  cag
```

TFIIIA MOLECULE AMINO ACIDS 235-253:

```
          H    M    K    T    H    A    P    E    R    D    V    C    R    C
    10321 cac  atg  aaa  act  cat  gcc  cca  gaa  agg  gat  gta  tgt  cgc  tgt

          P    R    E    G    C
    10363 cca  aga  gaa  ggc  tgt
```

*LOOP THETA BINDING TO TRANSCRIPTION FACTORS

TFIIIA MOLECULE AMINO ACIDS 254-265:

```
          G    A    T    A    T    T    V    F    A    L    G    A
    10378 ggc  gcc  acc  gca  aca  act  gtg  ttt  gcc  ctc  ggc  gcg
```

TFIIIA MOLECULE AMINO ACIDS 266-284:

```
          H    I    L    S    F    H    E    E    S    R    P    F
    10414 cat  atc  ctc  tcc  ttc  cat  gag  gaa  agc  cgc  cct  ttt

          V    C    E    H    A    G    C
    10450 gtg  tgt  gaa  cat  gct  ggc  tgt
```

*LOOP IOTA BINDING TO TRANSCRIPTION FACTORS

TFIIIA MOLECULE AMINO ACIDS 285-291:

```
         G    A    T    F    A    M    A
10471  ggc  gcc  acc  ttt  gcc  atg  gcc
```

GENE INTRON SEVEN

```
10492 gtaagcact
10501 caccctcata ctcatggtcc tatagtctat gctttcacaa catggttttc atattaatat
10561 ttcattaata actttctctt tcattgtag
```

*LOOP IOTA (CONTINUED) BINDING TO TRANSCRIPTION FACTORS

TFIIIA MOLECULE AMINO ACIDS 292-296:

```
         Q    A    L    T    A
10590  caa  gcg  ctc  acc  gca
```

TFIIIA MOLECULE AMINO ACIDS 297-311:

```
         H    A    V    V    H    D    P    D    K    K    K    M    K
10605  cat  gct  gtt  gta  cat  gat  cct  gac  aag  aag  aaa  atg  aag

         L    K
10644  ctc  aaa
```

GENE INTRON EIGHT

```
10650 gtaagttgaa actacttagg caagcttagt t
10681 ttcaagtgga aattgtttaa ggccagaagg agtctgtttg gaattctttt cacctgcttt
10741 actgtttgag tctgcactac tgttgaagac tttacttcct cataaagcaa tgttgtacac
10801 tatatctgct ggtacatatg actatcgtaa aattaactca gacagttttg attttgaatt
10861 ctaatcgtgt gtcttcctta ttcccaaag
```

3' END OF THE TFIIIA MOLECULE

TFIIIA MOLECULE AMINO ACIDS 312-365:

```
         V    K    K    S    R    E    K    R    S    L    A    S    H
10890  gtc  aaa  aaa  tct  cgt  gaa  aaa  cgg  agt  ttg  gcc  tct  cat
         L    S    G    Y    I    P    P    K    R    K    Q    G    Q
10929  ctc  agt  gga  tat  atc  cct  ccc  aaa  agg  aaa  caa  ggg  caa

         G    L    S    L    C    Q    N    G    E    S    P    N    C
10968  ggc  tta  tct  ttg  tgt  caa  aac  gga  gag  tca  ccc  aac  tgt

         V    E    D    K    M    L    S    T    V    A    V    L    T
11007  gtg  gaa  gac  aag  atg  ctc  tcg  aca  gtt  gca  gta  ctt  acc

11046  L    G
       ctt  ggc
```

```
11052 taa (STOP)
```

TFIIIA GENE 3' DOWNSTREAM REGION

```
11055 gaactg      cactgctttg tttaaaggac tgcagaccaa ggagcgagct
11101 ttctctcaga gcatgctttt ctttattaaa attactgatg cagaacattt gattccttat
11161 catttc
```

TNF alpha GENE 3' DOWNSTREAM REGION:

```
4520 a catggtctcc ttcttggaat taattctgca tctgcctctt
```

```
4561 cttgtgggtg ggaagaagct ccctaagtcc tctctccaca ggctttaaga tccctcggac
4621 ccagtcccat ccttagactc ctagggccct ggagacccta cataaacaaa gcccaacaga
4681 atattcccca tcccccagga aacaagagcc tgaacctaat tacctctccc tcagggcatg
4741 ggaatttcca actctgggaa ttccaatcct tgctgggaaa atcctgcagc tcaggtgaga
4801 tttccggctg ttgcagctgg ccagcagtcc ggagagagct ggagaggagc cgcattctca
4861 ggtacctgaa tcacacagcc aagggacttc cagagattcg ggtgtctagg cttcaaatca
4921 ccctgtccta actctgcaac ctgaaccagc cacttaacct atctatccaa tggggatagg
4981 aatgtccacc acacataggg catgtgagag aaggcctgac ctccatcaga ggacctcact
5041 cagcccttgg cacagtgggc acttagtgaa ttctggcttc cttcaaccag tttccagctg
5101 ttctatcccc ttccattctc tcagtgggtg aaatcgaaga gactgaggac aataaagaac
5161 aaggaaccga actgccggac gtggtggcat gcacctgtaa tcctaccact ttgcaaggcc
5221 aagtgagag gatcgcttga acccaggagt tccagacaa cctgggcaac atagtgagat
5281 cctgtctcta tttttttaaaa aagaatgaaa cataggaata agatgtgggt gaaggactca
5341 catgccggct tggtcccact ggtctttgtg gtgaaggagg ggagaggtga gaggtgggta
5401 atccggaaag agaaaagcac ccctccctg gatgaaggct cttctggaga gagtcaaaga
5461 caaataaggg tggggcgcag tggctcatgc ctgttatccc aacactttgg gaggctgagg
5521 tgggaggacc acttgagccc actagttcaa gaccagcctg tgcaacatag caagaccttg
5581 tttctagaaa aaaaattaaa gattagtcag gtgtagtggt gcatgcctgt aatcctagct
5641 cctcaggagg ctgaggcagg aggatcactc aagcccagga gtttgaggtt acagtaagct
5701 atgatcatgc cactgtaccc ccgtctgggt gacagaacga gaccctgtct caaaaaaata
5761 ataattccaa aaacaaatat ggagacggaa attgagcccc cctagactgg gagcccccac
5821 tgagttcgga aattaggctt tacctccagc cctggggtgc caggcaggag aaaaccatgt
5881 ggtaggctga gggggtaggg tgacccattg gggtgaccta gataggcct tgggtcaccc
5941 tctgcctcct ccagcctgtg gctgaaagtc agccatgaag taatggggga cactgttact
6001 catcccagaa gcacccacac ttactcactt ttgggaaggg ggacctaaag tgtgaaaaaa
6061 aggtgaggat tttccgtctc accctaaatg ggacacccta agtggggcat cggttttttcc
6121 tcctccccag aacttcctgg tgttttcagg caccacaggc tccttcctgc catccccatc
6181 tctctctaat attctcccct tctttctcct tcagcctcct ccccttcagac cccatgagcc
6241 ttgaattaag ctccttggag gagaagagtt gactgtcggg taggagacag agaggccttc
6301 aggcagctct aggggagaa gtgcgggccc cctccaggct tcattcctct gtcatgatag
6361 gggcttactc tgctgctggg cctttctgag tggtgcttgc tgggctctgt aatgacccct
6421 ctcactgttg gggggtaccc aagagaaaag agtatggtgc agagtctggt tgggaccatg
6481 tggccctgaa aatcaggatg cctagagaag cttcggagtt tgagaagtcc cccttcctcc
6541 caccctccaa ctgggctaat ggtggggcct ggccattcag aggcagggag ggggtgggac
6601 aggcagacca tcatccctag gagcaaaggc catacactgt gttgtgatga attgtttcaa
6661 gcaaccagaa gagtactgag aatatttaac ccgcacccgt gcacccaccc tgaattaaga
6721 cgtgtgtcgc aactcagcat ctttatcggc agcactgaag ctttccattc tttattttca
6781 tcaggttcaa aatcaatttc caaacagtct cctacatttt tcccactgcc atggggtcct
6841 gggcgtccgg gcccccaata ttcacgcact cgcaccacgc actcatattc cctcaccca
6901 ccatcacggc cccaaagaag gtcttccctc tcgcgaagtc caccatatcg gggtgactga
6961 tgttgacgta caccctctcg ccctccggga gctgcaccag gccgccgaac cccacgctcg
7021 tgtaccagag aggcccgtac ccttgtctcc tggccgggtc cagcactgga gtcaccgtct
7081 cggcgccctc gagcagcagc tcgggagtgc ccggcccgta ggcgccccc gcccggtaca
7141 gagagctgcg cagcgtgacc gagcggccct ggggtcccc gccgccaggg ggcgcccggc
7201 cccggtagcc gacgagacag tagaggtaat agaggccgtc
```

CHAPTER 14

COMMANDS EMBEDDED IN THE 3' REGION OF A GENE

At the time of the writing of this text, only limited knowledge of the role of the 3' region of a gene is understood. The 3' region of a gene is obviously responsible for indicating to the transcription complex the position to cease transcription of the pre-mRNA. It has been speculated that embedded in the 3' region of a gene that there is a function such as a REPEAT command present. If a REPEAT code is embedded in the 3' region, this signal causes the transcription complex to read the transcription region of the gene a second time.

At the time of the initial design of the synthetic gene presented in this text it was thought that the most efficient approach to creating a functional synthetic gene would be to insert the transcription segment of the modified TFIIIA molecule inside the 5' region and the 3' region of the TNF gene. The justification was that the nuclear transcription machinery would see and respond to the functions present in the 5' region and the 3' region of the TNF gene, while simply transcribing the modified TFIIIA transcription region. The design was contrived by theorizing that this design would function the smoothest of the potential options at the time. Given that there is lack of concrete understanding of the functional behavior of the 3' region of a gene, the above approach is still considered the most valid approach at the time of publication of this text.

Further speculation lead to a logic that suggests that additional critical command instructions may be present in the 3' region of a gene. One concept is that for every mRNA that is generated by a gene, a specific rRNA is generated by the same gene to efficiently effect the translation of the mRNA produced by the transcribed gene. A small molecule RNA (smRNA) may be generated by the gene that triggers a rRNA gene to generate a rRNA to specifically translate a specific mRNA. If the 3' region of a gene is indeed responsible for generating a rRNA that is specific to and directed at the mRNA the gene has generated, then the above synthetic gene design may need to be modified such that the 5' region from the TNF gene remains the same, but following the modified TFIIIA transcription sequence, the 3' region of the original TFIIIA molecule is attached, instead of the 3' region of the TNF gene. It may be necessary to attach the 3' region of the original TFIIIA gene in order to insure that the mRNA of the modified TFIIIA molecule is' translated properly once the mRNA migrates to the cytoplasm of the cell.

Other command instructions may be present in the 3' region of a gene. Instructions such as how to assemble complex protein molecules consisting of more than one of the same amino acid chain or complex protein molecules consisting of multiple differing amino acid chains. The smooth endoplasmic reticulum, directly attached to the nucleus, may act at the cell's processing unit. Small molecule RNAs (smRNA) may act as signals to the smooth endoplasmic reticulum to indicate to the smooth endoplasmic reticulum the instructions as to how to construct the macromolecules the cell requires.

The 3' region may contain a number of differing small molecule RNAs, each smRNA acting as a separate signal. In the case of more than one smRNA being generated by the 3' region of a gene, each smRNA would travel to a different location in the nucleus and act as a distinct command instruction.

The proposed differing functions of the 3' region of a cell suggest differing STOP codes. Like the three different STOP codes present in mRNA molecules, the DNA may also have different STOP codes that represent different functional assignments. Certainly the stop command of STOP and DETACH would be likely, instructing the transcription complex to stop transcription and disassemble. STOP and REPEAT would also be a likely instruction, directing the transcription complex to stop transcription and return to the Transcription Start Site to repeat transcription of the gene; note in this case the STOP could would need to somehow convey to the transcription complex how many times to repeat the transcription process. STOP and RESTART would be a third instruction if there are one or more small molecule RNAs that need to be generated in the wake of the pre-mRNA being transcribed. Other STOP codes may be present to direct alternative functions when necessary.

At the time of the original publication of this text, given the lack of concrete evidence to the contrary, the Courier Gene design as described in this text, is theorized to be the most likely design to generate an effective modified TFIIIA molecule to neutralize the HIV genome.

CHAPTER 15

DESIGN OF A DELIVERY SYSTEM TO TRANSPORT MODIFIED TFIIIA GENES

One of the challenges is to deliver the modified TFIIIA gene to their proper cellular target. Naturally occurring TFIIIA molecules are constructed in the cytoplasm of a cell. Once constructed, the TFIIIA migrates from the cytoplasm to the nucleus of the cell. The TFIIIA molecule binds to the DNA.

Medically therapeutic protein products include insulin to treat diabetes mellitus, Calcitonin to manage osteoporosis, and biologic agents to manage inflammatory arthritis. Such protein products are either injected or infused through an intravenous access, or sniffed up the nose to be absorbed by the mucosal lining of the nares. The hydrochloric acid secreted by the gastric cells in the stomach is meant to break down proteins for digestive purposes. Medically therapeutic proteins that are ingested are generally made ineffective due to destruction by the hydrochloric acid present in the stomach.

Once a therapeutic protein enters the blood stream per injection, intravenous access, or nasal absorption, passage of the protein from the blood to the cell is dependent upon the compatibility of the protein with the cell membrane transport mechanisms and the configuration of the cell surface receptors fixed to the external membrane of the cell.

Cells comprising human tissues are comprised of a cell membrane as the exterior boundary. The cell membrane is a lipid bilayer comprised of lipoproteins molecules. Lipoproteins have a hydrophilic end to the molecule and a hydrophobic end to the molecule. The bilayer is configured with hydrophilic ends of the lipoprotein molecules pointed to both the exterior and the interior of the cell. The hydrophobic ends of the lipoprotein molecules is pointed toward the center of the bilayer. Mounted in the exterior lipid layer are receptors that act to sense the characteristics of the environment outside the cell. Some receptors are utilized by the cell to detect which proteins are beneficial to the cell and should be absorbed into the cell. Some of the receptors are meant to be triggered, which then generates a chemical reaction inside the cell.

Depending upon the type of protein, some therapeutic proteins will remain extracellular and generally not directly interact with cells, some proteins will interact with cell surface receptors, and some proteins will be absorbed through the cell wall into the interior of the cell. Tumor Necrosis Factor (TNF) blocking biologic agents generally act extracellularly to deactivate tumor necrosis factor alpha molecules, which is a pivotal molecule implicated in inflammatory joint disease such as rheumatoid arthritis. Insulin interacts with cell surface receptors to regulate and facilitate the absorption of glucose molecules into cells. Some proteins such as albumin pass through the cell membrane and are absorbed into the interior of the cell to act as a form of nutrient for the cell.

Some proteins such as insulin, engage cell surface receptors, stimulating action on the cell surface or stimulating an action to place inside the cell, but the protein never enters into the cell.

Further study will determined if a molecular virus killer circulating in the blood stream will be absorbed into the target cell infected by a virus.

If it is determined that a pharmaceutical synthetic gene that would generate a molecular virus killer protein cannot traverse the lipid bilayer cell membrane on its own accord, then possibly a transport vehicle may need to be employed.

The viral genome is already adapted to targeting the host cell the virus infects and uses as a resource for replication.

A virus virion is equipped with surface probes that are fashioned to seek out and engage specific surface receptors on the exterior of the target cell's membrane. Once a virus virion's exterior probes engage the appropriate cell surface receptor on the exterior of a target cell, either a passage is opened up traversing through the cell membrane and the viral genome is inserted into the host cell, or the target cell engulfs the viral virion along with its genomic contents. Once the viral genome breaches the cell membrane, the viral genome embeds into the nuclear genome of the cell or in the case of an RNA virus such as Hepatitis C, the RNA viral genome bypasses the nucleus and mimics a messenger RNA molecule to directly be translated to produce viral proteins to be utilized in the construction of copies of the viral virion and genome.

Since the virus virion is designed and very well adapted to seek out its target cell, the virus virion could be enlisted to act as a transport vehicle to carry the synthetic modified TFIIIA gene to viral infected host cells in the body. See Figure 45.

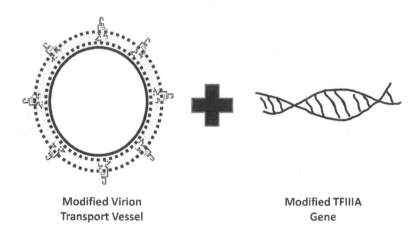

Modified Virion
Transport Vessel

Modified TFIIIA
Gene

Figure 45 Virus shell enlisted as a transporter
of TFIIIA molecules to target cells

A process could be designed to utilize hybrid cells where the gene to produce modified TFIIIA molecules are manufactured and packaged into a viral vector that is a replica of a naturally occurring viral virion, the viral vector being void of the viral genome payload.

A sufficient amount of hypoallergenic viral vectors carrying a payload consisting of a modified TFIIIA gene would be injected into a patient. See Figure 46. The viral vectors would seek out host cells both infected with the virus and not infected with the virus. The viral vectors would engage host cells and deliver modified TFIIIA gene into the intracellular cytoplasm of the host cells. The TFIIIA gene would migrate from the cytoplasm to the nucleus of the host cell. Once in the nucleus of the host cell the modified TFIIIA would be embedded into the cell's nuclear genome. The gene would be transcribed and generate an mRNA that would code for modified TFIII A molecules. The modified TFIIIA molecules would enter the cell's nucleus and seek out the unique identifier of the critical gene of an embedded viral genome that it is meant to silence. If the viral genome is present, the modified TFIIIA molecule would attach to the viral gene's unique identifier and prevent transcription of the gene. In the case of a viral RNA genome, the modified TFIIIA molecule should silence the unique identifier of the viral negative sense RNA or viral mRNA. If the viral genome is not present, since the TFIIIA is specifically designed to engage only the unique identifier associated with the viral genome, the TFIIIA molecule will migrate harmlessly until degraded by intracellular enzymes.

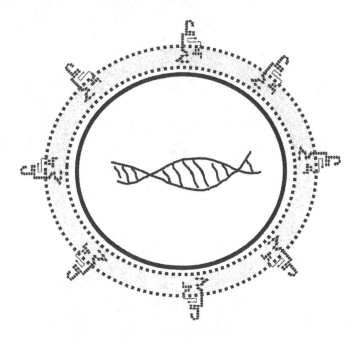

Figure 46 Virion carrying a modified TFIIIA molecule

An alternative treatment strategy would be to employ viral transport vectors to carry messenger RNA that are designed to generate modified TFIIIA molecules once inside the cytoplasm of the target cell. Possibly the virus virions could be utilized to transport modified TFIIIA molecules directly to infected cells. The HIV life-cycle represents a model of how this could be done, since HIV introduces RNA into its host, which becomes integrated into the cell's nuclear DNA.

CHAPTER 16

UNDERSTANDING HOW TO BUILD
A FULLY SYNTHETIC GENE

The human gene presented in the first part of this text is a synthetic gene. It is a splicing of a TNF gene and a TFIIIA gene. The protein coding portion of the TNF alpha gene is removed and in the place of the TNF alpha protein coding segment is inserted the protein coding segment of the TFIIIA protein where the nucleotide coding has been modified to produce a protein intended to seek out the unique identifier of the HIV genome.

Admittedly, though this is a manmade gene, this is not a fully synthetic gene. The 5' upstream region and the 3' downstream regions were borrowed from the TNF gene. In addition, the modified gene was comprised of introns that were borrowed from the original TFIIIA gene. To date, there is a fundamental lack of understanding what the nucleotides comprising the 5' region and the introns and the 3' region actually mean.

From a practical standpoint, the 5' region of a gene is the section of the gene that acts as the anchor segment that transcription factors attach to upstream from the protein coding segment to facilitate assembly of the transcription complex. In general, the 5' region is comprised a TATA box, approximately 25 nucleotides between the TATA box and the Transcription Start Site, a promoter region and an enhancer region. All of these subsegments appear to assist in the assembly of a transcription complex.

The 3' Downstream region appears to have at least three functions. The 3' region signals to the Transcription Complex that the transcription process has been completed. The 3' region also signals the component proteins comprising the Transcription Complex to disassemble. In some cases, the 3' region directs the Transcription

Complex to repeat transcription of the coding region of the dame gene.

The 5' Upstream region appears to possess a role of sole physical bonding functions. Some segments of the 5' Upstream region simply act as physical targets to enable specific transcription factors to bind to in order to facilitate proper construction of the Transcription Complex upstream from the Transcription Start Site.

The 3' Downstream region in contrast must possess segments of nucleotides that act as signals to the Transcription Complex to first stop transcription and then to disassemble. The 3' Downstream segment possesses elements that are reminiscent of intelligence. Unintelligent random circumstances do not create signals such as STOP, DISASSEMBLE and REPEAT.

The presence of introns in the DNA has posed a puzzle due to their apparent uselessness. Introns are the portions of the coding region of a gene that are removed during the transcription process and do not appear in the messenger RNA that migrates to the cytoplasm to be translated.

Introns represent proof of an intelligent design being responsible for the construct of the human genome. Proper construct of proteins requires not only the presence of mRNA to act as a template with which to generate amino acid chains, but also requires the precise orchestration of numerous auxiliary factors. To successfully produce proteins there must be present the proper tRNA molecules, the proper rRNA molecules, an adequate amount of amino acids (some of which are essential, while some are required to be assembled), the proper assembly instructions to bond multi-amino acid chains together into a macromolecule, the proper assembly instructions to bond an amino acid chain to other types of molecules including lipids and sugars, and instructions regarding the exact location the final molecule is to end up inside the cell responsible for assembly or outside the cell responsible for assembly, and instruction regarding how many molecules are to be assembled together in a specific location and whether a particular three dimensional shape is to be created by the assembly of the proteins.

The introns are responsible for creating intracellular signals that dictate assembly of tRNA molecules, rRNA molecules, nonessential amino acid molecules in order to insure that there exist the proper materials to generate the protein dictated by the mRNA molecule once the mRNA molecule migrates to the cytoplasm to be utilized as a template. Subsegments of the introns act as signals to the smooth endoplasmic reticulum to coordinate assembly of macromolecules and complex molecules.

A fully synthetic human gene will be achieved when all of the nucleotides comprising the manmade gene are coordinated together, each with a specific and known purpose. Understanding the programming language of the DNA that acts as the instruction code to oversee assembly requirements of protein construction is not that far in the future.

CHAPTER 17

SUMMATION

Background – Stopping HIV

HIV is a worldwide crisis, which gets worse as each day passes. Once infected, the virus stays with the patient for the rest of the person's life, as currently there is no cure. HIV interferes with one's immune system, making the infected individual susceptible to other common diseases, which ultimately may lead to a premature death. The problem with treating HIV is that the viral operations are carried out within the interior of the host cell and medicine does not have treatments directed at intracellular operations. A new approach is needed. This book describes such an approach.

In treating an intracellular disease, the strategy needs to take in to account the complexity of the internal operation of the cell and the differences between cell types; specifically the idiosyncrasies of the cell type targeted for treatment. HIV's virion attaches to a T-Helper cell and inserts the HIV genome into the cytoplasm of the cell. Once in the cell's cytoplasm, the HIV genome is converted from its RNA form to a DNA sequence. The HIV DNA genome is then transported into the cell's nucleus where it is inserted into the cell's native nuclear DNA. When activated, the genes in the HIV genome take over the cell's operation and dedicate cellular machinery to producing HIV virions, a process which generally results in the T-Helper cell being destroyed.

One means of inhibiting the HIV genome from being transcribed is to have a protein attach itself to a sensitive spot on the genome: a spot that will prevent the HIV genome from being transcribed. Proteins that attach themselves to the DNA are called DNA Binding Proteins. Each cell type only uses a limited number of the genes in its DNA. In some situations, cells use DNA Binding Proteins to inhibit the transcription of genes they do not use.

Our research showed that the HIV genome has a sensitive spot for the DNA Binding Protein to attach to between its TATA box and the beginning of its transcription start site. It consists of a unique set of 25 nucleotides, which we refer to as the HIV genome's ID. With the DNA Binding Protein attached there, the HIV genome cannot be transcribed.

Our research has indicated that a suitable protein to modify so that it will attach itself to the HIV genome's ID is the Transcription Factor III A DNA binding protein. The TFIIIA DNA binding sites contain 30 well-spaced amino acids, more than enough to cover the 25 nucleotides of the HIV ID. In a previous text, Volume 4 of this series, we reported on a Transcription Factor IIIA protein optimally designed to attach to the HIV ID. We refer to such a modified TFIIIA molecule as the HIV Killer Protein.

Current Work – Eradicating HIV

Our current work, as reported in this book, is to provide a means for the HIV Killer Protein to be available to silence the HIV genome should it enter the cell's cytoplasm. More directly, we designed a gene that contains the HIV Killer Protein, which is produced if the HIV genome enters the cell's cytoplasm. That is, the gene, once placed in the T-Helper cell's DNA, becomes an intracellular vaccine in that it stands guard ready to kill the HIV genome should it attack the cell.

We used a three-step process to design the gene. First, using the data from Volume 4, we show how to create the nucleotide sequence that will produce the HIV Killer Protein. Next, we show how to place that sequence into an mRNA, which could be used to carry out the production of that protein.

The next step was to design a gene to contain the DNA sequence, which when transcribed and the results processed, would produce the required mRNA. However, there is the additional requirement that the gene must undergo transcription and the killer proteins produced if HIV ever penetrated the cell's wall. Given the lack of an existing methodology with which to design genes, we sought a model for our effort. We found a suitable model in the Tumor Necrosis Factor alpha (TNF) gene that is transcribed whenever a pathogen enters the cell's cytoplasm. Thus, this step consists of configuring the current nucleotide sequence of the TNF gene into a sequence that will, when transcribed, produce a pre-mRNA that, when processed, will produce the desired mRNA.

Although this produced the gene we were seeking, two other issues came to mind. The first was on how to get the newly designed gene into the T-Helper cell's DNA, the only cells impacted by the HIV genome. The solution to this was relatively straight forward. We followed the process by which HIV itself is inserted into the T-Helper cell's DNA. One advantage of this approach is minimal side effects.

The second issue is that of the possibility that some of the patient's T-Helper cells might already be infected with HIV. There are two solutions to this. First, one might include some HIV Killer Proteins in the virion that carries the gene to the T-Helper cells. Or, one might, after the gene is inserted into the cell's DNA, trigger the transcription of the gene. Either way, we have equipped the DNA Killer Protein with a badge to allow it to enter the nucleus in case it cannot find the HIV genome in the cytoplasm.

The Next Steps

The intercellular therapies described in this book act like a platform, a springboard, from which changes to the global approach to medicine will begin to take place. Included are treatments for pathogens as well as DNA defects and desirable adjustments. The concepts are applicable to all forms of life including animal (human), the food supply including trees and plants, and those aspects which impact our environment.

An attack on pathogens would seem like a reasonable place to start given that eradicating HIV was used as the example in the book. Modifying the approach used for HIV to eradicate Ebola as well as the other four viruses described in Volume 4 would certainly improve the lives of tens of millions around the world.

A far richer set of opportunities lies in the development of means to correct or compensate for defects in the patient's DNA as well as to make adjustments to compensate for our longer lives and more active life styles. A short list of diseases that might be treated with this technology includes osteoarthritis, diabetes, cartilage wear out (like that of the knee), and at least some cancers.

Cartilage wear out is a prime example. The longer we live the more likely it is that we will end up wearing down the cartilage of our knees to the point of needing a walker, a wheelchair, or a knee replacement. The objective here is to develop a therapy that will cause the cartilage to be replenished at its current wear out rate. Challenges include the development of an improved understanding of the cartilage's replenishment command and control mechanism, and the genes that provide the proteins that support that process. For us, this is a very interesting problem and one of the focuses of our future work.

Our food supply is another area where this technology can provide considerable help. Life forms like trees and plants that support our food supply are constructed of cells with DNAs that are very much like those in our bodies. Also, like our cells, trees and plants have diseases associated with pathogens and DNA errors. Overcoming these diseases would be a big step in reducing the projected shortfall in our food supply to feed our expanding population.

As one undertakes the design of genes for different purposes and different species one becomes critically aware that the sequence of nucleotides that the gene contains to generate the protein ends with a stop codon. Confounding this is the knowledge that the sequences in some of the genes produce more than one protein. Still, each protein's sequence ends with a stop codon, but they are not all the same. In fact, there are three stop codons, some of which appear in prokaryotic cells and some in eukaryotic cell.

Given the critical importance of having the correct stop codon in each position, we under took a research effort to determine the specific functions of each stop codon. We found that each stop codon has a unique set of functions it triggers when it is read, and that the stop codons are not interchangeable. We report these findings in Addendum Two *Unique Functions of Each Stop Codon in the Genetic Code.*

ADDENDUM ONE

ANALYSIS OF NUCLEOTIDE-AMINO ACID BONDING CHARACTERISTICS

Basic Binding Processes

With the DNA target site defined, the next step is to define an amino acid sequence that will bind to it. This requires some knowledge of how the binding process works. For example, which amino acids bind to which nucleic acids and how does the binding process take place? Further, a protein is made of a string of amino acids. As it is being made, its form changes. What are the possible forms and how do they impact the possible binding capability of the resulting molecule? We will cover these aspects in the next few parts of this section. Once the basics are in place, we will be in a position to begin the design of the DNA binding molecule.

a) How do Amino Acids Bind to Nucleic Acids?

There are two main binding processes that occur between these two sets of acids: the sharing of electrons, generally referred to as hydrogen bonds, and van der Waals (a sort of mutual attraction). In the following we will have a close look at these. We start with the hydrogen bonding process and what the binding process has to work with in both the nucleic acids and the amino acids.

Nucleic Acids

Figure 47 shows the types of hydrogen bonds associated with each type of nucleic acid for both the major and minor groves of the DNA. An inward pointing arrow indicates the ability to accept an electron to be shared while an outward pointing arrow indicate the availability of an electron to be shared. Thus, for example, the oxygen atom at the 4 position in the major grove of Thymine (t) can accept an electron while the hydrogen atom in the 4 position of Cytosine (c) can provide or donate one. Table 7 shows the complete set of hydrogen bond possibilities with which the binding process has to work with. The dash symbol indicates no elements are available.

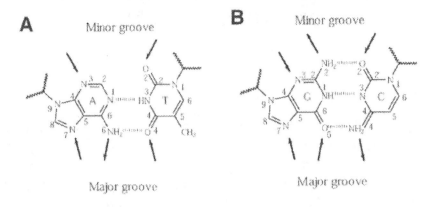

Figure 47 Electron Acceptors and Donators

Right away we can see the possibility of selectivity. That is, 'a' can both provide and accept electrons, 't' can accept one, 'c' can donate one and 'g' can accept two. In the next section we will see how these characteristics marry up with the capabilities of the amino acids.

Nucleic Acid	Accept/ Donate	Major Grove		Minor Grove	
		Number	Elements	Number	Elements
A	A	1	N	1	N
	D	1	NH_2	-	
T	A	1	O	1	O
	D	-		-	
C	A	-		1	O
	D	1	NH_2	-	
G	A	2	N & O	1	N
	D	-		1	NH_2

Table 7
Hydrogen bonding possibilities.

b) Which Amino Acids Bind to Which Nucleic Acids and other elements of the DNA?

The 20 amino acids used in the construction of proteins have a number of characteristics that a designer needs to understand. These characteristics include the number of electrons that each can accept or donate, the type of amino acid e.g., polar, the charge that is on it and its reaction to water to name a few. First, we investigate the electron sharing capability and match it to the corresponding capability of the nucleic acids.

From Appendix A, we note that Arg (R) has a strong affinity for 'g' while Asn (N) has a strong affinity for 'a'. Further, Lys (K) has an affinity for 't' and Glu (E) for 'c'. While there are other possibilities, to keep the discussion as clear as possible we will take these to be our primary amino acids, the ones that we will use in the design to bind to specific nucleic acids.

We also note that Ser (S) does not have an affinity for any of the nucleic acids, but binds very well with the DNA backbone or rail. We will use it as our spacer/stabilizing amino acid. These selections are summarized in Table 8.

Bonds To Basis		
Amino Acid	**Base**	**Bond Type**
Arg R	G	Multiple Donor
Asn N	A	Accepter + Donor
Lys K	T	Single Hydrogen Bond
Glu E	C	Single Hydrogen Bond
Bonds To Backbone		
Ser S		Van der Waals attractions generally appear to be used for stability and Serine has a large attraction for the phosphate elements in the DNA backbone[9].

Table 8
Bonds to Basis and Backbone.

[9] See for example Table 6 in Nichoias M. Luscombe, Et Al, Amino acid-base interactions: a three-dimensional analysis of protein-DNA interactions at an atomic level.

c) Basic Protein Structures

In this section we look at the configuration sequences that amino acids go through as they transitions from the manufacturing process, as a string, to a DNA binding protein configuration. We first look at the basic protein structures and then how some of those structures facilitate the binding of the amino acids they consist of to the elements of the DNA.

Proteins have many different shapes. When they are first manufactured they are just a one dimensional string of amino acids, which is called the primary structure. It is also the backbone of the protein. However, in this form it actually consists of amino acid residues as opposed to amino acids because as the amino acids are connected together a water molecule is lost at the point where the connection occurs.

As an illustration[10], let's suppose that we are going to connect an alanine amino acid to a glycine amino acid. Figure 48a and 48b show the equations for glycine and alanine, respectively, while Figure 48c shows the equation when they are connected together. As can be seen in the figures, the water molecule at the site of the connection is lost. What remains of the amino acid is called the residue and it is the string of residues that make up the backbone of the protein. Although not quite evident yet, the backbone consists of a repeating sequence of the elements **CH-C-N**. Note: C = carbon atom, H = hydrogen atom, and N = nitrogen atom. This will become important in the following.

---

[10] For a more detailed discussion see Chemguide's 'The Structure of Proteins' at http://www.chemguide.co.uk/organicprops/aminoacids/ proteinstruct.html.

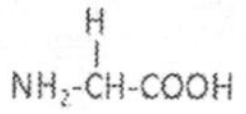

H
|
NH_2-CH-COOH

Figure 48a Glycine

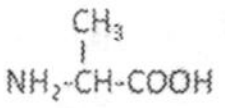

CH_3
|
NH_2-CH-COOH

Figure 48b Alanine

H CH_3
| |
NH_2-CH-COOH NH_2-CH-COOH

Amino Acid H_2O Amino Acid

→

H   H CH_3
| | |
NH_2-CH-C-N-CH-COOH
        ‖
        O

Residue   Residue

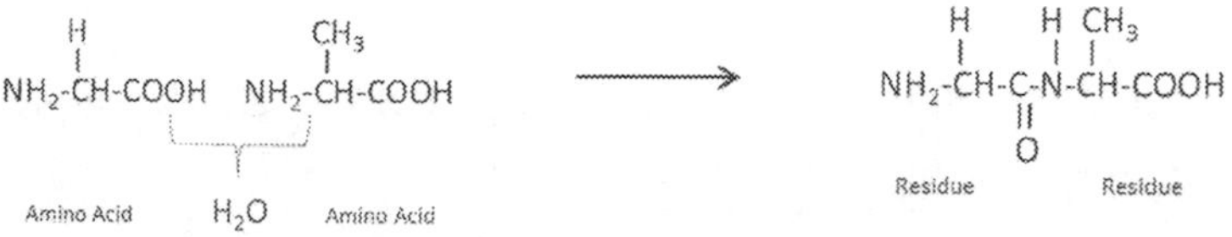

Figure 48c Glycine connected to Alanine

Figure 48 Creation of protein backbone

Although this string is indeed a molecule, it is not a functional protein. For it to become a functional protein the string must have starting and ending sequences and the entire sequence must be folded into a three-dimensional shape. Three steps are used to describe the process of folding. Level is sometimes used in place of step. Level 1 is the string as it is manufactured. Level 2 is a two-dimensional view of the first fold. Level 3 is the three-dimensional configuration.

At the second level most proteins, or parts thereof, fold into one of two shapes called alpha helix (α-helix) and beta sheet (β sheet). The α-helix form tends to fit into the major and minor grooves of the DNA, while the β sheet tends to attach to the DNA's backbone. Thus, herein we will describe the alpha helix form since we are designing a protein to bind to DNA bases as opposed to its backbone.

We will use conventional biological symbols and abbreviations. For example, when discussing the backbone we will use the letter R in place of the amino acids side chain when the makeup of the side chain has no impact on the discussion[11]. Thus, glycine would be shown as:

---

[11] The amino acid proline is an exception as in it the hydrogen on the nitrogen nearest the "R" group is missing, and the "R" group loops around and is attached to that nitrogen as well as to the carbon atom in the chain.

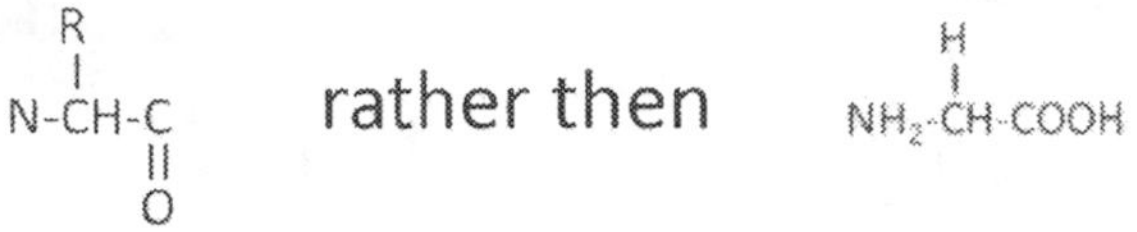

$$N-CH-C \overset{R}{\underset{\overset{\|}{O}}{|}}$$ rather then $$NH_2-\overset{H}{\underset{}{CH}}-COOH$$

Figure 49

Or for a string of residues making up a portion of a protein we might simply write what is presented as:

$$\underline{N_H\text{-}C_R\text{-}C_O}\text{-}\underline{N_H\text{-}C_R\text{-}C_O}\text{-}\underline{N_H\text{-}C_R\text{-}C_O}\text{-}\underline{N_H\text{-}C_R\text{-}C_O}\text{-}\underline{N_H\text{-}C_R\text{-}C_O}\text{-}\underline{N_H\text{-}C_R\text{-}C_O}$$

  1   2   3   4   5   6   7   8   9   10 11 12 13 14 15 16 17 18

Figure 50

Where N_H is the NH complex, C_R is the CH with the side chain attached, C_O is the Carbon with the Oxygen attached and $\underline{N_H\text{-}C_R\text{-}C_O}$ represents the residue of a single amino acid. In the literature this is often written as NCO and, from time to time when the context makes it clear, we may use that form as well.

d) The Alpha Helix Structure - Overview

In an alpha helix amino acid residue string there is a slight right hand twist at the point where one amino acid residue attaches to the next. This leads to the alpha helix having a shape like a coiled spring. The right hand twist causes the sequence of atoms to be coiled in the clockwise direction when looking in the direction of the protein build[12]. Each loop consists of exactly 11 atoms[13] – the C_R combo with the side chain attached is counted as one atom. Thus, each turn has 3 complete amino acid residues and two atoms from the next residue. That means that the residues in each turn are offset from

---

[12] That is, an α-helix is right-handed. It turns in the direction that the fingers of a right hand curl when its thumb points in the direction that the helix rises.

[13] See numbers in Figure 30.

the ones above and below by two atoms. How this fits together can be seen in Figure 51.

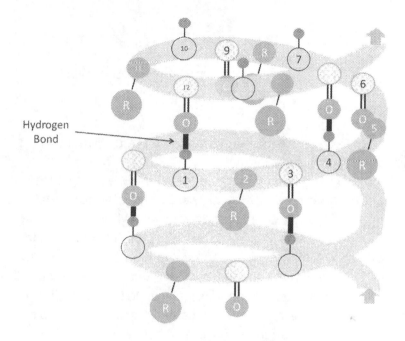

Figure 51 Alpha helix structure

This diagram shows several important features of the alpha helix structure. First, the N_H elements[14], with their hydrogen atoms pointing up, occur just before the carbon atoms to which the side chains are attached and the C_O elements, with their oxygen atoms pointing down, occur just after the carbon atoms. Since it is the hydrogen bonds between the N_H and C_O elements that hold the alpha helix in its coiled configuration, these elements need to be brought into alignment. The two extra atoms in a coil bring these elements into the proper orientation so the hydrogen bonds can take place. A solid line is used to show that the hydrogen atom in the N_H element points in the up direction. The dashed line shows that if it pointed in the down direction there could not be 11 amino acids in each coil.

---

[14] N_H elements are light gray, C_O elements are dotted with double lines to oxygen, hydrogen bonds are black, and Carbons are solid with attached side chains marked R.

The positions of N_H and C_O in the coil results in a strong hydrogen bond between them that has the nearly optimum N to O distance of 2.8 Å[15],[16].

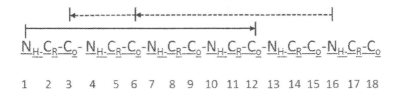

$$\underline{N}_{H}\text{-}\underline{C}_{R}\text{-}\underline{C}_{O}\text{-}\ \underline{N}_{H}\text{-}\underline{C}_{R}\text{-}\underline{C}_{O}\text{-}\underline{N}_{H}\text{-}\underline{C}_{R}\text{-}\underline{C}_{O}\text{-}\underline{N}_{H}\text{-}\underline{C}_{R}\text{-}\underline{C}_{O}\text{-}\underline{N}_{H}\text{-}\underline{C}_{R}\text{-}\underline{C}_{O}\text{-}\underline{N}_{H}\text{-}\underline{C}_{R}\text{-}\underline{C}_{O}$$

1 2 3 4 5 6 7 8 9 10 11 12 13 14 15 16 17 18

Figure 52 Hydrogen atom points in the up direction

This shows, if one looks along the left side for example, that the alignment of the atoms in the vertical direction is such that C_O is always above N_H while C_R is always below it. What this is telling us is that if a residue's side chain is pointing in a particular direction that three coils above or below it is another residue which may have its side chain pointing in the same direction. Since residues are all of the way around each coil, we need to determine the direction of each as some, it would seem, will be in a better position to bind to bases than others. Thus, the angular position of the amino acids around the coil must be considered as one of the design constraints. Further, the amino acid side chains project outward and downward from the helix thereby avoiding steric interference with the polypeptide backbone and with each other. If the side chains did not stick out away from the internal structure of the alpha helix they would not be able to bind to the nucleotides as the core of the helix is tightly packed; that is, its atoms are in van der Waals contact[17]. Why they stick out is discussed below.

In addition to the α-helix having 3.6 residues per turn, it has a pitch (the distance the helix rises along its axis per turn) of 5.4 Å. The α-helices of proteins have an average length of 12 residues, which corresponds to over three helical turns, and a height of 18 Å.

---

[15] Å = 0.1 nm

[16] See for example Proteins: Three-Dimensional Structure at http://biochem118.stanford.edu/Papers/Protein%20Papers/Voet%26Voet%20chapter6.pdf.

[17] See for example Proteins: Three-Dimensional Structure.

1. Design of a α-Helix DNA-Binding Protein

Proteins are very complex molecules. Before a molecular architect attempts to design one, the design parameters and constraints need to be well in mind. While we will introduce the major parameters, resources do not permit all of them to be covered in detail. Thus, in this section we will first cover the parameters associated with the protein and then those associated with the DNA. We include those introduced above for completeness. This will be followed by a discussion of how these two sets of parameters interact, e.g., generate constraints.

A. Design Parameters and Constraints

1) Associated with the Binding Structure of the Protein

a) Amino Acids

Amino acid characteristics which need to be considered in the design of a protein include:

- Type – Polar, charge, etc[18].

- Length of side chain.

- DNA elements to which they tend to bind.

- Types of binding – Hydrogen and van der Waals (vdW)

- Interaction with other amino acids. For example, in α-helixes the amino acid side chains project outward and downward

---

[18] To address the question as to "What causes polypeptide chains to fold into functional protein?" one notes that the amino acids in proteins can be divided into four groups: acidic, basic, polar and non-polar. Based on these classifications, the amino acids have varying affinities to bond with other amino acids. The specific tertiary structure is the result of such bonding between amino acids. For example, two polar amino acids may create hydrogen bonds, while an acid and a base may bond based on electron charges. Polar amino acids are those with side-chains that prefer to reside in a water environment. For this reason, one generally finds these amino acids exposed on the surface of a protein.

from the helix thereby avoiding space interference with the polypeptide backbone and with each other.

- Function – e.g., C and H binding to zinc ion in zinc fingers.

b) Alpha Helixes

In designing an α-helix protein characteristics that need to be taken into account including:

- Alpha helixes are right-handed; that is, they turn in the direction that the fingers of a right hand curl when its thumb points in the direction that the helix rises.

- An α-helix has 3.6 (more precisely 3.67) residues per turn and rises about 5.4 Å along its axis per turn (called pitch).

When the backbone of a protein is generated there are angles formed at the N_H-C_R and C_R-C_O junctions called torsion or dihedral angles. The magnitudes of the angles are 57.8 degrees at the N_H-C_R junction and 47.0 degrees at the C_R-C_O junction[19]. The total is 104.8 degrees which is a bit more than a quarter of a turn (90 degrees). Thus, the change in direction of the protrusions of the side chains from the α-helix, from one side chain to the next, is about 105 degrees.

2) Associated with the DNA Structure

The DNA helix can assume one of three slightly different geometries, of which the "B" form described by James D. Watson and Francis Crick is believed to predominate in cells. It is 20 Å wide and extends 34 Å per 10 bp of sequence (rises 3.4 Å from the center of one nucleic acid to the next).

The B form of the DNA helix twists 360° per 10.6 bp in the absence of strain. But many molecular biological processes can induce strain. A DNA segment with excess or insufficient helical twisting is referred to, respectively, as positively or negatively 'supercoiled'.

---

[19] See for example Figure 6-4 in Proteins: Three-Dimensional Structure.

B. Design Aspects

1) General

Aspects that might make the molecule being designed fold further than the α-helix form are intentionally avoided. For example, cysteine amino acids are not used as they make the disulfide bonds which result in molecules folding to the third level.

Certain amino acids are specified as primary because they are known to bind to nucleic acids. However, others do as well and could be used instead of those used herein.

It may not be necessary to have an amino acid attached to each and every nucleic acid. That is, having some of the primary positions (those facing the DNA) filled with non-nucleic acid binding amino acids may not matter so long as the binding attraction of the protein sequence is sufficient to cause the protein to bind permanently to the HIV binding site.

2) Twist of the DNA

In an unstressed state, the DNA twists along its central axis at the rate of one complete turn about every 10.4 nucleotides or 34.46 degrees between each nucleic acid. This is referred to as twist w[20]. As the α-helix is pulled into the major groove of the DNA by the amino acid to nucleotide attraction (binding), there may be some distortion. This distortion may occur in the DNA twist, other parts of the DNA structure, in the structure of the α-helix or in all of the above. While we make note of these possibilities, in the following analyses and design we assume that the α-helix structure remains unchanged and that the DNA twist is unchanged (w = 34.46 per nucleotide).

3) Rotational Position of the Primary Amino Acids

The α-helix fits into the major groove of the DNA. The direction of the α-helix at its closest point to the center of the major groove is taken

---

[20] The twist is in the same direction as that of an α-helix (which is right-handed). That is, it turns in the direction that the fingers of a right hand curl when its thumb points in the direction that the DNA strand rises.

to be zero degrees. To provide for the maximum potential binding between the targeted nucleic acids and the amino acids side chain direction, as measured around the α-helix, we will restrict it to ± 90 degrees which might sometimes be referred to a 0 to 90 degrees and 270 to 360 (or 0) degrees.

4) Stabilizing the Structure

Given that some of the amino acids will be beyond ± 90 degrees described above as our imposed angular condition for an amino acid to attach to a nucleic acid, one might chose amino acids for those positions that tend to bind to the rails of the DNA structure, either the sugar or the phosphate elements, which would provide stability for the binding process.

C. The Design Process

The design of a DNA binding molecule is a problem involving the simultaneous optimization of a number of parameters such as selecting the targets for the amino acids, matching the height of the amino acids with their targeted nucleosides along the DNA helix, and positioning the amino acids such that their side chains point in the direction of their intended targets. In this section we describe our approach to this multidimensional problem. From the above the nucleotides are already known as are the amino acids that we expect to bind to them.

In this initial design we will consider a single α-helix. However, if need be, it could be broken up into a number of connected α-helixes.

1) Matching the Heights

Along the DNA helix the nucleotides rise 3.4 Å from the center of one nucleic acid to the next while the amino acids in the α-helix rise at rate of 0.49 Å from one atom to the next.

As a first step we layout the protein backbone in a linear fashion. This is done by making a table listing the atoms in the backbone of the α-helix structure using the sequence NCO with the C, representing the atom with the side chain.

The list is made sufficiently long to include the expected number of amino acids in the α-helix. The heights of the atoms are added in the α-helix. In the general case, zero height is taken to be the position where the first amino acid's side chain is directly in line with the center of the first target nucleotide. However, the zero position could be defined as occurring in other places including the middle of the target sequence or at its end.

An angle is added to each atom. The angle of interest is its rotation about the zero point of the α-helix. The reason for this will become apparent later.

Using the height of the atoms, we then note on this list the height of each nucleotide along the DNA. The twist of the DNA at the position of each of the nucleotides is added. We refer to this list as the Protein Design Template an example of which is shown in Table 6.

2) Add the Names of the Nucleic Acids in the Target Sequence

Since we know the names of the nucleic acids in the target nucleotide sequence these are added to the list.

3) Identifying the Amino Acids

In a DNA binding protein the amino acid side chains have two basic purposes: bind to the target nucleotide sequence and bind to the DNA backbone to enhance stability of the attachment of the α-helix to the DNA helix. In designing an efficient layout of the α-helix structure it is necessary to position the amino acid side chains around the curve of the α-helix such that they point, as near as possible, in the direction of their intended targets. Our current guiding rule for this is that a side chain intended to bind to a selected nucleotide should not exceed ± 90 degrees from the perpendicular direction to the nucleotide and should not be above or below it by more than 1 Å.

Thus, the position of each C atom is examined in relationship to the nearest nucleotide to see if it meets the above angular and height rules. If it meets these two criteria, the appropriate binding amino acid for the nucleotide is entered from Table 7. If it does not, we enter the stability amino acid from the table. Table 9 is used to show the results of the analysis.

Atom No	Atom Sym	Residual Side Chain	Coil Number	Side Chain Angle Deg	Residual Atom Height in Å	Amino Acid	Nucleotide Height in Å	DNA Twist ω	Nucleo-tide Name
1	N		1	-35					
2	C	1		0	0		1 @ 0	0	
3	O			35	0.49				
4	N			70	0.98				
5	C	2		105	1.47				
6	O			140	1.96				
7	N			175	2.45				
8	C	3		210	2.94				
9	O			245	3.43		2 @ 3.4	34.46	
10	N			280	3.92				
11	C	4		315	4.41				
12	O		2	350	4.9				
13	N			25	5.39				
14	C	5		60	5.88				
15	O			95	6.37				
16	N			130	6.86		3 @ 6.8	68.92	
17	C	6		165	7.35				
18	O			200	7.84				

Table 9
Example of a Protein Design Template.

The first nucleotide is noted in the target sequence is A (adenine). Since there is an amino acid with a side chain angle of zero and it is at the same height as the nucleotide[21], there is a binding opportunity. From Table 8 we see that Asn is the amino acid that we have selected to bind to A. We enter Asn into our results table for the amino acid. We also color that row light gray to provide an indication as to where binding strategies have been setup.

The C atom is investigated for the second amino acid and it is found to fail the height test for the second (G) nucleotides: 1.47 Å vs. 3.4 Å for G. We enter the stabilizing amino acid (Ser S) from Table 8 in its cell in the amino acid column. We also mark its row with dots, to indicate that the amino acid provides stabilization, and its cell in the Residual Atom Height column we make dark gray with white letters

---

[21] Both deltas are zero since we selected this as our starting condition. Each of the remainder alignments we will have to check.

to indicate height is the reason it is not binding to a nucleotide. Since it would meet the angle test for G (105 vs. 34.64 for a delta of 70.36 degrees) we leave the marking of its Side Change Angle cell unchanged.

The third amino acid's side chain is more than 90 degrees displaced from the second nucleotide (210 vs. 34.64 degrees). It is treated the same as the second amino acid with the exception that we mark its Side Chain Angle cell to indicate that it fails the angle requirement. Its height is within 1 Å of the G nucleotide so we leave its height cell unchanged.

Atom No	Atom Sym	Residual Side Chain	Coil Number	Side Chain Angle Deg	Residual Atom Height in Å	Amino Acid	Nucleotide Height in Å	DNA Twist ω	Nucleo- tide Name
1	N		1	-35					
2	C	1		0	0	ASN N	1@0	0	A
3	O			35	0.49				
4	N			70	0.98				
5	C	2		105	1.47	Ser S			
6	O			140	1.96				
7	N			175	2.45				
8	C	3		210	2.94	Ser S			
9	O			245	3.43		2@3.4	34.64	G
10	N			280	3.92				
11	C	4		315	4.41	ARG R	ΔH = 1Å	Δω=79.64	
12	O		2	350	4.9				
13	N			25	5.39				
14	C	5		60	5.88	GLU E	ΔH = 1Å	Δω=9.28	
15	O			95	6.37				
16	N			130	6.86		3@6.8	69.28	C
17	C	6		165	7.35	Ser S			
18	O			200	7.84				

Table 10
Initial Portion of the Design of a DNA Binding
Molecule for HIV Killer Protein.

The fourth amino acid meets both the height and the angle conditions, ΔH = 1Å and Δω = 79.64 degrees respectively. From Table 10 we see that Arg binds to G. We enter it into our results table along with the delta values and then color the appropriate cells gray.

The remaining amino acid/nucleotide/stability combinations for our DNA binding molecule are established in the same manor. The binding molecule has 57 amino acids. The alignment of the amino acids with the nucleotides they are designed to bind to is shown below. The small letters in the figure indicate nucleotides to which the molecule is unable to bind.

```
N S S R E S S N S S R E S S K S S R S S E K S S K S S K
a     g c     a     g c     t     g     c t     t     t

K S K S S R S E S E S S K S R S K S S N S E S K S S R R
t   t     g   c   c     t   g   t     a   c   t     g g
```

DNA binding molecule

4) Observations on the Design of the HIV Binding Molecule

An examination of the data shown above for the HIV binding molecule provides the following points about the design:

- 56 amino acids are needed to cover the nucleotide sequence of about 82 Å.

- Amino acids are positioned to bind with 21 of the 25 nucleotides.

- Of the 4 nucleotides which are not bound to amino acids none are adjacent.

- 35 of the amino acids bind to the DNA backbone.

We might get a somewhat different amino acid sequence if we chose a different amino acid/nucleotide combination as the starting point. In fact, we might be able to select a starting point that provides an optimum amino acid sequence. One approach is to use the center of the amino acid binding sequence and the center of the DNA binding target as the starting point. We call this technique 'Centering'.

5) Examination of Variations of the Design Parameter Constraints

As part of this engineering analysis, one always examines variations in the design parameters used to determine their impact on the results. Here we report two results.

- First we look at increasing the Height Limit of 1 Å.

  - Three additional amino acids would bind with their target nucleotides if the vertical distance limit was raise from 1 to 1.5 Å.
  - Increasing it 2 Å permits all of the amino acids to reach a nucleotide.

- Next we examine to see if there is an advantage of the protein binding to the DNA before or after the current design position. Since there are only three amino acids per residue in the proteins backbone, we look one amino acid (0.5 Ås) in each direction.

  The data derived in the analysis indicates that there is no significant difference among the three positions.

6) Multi Section Options for Alpha Helix Approach

There may be situations where a large binding section (for example, 56 amino acids in the discussion above) exceeds the physical limits of DNA binding protein to DNA binding site process. To accommodate these limitations, we describe several alternatives to the single alpha helix design. We refer to them as Sectioning, Sectioning with Centering, Sectioning with Gaps, and Sectioning with Change of Direction.

a) Sectioning

   Sectioning simply refers to breaking the string of amino acids constituting a single alpha helix into a set of amino acids, each constituting an alpha helix of its own. For example, one might want to use a zinc finger approach and spread the binding molecule across several of its fingers.

b) Sectioning with Centering

   Sectioning an alpha helix binding molecule provides the potential to slightly modify its binding arrangements, especially in the sequence of the amino acids. One way to do this is to treat each section as a separate alpha helix and use centering as described above.

c) Sectioning with Gaps

Sectioning an alpha helix binding molecule provides the potential to alter the sequence of nucleotides that are bound to. For example, if the binding becomes constrained by insufficient space, the space between fingers could be used to inject gaps. That is, by adjusting the number of binding amino acids placed in each finger and the positions within the fingers as to where the binding starts and ends.

d) Sectioning with Change of Direction

Sectioning an alpha helix binding molecule provides the potential to reverse the sequence of nucleotides that are intended to bind to a specific DNA binding site. This might occur, for example, if the binding becomes constrained by insufficient space for the linking molecules. One solution is to turn one or more of the sections around to give the linkers more room. If a section is intended to be turned around, then its sequence might have to be reversed.

e) Combinations of the above

Most of the above can be used in combination to optimize the intended binding.

2. Designing the HIV Killer Protein – Level 1

Having a molecule that can bind to a particular nucleotide sequence is necessary but insufficient in the development of our protein to kill HIV. Once the molecule gets into the cell's cytoplasm it must be able to get into the nucleus so that it can get to the HIV's genome. That is, it needs a transport mechanism that is acceptable to the cell, otherwise the cell may just disassemble it and reuse the amino acids elsewhere. This transport mechanism is referred to as the Intracellular Transporter.

This transporter must have several aspects to carry out its mission. First, it must appear to the cell to belong in the cell. Second, it must have the characteristic of a molecule that the cell normally transports to its nucleus. Third, it must be able to carry the binding molecule in such a way that the binding molecule's amino acids can locate and attach to the intended nucleotides. Finally, the transporter must in itself support the mission of stopping the transcription of the HIV genome.

Other aspects of the overall design mentioned in the Approach include the intercellular transporter and the manufacturing process. The intercellular transporter is the mechanism that transports the killer protein from the outside world to the cytoplasm of the cell. That is, it is available in some form like a pill or injectable fluid such that it can be placed in the body in such a way that it enters the blood stream and that the blood stream carries it to the intended cell type, the T-Helper cell. Once finding a T-Helper cell, the transporter must attach to it in such a way that the killer protein it is carrying is injected into the cytoplasm of the cell.

The design must also consider how the killer protein and its transporters are to be manufactured. Generally, one would consider each of the steps necessary in the manufacturing process. For example:

- The building the killer protein with the binding molecule

- The building of the transporter

    - Including the killer protein in the transporter
    - Affixing the appropriate molecules to the surface of the transporter which will allow the transporter to insert the protein into the cell

Summary of Amino Acid Characteristics and Bindings to Nucleic Acids

In designing a protein, one selects the amino acids that make up the protein to cause the protein to carry out specific tasks. The specific task at hand is to design a specific area of a protein to bind to a specific area of the DNA which is defined by a specific nucleotide sequence. The DNA is made up of nucleic acids. Thus, as a first step, we examine the binding of amino acids to nucleic acids of which there are, in general, three types; hydrogen bonds, van der Waals contacts and water-mediated bonds. We note that in the design of a protein, at least those associated with binding, to prevent transcription the objective is to select the amino acids which make strong bonds with specific nucleic acids. Thus, van der Waals contacts and water-mediated bonds, both of which are generally not specific in their bindings, are of less interest than hydrogen bonds. That is, hydrogen bonds are much stronger that either van der Waals contacts or water-mediated bonds. Thus, in the following we shall emphases hydrogen bonds[22].

From the literature, points that might be worth keep in mind from a 'trying to understand the bonding process' point of view include:

- Greater specificity is more likely to occur in major groove than minor.

- Protein-DNA interactions are at the atomic level.

- Some amino acids can bind using multiple donor or accepter plus donor configurations. Amino acids binding with two sites show more specificity for specific bases.

- Single hydrogen bonds are usually not indicators of specificity, more in the role of stabilization of the structure.

---

[22] For more on this see for example Nicholas M. Luscombe, Et Al, Amino acid-base interactions: a three-dimensional analysis of protein-DNA interactions at an atomic level.

- On protein side, polar and charged residues play a central role in hydrogen bonds.

- Arginine and lysine hydrogen bonding strongly favor guanine while hydrogen bonds of asparagine and glutamine favor adenine.

- Where hydrogen bonds are considered, amino acids with short side chains, like serine and threonine, have limited access to bases and therefore generally contribute to stability rather than specificity.

- Cys, Met & Trp have no base contact.

- Some amino acids such as A, C, F, I, L, M and V are hydrophobic and tend to move away from water. Others like E, G, H, K, N, Q, R, S and T are hydrophilic and tend to move toward water. Others are neutral about water. In developing a protein that binds to the DNA one observers that the side chains of the hydrophobic amino acids tend to force their way inside the three dimensional protein which is fine for developing the correct structure, but of no value in actually binding to the DNA. The side chains of the amino acids that are used to bind to the DNA need to stick out of the protein. Thus, they need to be hydrophilic or at least neutral.

Hydrogen bonds result when a hydrogen atom shares electrons with another atom, usually nitrogen or oxygen. The acid containing the hydrogen atom is referred to as the donor and the molecule it bonds to is referred to as the acceptor.

Examining the data in the literature[23] we see the following:

- Amino Acids

  - Only Asn, Gln and His have both acceptors and donors
  - Arg, Lys, Ser, Thr and Tyr only have donors
  - Glu and Asp have only acceptors
  - None of the rest have acceptors or donors

---

[23] See for example Luscombe.

- Nucleic Acids

  - Adenine has both a donor and an acceptor
  - Cytosine only has an donor
  - Guanine has two acceptors and no donors
  - Thymine has only an acceptor

Next we make the following selections of amino acids to bind to specific nucleic acids.

- Asn (N) will be used to bind to Adenine (a)

  - Gln (Q) is one link longer than Asn and the literature indicates it does not bind to Adenine as well as Asn. It is a possible alternative.
  - His (H) is one of the atoms that create the zinc fingers. Thus, we hesitate to use it in case fingers become involved even though nature does to some degree.

- Glu (E) will be used to bind to Cytosine (c)

  - No nucleotides have two donors that can bind to Glu's two acceptors. Further, no normal paring of nucleotides (a-t or g-c) have major grove donors that can bind to these acceptors.
  - Asp (D) seems similar to but shorter than Glu, but maybe an alternate.

- Arg (R) will be used to bind to Guanine (g)

  - Only amino acid with two donors to bind to G's two acceptors.

- Lys (K) will be used to bind to Thymine (t)

  - Thr (T) has shorter side chain, seems to bind well with rails.
  - Tyr (Y) has complex side chain.

- Ser (S) will be used in positions on the backside of the alpha helix to add stability

  - It has short side chains.
  - The literature indicates it attaches very well to the rails.
  - Thr (T) is similar, but with more baggage – 2nd CH_3.

These selections and additional information on the other amino acids is provided in Table 11.

Nucleic Acids →				Adenine		Thymine		Guanine			Cytosine	
Donate/Accept →				A	D	A	D	A_1	A_2	D	A	D
Amino Acid		Donate/ Accept		N	NH_2	O	-	N	O	-	-	NH_2
N	Asn	D	NH_2	x								
		A	O		X							
K	Lys	D	NH_3^+			X						
		A	-									
R	Arg	D_1	NH_2^+					X				
		D_2	NH_2						x			
		A	-									
E	Glu	D	-									
		A	O	No nucleotides have two donors that can bind to Glu's two acceptors. But it seems to bind well to cytosine.								X
		A	O⁻									
S	Ser	D	OH	Short side chain (2 elements). Binds well with DNA rails.								
		A	-									
T	Thr	D	OH	Short side chain (2 elements). Binds well with DNA rails. Seems equivalent to Ser, but has second CH_3. Possible alternative.								
		A	-									
Q	Gln	D	NH_2	One link longer than Asn. Reference 12 indicates it does not bind to A as well as Asn. Possible alternative.								
		A	O									
Y	Tyr	D	OH	The hydrogen it has available for bonding is off its 6 carbon molecule, a more difficult side chain to work with.								
		A	-									

D	Asp	D	-	Similar to Glu. Note that no nucleotides have two donors that can bind to Asp's two acceptors. Further, no normal paring of nucleotides (A-T or G-C) have major grove donors that can bind to these acceptors.
		A_1	O	
		A_2	O⁻	
H	His	D	NH⁺	Second part of Zinc connecter.
		A	NH	
P	Pro	D	-	Nonpolar side chains. No As or Ds to share.
		A	-	
L	Leu	D	-	Nonpolar side chains. No As or Ds to share.
		A	-	
M	Met	D	-	Nonpolar side chains. No As or Ds to share.
		A	-	
V	Val	D	-	Nonpolar side chains. No As or Ds to share.
		A	-	
I	Ile	D	-	Nonpolar side chains. No As or Ds to share.
		A	-	
C	Cys	D	-	Nonpolar side chains. No As or Ds to share.
		A	-	
W	Trp	D	-	Nonpolar side chains. No As or Ds to share.
		A	-	
F	Phe	D	-	Nonpolar side chains. No As or Ds to share.
		A	-	
G	Gly	D	-	Nonpolar side chains. No As or Ds to share.
		A	-	
A	Ala	D	-	Nonpolar side chains. No As or Ds to share.
		A	-	

Table 11

Rational for Selecting Amino Acids to Bind
to Nucleotides and DNA Rails.

UNIQUE FUNCTIONS OF EACH STOP CODON IN THE GENETIC CODE

Summary

The fact that the genetic code contains three stop codons, but only one start codon has troubled researchers ever since the code was uncovered. Many seem to proceed as if there is no difference in their functions. However, the results of this study, which examined stop codon usage in prokaryotic, eukaryotic and viral genomes, indicate that each stop codon, in addition to its command to release the emerging protein, has one or more additional functions that are both necessary and unique. Thus, the stop codons are not interchangeable.

Briefly, the functions of the stop codons are:

The UGA stop codon specifies that the ribosome reader is to release the emerging protein and disassemble. It is used to specify the end of the code for the last, or only, protein in the mRNA. It does not specify any alteration to the mRNA's 3' end. It is used in prokaryotic and viral genomes.

The UAA stop codon specifies that the ribosome reader is to release the emerging protein and then continue reading the mRNA's code and look for another start codon. UAA is used in mRNAs in all three domains which contain code for multiple proteins in sequential order. It is used to specify the end of each protein's code, except the last.

The UAG stop codon specifies that the ribosome reader is to release the emerging protein and disassemble. The ribosome reader is also to cause a portion of the Poly(A) tail attached to the mRNA is to be removed. This codon is used in the human genome, and perhaps other genomes in eukaryotic cells, to specify the end of the code for the last, or only, protein in the mRNA.

Prokaryotic and eukaryotic cells use different means of controlling the lifespans of their mRNAs. In prokaryotic cells a Poly(A) tail is attached to an mRNA to order its destruction. In eukaryotic cells it is used to keep track of the number of times the mRNA has been read. The UGA stop codon does not specify any alteration to the mRNA's 3' end which is what is needed in prokaryotic cells. However, eukaryotic cells require that an action to the Poly(A) tail be specified which is what the UAG stop codon requires.

Discussion

The Genetic Code identifies the codons used by the ribosome readers to translate the RNA code in the mRNAs into proteins. It has been a point of interest as to why nature needs three stop codons, but only one start codon. In this study we begin to address that question. Our hypothesis is that nature would only have multiple stop codons if each had a different function.

As one attempts to understand the intent of different sequences of DNA and RNA code one is faced with trying to understand what the creator of the sequence had in mind. Further, when one attempts to create a sequence for a specific purpose, like an mRNA to produce a particular protein, one is also placing nucleotides into the sequence at precise locations to instruct the reader, as well as other molecules, to carry out specific functions in a defined order. Thus, in examining or creating a sequence the reader's response to each nucleotide or set of nucleotides must be precisely known; in examining the sequence to determine the reason it was used in a specific position, and in creating a sequence to ensure that the desired functions are carried out at each specific position. That is, each nucleotide or set of nucleotides in a sequence represents a command or set of commands to the reader and, in some situations, other molecules. With that in mind it is easy to see that sequences of nucleotides can be viewed as a machine language, base-4, digital computer program, or parts thereof, including subroutines.

Material

For this study we selected genes from genomes in all three domains: Prokaryotes cells, Eukaryotes cells and Viruses. To be sure we are clear on the stop codon usage, we take our data from the DNA portions of the genes and genomes to be analyzed. By doing this we can show the exact locations of the start and stop codons as they appear in the genes and genomes themselves. However, in doing the analysis, one must remember that in the 'U' in the RNA form of the Genetic Code is replaced by a 'T' in the DNA form[24].

For the Prokaryotes cells we used the E. coli genome. In this genome we selected the lactose operon in the NCBI GenBank, reference number J01636.1, which can be found at http://www.ncbi.nlm.nih. gov/nuccore/146575.

For the eukaryotes cells we used a random assortment of genes from the homo sapiens genome in the NCBI database[25].

For viruses we used the HIV genome we cited in Volume III of the series Changing the Global Approach to Medicine, NCBI K03455.1, which can be found at http://www.ncbi.nlm.nih.gov/nuccore/k03455.1 .

---

[24] Both the DNA and RNA forms are given where it would seem to be helpful.
[25] The specific reference for each gene selected is shown in the text.

Analyses[26]

1. Lactose Operon

The lactose operon genes are translated in two parts: LacI is translated alone while LacZ, LacY and LacA are translated as a sequential group. We start our analyses by extracting the information shown in Figure 53 for the four genes of the operon from the DNA portion of the lactose operon data in GenBank reference j01636.1. Section A contains the information for the LacI gene and Section B the information for the three sequential genes. The small arrows and dots represent reader continuation. Dots without an arrow indicate code continuation which is not read. The numbers given are the DNA locations, in the GenBank reference, of the nucleotides to which the arrow points.

The code for the LacI gene starts at position 79[27] and ends at position 1161. Proceeding from the start codon in positions 79-81 one finds the first stop codon, the TGA (UGA), in positions 1159-61. That stop codon instructs the ribosome reader to end the emerging protein and to disassemble since there are no more proteins to be translated in this reading.

The code for the for the LacZ, LacY and LacA proteins is contained in positions 1284 to 6356. Proceeding from the start codon in positions 1284-86 one finds the first stop codon in positions 4356-58. However, it is not a TGA (UGA). That stop codon would cause the reader to disassemble which would prevent the remaining protein code from being translated. Here the TAA (UAA) stop codon is

---

[26] In this study the DNA is viewed as a base 4, machine language digital computer program. Genes are sbroutines. The mRNAs are transformed snippets of that code. The codons shown in the Genetic Code are viewed as commands for RNA ribosome, the biological complex that reads the mRNA code. That is, the Genetic Code is the operational code (opcode) for the mRNA processor. The readers of the DNA use a different processor or processors, which has or have a different opcode or set of opcodes.

[27] NCBI reference specifies lac repressor protein, LacI, uses a GTG start codon.

used. This stop codon instructs the ribosome reader to end the emerging protein and continue to the next start codon, which it finds in positions 4410-12, and which happens to be the start codon for the LacY protein.

The same is true at the end of the code for the translation of the LacY protein except the next start codon is for the LacA protein.

The same TAA (UAA) stop codon appears at the end of the LacA protein code. However, six codons later a TGA (UGA) stop codon is found which instructs the reader to disassemble. This arrangement is actually expected in an evolutionary environment where code is reused without change. For example, programmers often use a subroutine for a number of purposes rather than writing a number of subroutines. They put code in the calling routines to adjust the output of the subroutine to fit the specific purpose of the part of the program that is calling the subroutine. Here, Nature simply added an instruction for the reader to disassemble rather than change the last TAA (UAA) stop codon. In any event, it is clear that two different procedures are required and the two stop codons provide for those procedures. It is also clear that these two stop codons are not interchangeable.

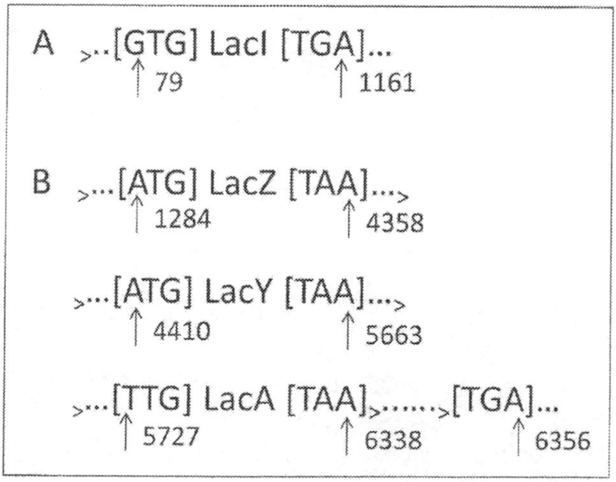

A >..[GTG] LacI [TGA]...
       ↑ 79   ↑ 1161

B >...[ATG] LacZ [TAA]...>
        ↑ 1284   ↑ 4358

   >...[ATG] LacY [TAA]...>
       ↑ 4410   ↑ 5663

   >...[TTG] LacA [TAA]>.......>[TGA]...
       ↑ 5727   ↑ 6338   ↑ 6356

Figure 53 Layout of Lactose Operon Genes

2. Homo Sapiens

The genes investigated in the Homo sapiens' genome are shown in Figure 54. They were not selected for any specific reason, except that they seem to be unrelated. It is noted that all three of the genes are monocistronic in that their mRNAs each produce a single protein. This is not to exclude polycistronic genes which occur in eukaryotic cells, which be dealt with later, but to concentrate on a new stop codon requirement which has been brought about by the emergence of the nucleus in the cell.

Figure 53 shows the start and stop codons for the genes presented in this section. It also shows the locations[28] of those start and stop codons as found in their DNA[29],[30],[31]. It is noted that each of the genes starts with the normal start codon. On the other hand they don't end with either of the stop codons shown in Figure 53, but end with the third stop codon TAG (UAG)[32]. Let us examine why.

---

[28] Using the locations specified by the Coding Sequence (CDS) where available.

[29] INS (Insulin): from NCBI sequence NC_000011.10 at http://www.ncbi. nlm.nih.gov/nuccore/nc_000011.10

[30] OCA2 (Eye Color): from NCBI sequence NM_000275.2 at http://www. ncbi.nlm.nih.gov/nuccore/NM_000275.2

[31] CYGB (Cytoglobin aka HGB): from NCBI sequence NC_000017.11 at http://www.ncbi.nlm.nih.gov/nuccore/nc_000017.11

[32] The stop codon in the NCBI reference is a TAA at locations 2625-27. The next codon at 2628-30 is the TAG stop codon. This is the same code reuse observation discussed with the lactose operon above.

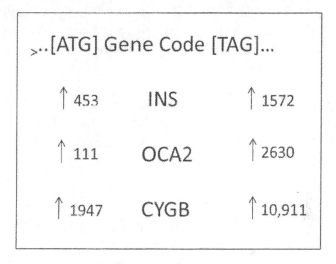

> ...[ATG] Gene Code [TAG]...

↑ 453	INS	↑ 1572
↑ 111	OCA2	↑ 2630
↑ 1947	CYGB	↑ 10,911

Figure 54 Examples of Homo Sapiens Genes

In prokaryotic cells there is a close relationship between the reading of the gene's code in the DNA and the translation of the code in the resulting mRNA which produces the protein. They are done together in the cell's cytoplasm. As eukaryotic cells emerged with their DNAs, as well as the operations done on them, in the nucleus, and their mRNA translations done separately in the cytoplasm, Nature added a Poly(A) tail to the mRNAs to provide an indication of wear out, i.e., the number of times the mRNA has been read. To facilitate this, Nature added a means to reduce the number of <u>adenine</u> acids in the tail each time the mRNA is read (Beelman, Tourriere). To help prevent an mRNA from being used past its projected useful life, Nature also add poly(A) ribonuclease (PARN) to initiate destruction of an mRNA when its Poly(A) tail reaches a specified minimum length.

But what can provide the signal to shorten the tail? The stop codon that ends the reading of the code for the last protein in the mRNA is an obvious choice. That lets out the TSS (USS) codon. The TGA (UGA) codon has potential, but would need to be modified to add the signal. Such a modification might have been deemed to cause confusion or harm in the case of mRNAs which don't use Poly(A) tails in this manner. In any event, it seems that Nature gave this task to the stop codon TAG (UAG). That is, the TAG (UAG) stop codon instructs the reader to end the emerging protein, provide a signal to remove a specific number of <u>adenine</u> acids from the mRNA's Poly(A) tail, and to disassemble.

This is not to claim that eukaryotic cells do not use the TGA stop codon as they do[33]. How the eukaryotic cells keep track of the usage of the mRNAs which utilize the TGA stop codons is beyond the scope of this report.

3. HIV

When one looks at the gene map of the HIV genome like the one shown in the Landmarks of the HIV-1 Genome, HXB2 strain[34], shown here in Figure 55, one gets the feeling that Nature just jumbled the genes together into a genome. The fact that some genes overlap others and some have parts at distant locations gives rise to the feeling that showing a consistent use of stop codons might be very difficult in this case. However, that is not true. In fact, it turns out to be very interesting.

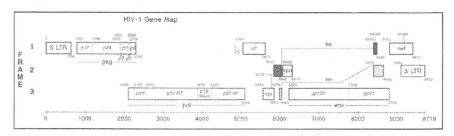

Figure 55 Gene Map for HIV-1 HXB2 Strain

Using material derived in the addendum, *Identifying the mRNAs in the HXB2 Strain of HIV-1*, which describes the seven mRNAs the T-Helper cells use to produce the HIV-1 proteins in the HXB2 strain, we extract the information shown in Figures 56 and 57.

---

[33] See, for example, the Homo Sapiens ACTN3 gene at NCBI reference sequence NM_001104.

[34] Landmarks of the HIV-1 genome, HXB2 strain which can be found at http://www.hiv.lanl.gov/content/sequence/HIV/MAP/landmark.html

Figure 56 shows that all seven of the mRNA start with the 'g' in position 456 and end with the 'a' in position 9719. That is, they all have the same initial set of code and the same tail. All but the first mRNA undergo significant splicing. For mRNAs two through seven, the initial set of code ends at the 'g' nucleotide in position 743. The code spliced out varies with the protein to be translated. Tat and Rev undergo additional splicing. The translation of Nef follows that of Env in mRNA 7.

```
1a  g--------------- Gag Group ------------------------------------------------------------a
1b  g----------------------------------------- Pol Group -----------------------------------a

2   g--------g    Spliced Out      ----------------- Vif -----------------------------------a

3   g--------g    Spliced Out          ----------------- Vpr --------------------------------a

4   g--------g    Spliced Out             --------------- Tat 1 ------- Tat2 --------------a

5   g--------g    Spliced Out                 -------------- Rev1 ------- Rev2 ---------a

6   g--------g    Spliced Out                     ---------------- Vpu -------------------a

7   g--------g    Spliced Out                         --------------- Env -------Nef----a
    ↑456  ↑743                    |<  Various  >|                          9719↑
```

Figure 56 Overview of HIV-1 HXB2 mRNAs

Figure 57 shows the stop codons used to end the translation of each of the genes along with their locations. Also shown for the mRNAs that have undergone splicing are the locations where the code is reattached to enable translation of each protein along with its start codon and the location of the start codon.

Figure 58 shows the data for the first mRNA. There are two possibilities in the translation of the code in the first mRNA depending on the location at which the reading begins. One position resulting in the translation of the gag group of genes and the other in the translation of the pol group of genes. As indicated in the figure, there are no stop codons internal to the gag complex of genes. This is also true of the pol group.

The gag group ends with a TAA (UAA) stop codon at 2292 with a TAG (UAG) following one codon later. This is the same code reuse observation discussed with the lactose operon above.

The translation of the pol group ends in a TAG (UAG) codon at 5096.

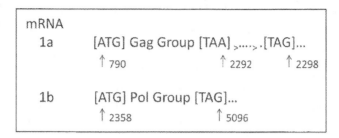

Figure 57 Data for mRNA 1

Figure 58 shows the data for mRNAs two through six. These mRNAs each contain code for a single protein as indicated. They all end with the UAG (TAG) stop codon. Tat and Rev are both further spliced as shown.

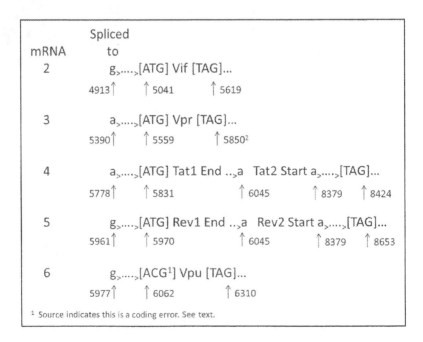

Figure 58 Data for mRNAs 2 through 6

Figure 59 shows the processing of the Env and Nef proteins. What is interesting here is that the Env code ends with a TAA (UAA) stop codon at 8795 which, according to our observations above, instructs the reader to end the emerging protein and continue to the next start codon. The next start codon is located two nucleotides later at 8797. It is the start codon for the Nef protein. The code for the Nef protein ends with a TGA stop codon at 9417.

Why a TGA stop codon? A better question might be - Why does Nature bother to use TAG stop codons in a virus that is probably going the kill the host cell before the mRNAs wear out? Both questions are beyond the scope of this effort.

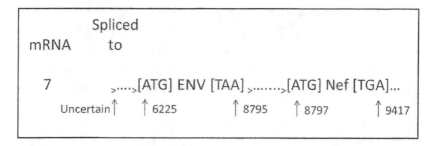

Figure 59 Data for mRNA 7

Observations and Rational

Although admittedly the size of our data set is as yet small, it contains some interesting points. Let's look at them.

Observation 1: The TAA stop codon.

Rational: The TAA command has two parts. It directs the processor to end the current protein and read on to the next Start codon. It appears in all three domains.

Observation 2: While a stop codon is needed to direct the processor to disassemble after ending the last protein in the mRNA, there exist two additional stop codons.

Rational 2: This is a two part rational:

1. There is another task that the processor needs to do in eukaryotic cells. The mRNA is a template and it has a predicted lifetime. That is, as the mRNA is read there needs to be an accounting of its use so that it is not used beyond its predicted lifetime which might results in the production of error filled proteins. Nature is well aware of this lifetime. The question is 'How does Nature ensure that the mRNAs are not used beyond their lifetimes? 'There are two ways to do this, one based on time and a second based on actual usage.

The literature does not contain information on a time-stamp being placed on mRNAs when they are created, but it does provide information on a potential usage strategy. That is, when mRNAs are created in eukaryotic cells, a Poly-A tail (Tourriere) is attached to its 3' end. Poyaderation places a sequence of 250 adenine nucleic acids (As) at a location at the 3' end (Wahle). These acids are removed by a deadenylation process do to some signal (Hoshino). As the mRNA is used the Poly(A) tail is shortened. When the tail becomes shorter than a specific length, it becomes a signal that specifies that the mRNA must be destroyed.

What provides the signal telling the deadenylation process to trim the mRNA's tail? The only entity that knows a reading of the mRNA has been made is the ribosome reader. Thus, it seems that the stop command used in the eukaryotic cells, the TAG (UAG), provides that signal. That is, when a TAG codon is reached by the ribosome reader, the codon is interpreted by the reader to provide, in addition to instructions to end the protein and disassemble, a third instruction. This third instruction is to provide a signal to a specific molecule, or set of molecules, to reduce the mRNA's Poly(A) tail by one or more As. This also appears to be a necessary step in the cellular command and control process.

2. In prokaryotic cells the Poly(A) tail is attached to mRNAs for a different reason. It is a signal to destroy the mRNA. Thus, while the TGA stop codon might be made to work in eukaryotic type of cells, it seems more appropriate to

use a different codon to prevent having to always check to ensure that the instructions are still appropriate every time changes are made to the DNA code. Thus, the use of the stop codon TAG.

Other Observations

The material for this study was specifically selected from three different entities with nothing in common, but the fact that all have DNA and molecules derived from them, and that all use the same nucleic and amino acids. It is striking that all entities operate the same at least as far as the currently available data permitted the study to go. Additional results, for or against the hypothesis, will be provided as new data becomes available.

The TAA followed by the TGA or TAG seems consistent with reusing code - inserting code from an outside source without change. In this case, not changing code that works, but putting a hard stop after the code to force the ribosome reader to disassemble.

It is interesting to look at the problem from two different ends: from an observer's point of view and from a needs point of view. An observer discovers three stop codons and sees three operations. Nature, looking at the requirements, sees three sets of functions and creates three stop codons.

References

Beelman, C., et al., Degradation of mRNA in eukaryotes, Cell, 4-21-1995.

Hoshino, S., et al., the Eukaryotic Polypepide Chain Releasing Factor (eRF3/GSPT) Carrying the Translation termination Signal to the 3'-Poly(A) Tail of mRNA. Direct Association of eRF3/GSPT With POLYADENYLATE-Binding Protein, J Bio Chem, 274, 16677-16680, 1999.

Tourriere, H., et al., mRNA degradation machines in eukaryotic cells, Biochimie, 2002.

Wahle, E., Poly(A) Tail Length control Is Caused by Termination of Processive Synthesis, Journal of Biological Chemistry, 1995.

POST SCRIPT 1

DECIPHERING THE CODON CODE
(Protein Building Instructions)

One of the most intriguing mysteries of molecular biology is the fact that there exist sixty-four codons used to identify twenty amino acids, and the three STOP codons. Given there are 20 differing recognized amino acids, a cursory view of the subject would suggest there should be only 23 differing codons with twenty codons coding for the 20 amino acids and three STOP codons. Therefore, 41 of the 64 codons should be nonfunctional. Nature tends to contrive systems that conserve energy requirements to produce the most efficient processes. Redundancy tends to occur only when there is a clear advantage to survivability of the life form that has been created. The most efficient approach to labeling the amino acids would have been to assign only one codon to identify one specific amino acid. Such an approach would have created the most precise means of identifying to the cell machinery the code to generate proteins by stringing together amino acid molecules. Excluding the three STOP codons, there are 61 differing codons that are used to identify the 21 amino acids. There exist three STOP codons due to each STOP codon represents a different STOP function when read by the ribosomes.

The key point in deciphering the reason behind why 64 codon codes exist rather than 23 codon codes directs attention to how the amino acid molecules are attached to a fledgling protein. The purpose of the codon code may be in identifying the spacial position of the amino acid as the amino acid is bonded to the protein molecule's amino acid chain.

Observation of how proteins are created as three-dimensional objects, that the functionality of many proteins are dependent of the spacial orientation of the amino acids comprising the protein. Many protein-protein interactions function as a lock-and-key mechanism. Lock-and-key protein interactions refer to one protein inserting a specific portion of the molecule into the binding site of a second protein. The inserting of a portion of one protein molecule into another protein molecule acts to (1) bond the two proteins together or (2) in the case of receptors or enzymes, causes a physical action or a chemical reaction to take place. The specifics of the three dimensional design of a protein act to either create a successful protein that is able to properly participate in a lock-and-key process. The successful design of a protein is dependent upon the amino acids being positions in space.

The basic equation of an amino acid is HN2-CHR-COOH. When one amino acid is attached to another amino acid position of the side chain (R) of the amino acids dictates the functional position of the amino acid. Some of the amino acids reach out their side chain (R) to bond to either other nucleotides in a separate protein molecule or to a nucleotide comprising a segment of DNA or an RNA. With respect to molecular architecture, both the type and position of an amino acid's side chain can influence bending and folding parameters of a protein's structure, in both positive and negative ways.

In Table 12 the Amino Acid are listed using IUPAC notation, with the name of each of the twenty-one amino acids in the left column. The three letter abbreviation and the one letter abbreviation for the amino acids are listed in the adjacent columns. In the right most column of Table 12 are listed the DNA Nucleotide Codes as described by convention.

The column listing the DNA Nucleotide Codes demonstrates: (1) three amino acids have six different codons, (2) five amino acids have four different codons, (3) one amino acid has three different codons, (4) nine amino acids have two different codons and two amino acids have one differing codon. Given the sixty-four possible combinations all amino acid codons described above are represented by a different three letter combination of nucleotides. The only codon that is used twice is the unique situation where the codon 'ATG' represents both the amino acid molecule 'methionine' but 'ATG' also represents the 'START' codon for purposes of transcription.

Review of the right most column of Table 12 demonstrates that other than the three amino acids of Arginine, Leucine and Serine which have six codons, the codons of the remaining amino acids have two of the three nucleotides are the same.

Further study of the codons shows that the three amino acids which have six different codons and the five amino acids which have four different codons contain a series of four codons where two of the nucleotides are the same and in each of the four one nucleotide represents either an A, C, G or T.

Regarding the nine amino acids that have two different codons review of the codons demonstrate that two letters are the first to nucleotides are the same for the amino acid the third nucleotide is either an 'A' or a 'G' or the third nucleotide is either an 'C' or a 'T'.

Amino Acid	Three Letter Abbreviation	One Letter Abbreviation	DNA Nucleotide Codes
Alanine	Ala	A	GC**A** GC**C** GC**G** GC**T**
Arginine	Arg	R	CG**A** CG**C** CG**G** CG**T** AGA, AGG
Asparagine	Asn	N	AA**C** AA**T**
Aspartic acid	Asp	D	GA**C** GA**T**
Cysteine	Cys	C	TG**C** TG**T**
Glutamine	Gln	Q	CA**A** CA**G**
Glutamic acid	Glu	E	GA**A** GA**G**

Glycine	Gly	G	GG**A** GG**C** GG**G** GG**T**
Histidine	His	H	CA**C** CA**T**
Isoleucine	Ile	I	AT**A** AT**C** AT**T**
Leucine	Leu	L	CT**A** CT**C** CT**G** CT**T** TTA, TTG
Lysine	Lys	K	AA**A** AA**G**
Methionine	Met	M	ATG
Phenylalanine	Phe	F	TT**C** TT**T**
Proline	Pro	P	CC**A** CC**C** CC**G** CC**T**
Serine	Ser	S	TC**A** TC**C** TC**G** TC**T** AGT, AGC
Threonine	Thr	T	AC**A** AC**T** AC**C** AC**G**
Tryptophan	Typ	W	TGG
Tyrosine	Tyr	Y	TA**C** TA**T**
Valine	Val	V	GT**A** GT**C** GT**G** GT**T**

START	---	---	ATG
STOP	---	---	TAA, TGA, TAG

Table 12. Amino Acid table using IUPAC notation.

If randomness was the basis of the design criteria, as suggested by the concept of Evolution, then there should be no order to the arrangement of the triplicate coding assignments to the amino acids. The fact that there is a consistent order, suggests reason and intent for the assignments of the triplicate codon codes to the twenty amino acids.

From a molecular design perspective, the four differing 'third' nucleotides in the codon code might dictate position of the side chain of the amino acid as the amino acid is attached to the protein's amino acid chain. A circle is 360 degrees in circumference. In essence an amino acid being attached to an amino acid chain can be attached to that amino acid chain with its side chain positioned anywhere in the 360 circumference about the axis of the protein molecule being built. Where an amino acid has assigned at least four codon codes, the codon codes have four differing nucleotides (the third nucleotide), the existence of these four codes may divide the circumference of a circle into four 90-degree quadrants surrounding the axis of the molecule. Such a coding system would dictate how proteins would be configured in relation to the position of the side chains of the amino acids comprising their structures. Position of an amino acid side chain would influence folding of the overall molecule and/or bonding capacity of the finished molecule. Where the codon code has only two assigned codons for an amino acid, the two codon codes may divide the circumference of the circle into 180 degrees about the axis of the molecule; that is binding the amino acid with its associated side chain R in one of two choices such as either the side chain is positioned right-handed or left-handed or the position of the side chain is positioned either top or bottom in relation to the axis of the molecule being constructed.

The amino acids with three, four and six codon codes assigned to them, are amino acids that have the smaller side chains. The smaller side chains are most likely amendable to positioning in quadrants around the circumference of the axis of the molecule. The amino acids with large side chains, most likely contain side chains of such a size that the end of the side chain moves so freely in space that it is only necessary to distinguish the position of the side chain in a range of a 180-degree sweep about the axis of the molecule. If such a format is true, this is a clever coding system to dictate the internal architecture of protein molecules.

As illustrated in Figure 60, some form of code must exist to set the R-side chain alignment of the amino acid being added to the existing chain in relation to the amino acids that are already present comprising the protein under construction.

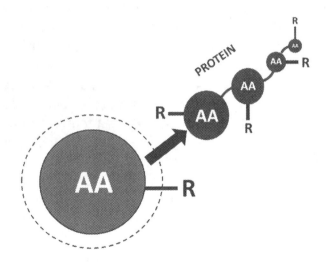

Figure 60 Amino acid to being added to a protein chain

As seen in Figure 61, one of the nucleotides comprising the codon code may act as a means of defining the orientation of the R-side chain of the amino acid being attached as the amino acid is bound to the protein under construction.

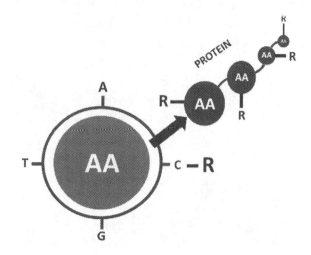

Figure 61 Codon code used to assign orientation of the R-side chain of an amino acid

As illustrated in Figure 62, the amino acids in one of the three codons may be assigned distinct degrees of orientation so that the R-side chain of an amino acid being added to a protein under construction will be oriented properly in relation to the amino acids already comprising the protein. Such precise orientation of the R-side chain of an amino acid facilitates folding of the protein and exposes potential bonding sites of the protein.

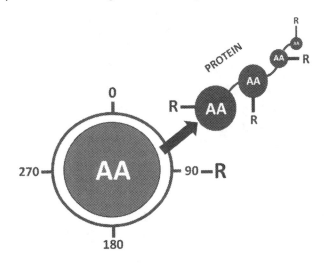

Figure 62 Distinct degrees of orientation assigned
to a nucleic acid in the codon code

The design secrets of creating the bends and folds in the special three dimensional structure of a protein may be as simple as deciphering the intent of the amino acid codon code. The codon code may act in the dual function of identifying both which amino acid to add to a protein chain as well as the spacial orientation the amino acid should have in relation to the primary axis of the protein as the amino acid is added to the protein molecule.

POST SCRIPT 2

INTERACTIVE 3D VIRTUAL MOLECULAR BIOLOGY LABORATORY

The molecular biology lab of the not too distant future will have no resemblance to the current biology research lab where specimens are cultured in a Petri dish and viruses and the cells they attack are viewed under high-powered microscopes.

In the future, the experimental molecular biology lab will be an empty room, void of pathogens, void of host cells, and void of benches and the microscopes where traditional laboratory workers would generally toil to study their research specimens.

The laboratory researcher of the future will dress in casual clothes, without the necessity of a having to dune on a cumbersome sterile jumpsuit and helmet. A DNA bioengineer will enter into a small gymnasium size room. The room will be windowless with four white walls, a tile floor and a blank white ceiling. There will be a petite waist high workstation in the center of the room.

Upon entering the interactive three-dimensional virtual biologic laboratory, the researcher will place a pair of virtual reality glasses over his or her eyes, resting them comfortable on their head. Peering through the lenses of the virtual reality glasses, the empty room will come alive. Within the confines of the unobstructed space within the gymnasium materializes the three dimensional holographic image of the human cell. The researcher will also put on specially designed gloves with sensors positioned on the fingertips to act as means to control and manipulate the imagery seen through the glasses.

The outermost boundaries of the human cell is the cell membrane dotted with an array of receptors. Within the boundaries of the exterior bilayer lipid cell membrane is the cytoplasm of the cell. Suspended in the cytoplasm rest the organelles of the cell. The largest of the organelles is the nucleus. Attached to the nucleus is the smooth endoplasmic reticulum.

The cell nucleus is defined by the nuclear membrane. Channels dot the nuclear membrane allowing molecules to transfer from the cytoplasm into the nucleus. Within the boundaries of the nuclear membrane, exist the spiral arms of the forty-six chromosomes dotted with histones. The nucleus represents a bustling ever active environment with proteins forming transcription complexes to engage and decode the DNA, spliceosomes modifying mRNAs, mature RNA molecules transiting the nucleus to the cytoplasm.

The virtual reality glasses will allow the laboratory researcher to physically maneuver through the human cell at will to gain the optimum advantage point of how a cell functions at any given point in the cell.

Future drugs will be designed and initially tested in such a virtual laboratory. A laboratory researcher will be able to view drugs and proteins that behave like drugs at the molecular level of the molecule. The laboratory researcher will be able to witness how a hypothetical drug would enter the cell and then transit the cytoplasm of the cell as it travels to its target inside the cell. Viewing the drug at the molecular level will allow the researcher to witness the exact manner of how the drug would engage the target structure in the cell. Modifications to the molecular structure of the drug can be made in real time by voice commands meant to allow the laboratory researcher the means to interact with the software generating the imagery being projected through the virtual reality glasses.

Nuclear signaling proteins will become important therapeutic molecules in the future. A nuclear signaling protein will engage a specific target segment of the DNA to activate transcription of a gene or prevent transcription of a gene.

The laboratory researcher will be able to view the nuclear signaling protein at the molecular level of the molecule. The researcher artificially immersed into the lab will be able to witness how the designer nuclear signaling protein would enter the cell and then transit the cytoplasm of the cell as it travels to its target inside the nucleus. The laboratory researcher would be able to witness the nuclear signaling protein transiting the nuclear membrane of the nucleus. Upon accessing the inner chamber of the cell's nucleus, the researcher will be able to study the nuclear signaling protein engage the DNA directly at the molecular level. Modifications to the molecular structure of the nuclear signaling protein can be made in real time by voice commands and hand gestures facilitating the means for the laboratory researcher to interact with the software generating the imagery being projected through the virtual reality glasses.

An interactive 3D virtual lab would vastly expedite the development of new drugs by allowing researchers to manipulate various combinations of molecular structure to determine the optimum molecular design prior to conducting animal studies.

POST SCRIPT 3

HIV GENOME EVIDENCE OF EXTRATERRESTRIAL INTERVENTION

For thousands of years much of the human race has believed in a deity of some form. This deity whether it be one entity or multiple entities has been expected to have been responsible for the creation and well-being of the human race. In 1859, Charles Darwin shattered the foundation of the age-old belief in God, by publishing his book titled Origin of Species By Natural Selection. Darwin's text dictated that life on the planet Earth was the result of 'Evolution' and not the creation of some Superbeing. The term 'Evolution' representing the concept that given enough time, randomness would result in the organization of atoms into organic molecules; then given enough time, randomness would produce enough various forms of life to populate the planet and Natural Selection (survival of the fittest) would dictate which of the random forms of life would flourish at any given time given the prevailing environmental factors of that time. The concept of Evolution, does not account for how water appeared in such abundance as to cover 72% of the planet's surface. Evolution also does not address how the Earth's atmosphere happens to be 79% nitrogen and 21% oxygen, the mixture necessary for nitrogen based life such as our own.

The concept of a God as creator of life meant that some form of thought was given to the design of the life forms that exist on the Earth. For the most part, Medicine and the community of Biosciences have followed Charles Darwin's teachings and adopted the concept of Evolution as the sole reason life exists on the planet. Though there has been numerous myths and beliefs in extraterrestrial intervention, no concrete scientific evidence has to date has surfaced to prove that the existence of life is related to anything but Evolution...until now.

The construct of the Human Immunodeficiency Virus (HIV) genome could not have been generated by chance occurrence. Like all messenger RNA producing nucleotide sequences, the coding represents a base-three codon code embedded into the base four nucleotide code. The codons are groupings of three nucleotides. As mentioned in Table 12 of Postscript One, there are 20 amino acids and there a sixty-one codon codes to represent these amino acids. The amino acids Methionine and Tryptophan have one three nucleotide code to represent their amino acids, but the remaining 18 amino acids have multiple possible codon codes. Nine amino acids have two possible codon codes, Isoleucine has three possible codon codes, five have four possible codes and three have six different codon codes.

The crux of the Central Dogma of Microbiology is that a gene is read linearly from the 5' end to the 3' end. A gene is generally comprised of three regions. The three regions of a gene are the 5' Upstream region, the Transcription region and the 3' Downstream region. At the 5' end is the 5' Upstream region which is where the transcription complex assembles. At the end of the 5' Upstream region and the beginning of the Transcription region is located the Transcription Start Site. Following the Transcription region is the 3' Downstream region, thought to be where the transcription complex disassembles. If the proper codes are embedded in the nucleotide sequence of the 3' Downstream the transcription complex may not disassemble, but instead repeat the transcription process for the same gene. It is generally considered a human gene is read from the 5' end to the 3' end producing one messenger RNA molecule.

The HIV genome has three distinct qualities which point at the viral genome being not the product of chance occurrence as would be dictated by the teachings of Evolution, but instead the genome represents a highly sophisticated biologic computer program that had to have been designed by some form of intelligence.

Within the construct of the HIV genome (1) there are eight genes utilizing overlapping coding regions; (2) overlap of four genes utilizing the same nucleotide sequence, (3) the eight viral gene sequence encodes for two messenger RNAs that accomplish this by utilizing two differing STOP codes to facilitate the construct of two differing mRNAs.

Minor variations in noncritical genetic coding may allow the genome of any biologic structure to be transcribed unimpeded and generate the intended biologic structure with variation. Any significant flaw in a biologic structure's genome will lead to ineffective transcription and failure of the biologic structure to be produced. Flaws that occur in sequences of genetic coding shared by two or more genes increase the odds a fatal flaw occurs preventing construct of the biologic structure.

In Figure 63 it is depicted the eight genes that comprise the HIV genome. As illustrated the eight genes have overlapping sequencing.

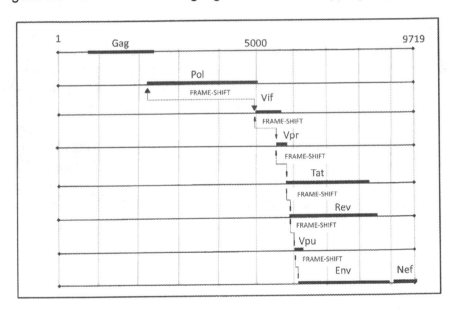

Figure 63 HIV genome with eight genes.

In Figure 64 it is illustrated the eight mRNAs that are produced with translating the HIV genome. Of note is that 5' Upstream region of each of HIV's mRNAs is identical for each of the nine mRNAs.

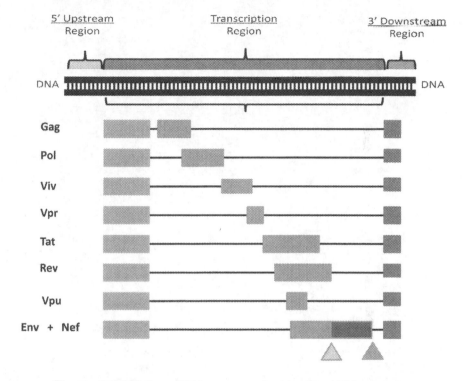

Figure 64 HIV's mRNAs generated by the HIV genome

HIV's 'gag' gene is presented in Figure 65 referenced from the National Center for Biotechnology Information (NCBI) website 'www. **ncbi**.nlm.nih.gov'.

```
CDS        336..1838

           /gene="gag"

           /note="Pr55"

           /codon_start=1

           /product="Gag"

           /protein_id="AAC82593.1"

           /db_xref="GI:2801504"

           /translation="MGARASVLSGGELDRWEKIRLRPGGKKKYKLKHIVWASRELERF

           AVNPGLLETSEGCRQILGQLQPSLQTGSEELRSLYNTVATLYCVHQRIEIKDTKEALD

           KIEEEQNKSKKKAQQAAADTGHSNQVSQNYPIVQNIQGQMVHQAISPRTLNAWVKVVE

           EKAFSPEVIPMFSALSEGATPQDLNTMLNTVGGHQAAMQMLKETINEEAAEWDRVHPV

           HAGPIAPGQMREPRGSDIAGTTSTLQEQIGWMTNNPPIPVGEIYKRWIILGLNKIVRM

           YSPTSILDIRQGPKEPFRDYVDRFYKTLRAEQASQEVKNWMTETLLVQNANPDCKTIL

           KALGPAATLEEMMTACQGVGGPGHKARVLAEAMSQVTNSATIMMQRGNFRNQRKIVKC

           FNCGKEGHTARNCRAPRKKGCWKCGKEGHQMKDCTERQANFLGKIWPSYKGRPGNFLQ

           SRPEPTAPPEESFRSGVETTTPPQKQEPIDKELYPLTSLRSLFGNDPSSQ"
```

Figure 65 HIV's 'gag' gene

Presented in Figure 66 is the genetic coding for the HIV genome to include nucleotides 1-1620.

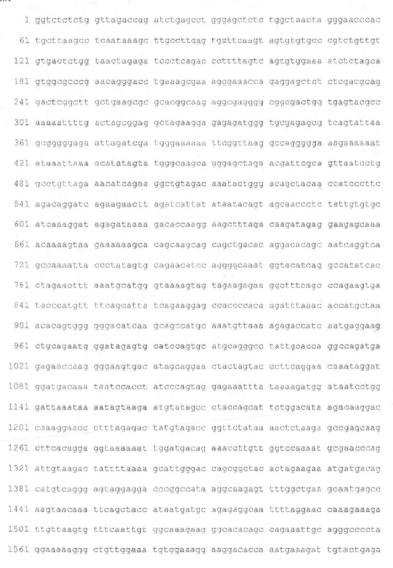

Figure 66 HIV genome nucleotides 1-1620

In Figure 67 is presented nucleotides 336 to nucleotide 660 of the 'gag' gene. The 'gag' gene is coded between nucleotides 336-1838 in the HIV genome. The HIV genome taken from the NCBI website. The codon 'atg' shows the start of the 'gag' gene.

HIV gene= "gag"   CDS: 336-1838.   Translation: MGAR.....

    1 ggtctctctg gttagaccag atctgagcct gggagctctc tggctaacta gggaacccac

   61 tgcttaagcc tcaataaagc ttgccttgag tgcttcaagt agtgtgtgcc cgtctgttgt

  121 gtgactctgg taactagaga tccctcagac cctttttagtc agtgtggaaa atctctagca

  181 gtggcgcccg aacagggacc tgaaagcgaa aggg   cca gaggagctct ctcgacgcag

  241 gactcggctt gctgaagcgc gcacggcaag aggc   ggg cggcgactgg tgagtacgcc

  301 aaaaattttg actagcggag gctagaagga gagagatggg tgcgagagcg tcagtattaa

  361 gcgggggaga attagatcga tgggaaaaaa ttcggttaag gccagggggga aagaaaaaat

  421 ataaattaaa acatatagta tgggcaagca gggagctaga acgattcgca gttaatcctg

  481 gcctgttaga aacatcagaa ggctgtagac aaatactggg acagctacaa ccatcccttc

  541 agacaggatc agaagaactt agatcattat ataatacagt agcaaccctc tattgtgtgc

  601 atcaaaggat agagataaaa gacaccaagg aagctttaga caagatagag gaagagcaaa

Figure 67 Gag gene nucleotides 336-660

Represented in Figure 68 is the latter portion of the 'gag' gene represented as nucleotides 1621 to nucleotide 1838. The three nucleotides 'taa' is the last codon of the 'gag' gene. The entire 'gag' gene sequence covers nucleotide 336 to nucleotide 1838 in the HIV genome.

HIV gene= "gag"   CDS: 336-1838.

```
1621 gacaggctaa ttttttaggg aagatctggc cttcctacaa gggaaggcca gggaattttc

1681 ttcagagcag accagagcca acagccccac cagaagagag cttcaggtct ggggtagaga

1741 caacaactcc ccctcagaag caggagccga tagacaagga actgtatcct ttaacttccc

1801 tcaggtcact ctttggcaac gacccctcgt cacaataaag atagggggc aactaaagga

1861 agctctatta gatacaggag cagatgatac agtattagaa gaaatgagtt tgccaggaag

1921 atggaaacca aaaatgatag ggggaattgg aggtttttatc aaagtaagac agtatgatca

1981 gatactcata gaaatctgtg gacataaagc tataggtaca gtattagtag gacctacacc

2041 tgtcaacata attggaagaa atctgttgac tcagattggt tgcactttaa attttcccat

2101 tagccctatt gagactgtac cagtaaaatt aaagccagga atggatggcc caaaagttaa

2161 acaatggcca ttgacagaag aaaaaataaa agcattagta gaaatttgta cagagatgga
```

Figure 68 Latter portion 'gag' gene nucleotides 1621-1838

Presented in Figure 69 are partial coding for both HIV's 'gag' gene and the 'pol' gene. The figure shows the latter portion of HIV's 'gag' gene from nucleotide 1621 to nucleotide 1838. The front end of the 'pol' gene includes nucleotides 1631-2220. The actual coding for HVI's 'gag' gene extends from nucleotide 336 to nucleotide 1838. The actual coding for HIV's 'pol' gene extends from nucleotide 1631 to nucleotide 4642. There is overlap of the 'gag' gene and 'pol' gene is show from nucleotide 1631 to nucleotide 1838.

HIV gene= "gag"   CDS: 336-1838. ⸺

HIV gene= "pol"   CDS: 1631-4642. ⸺⸺·

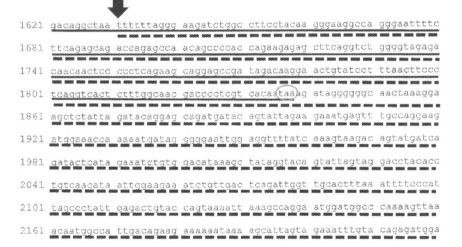

Figure 69 HIV's 'gag' gene and 'pol' genes
overlapping coding sequences

Presented in Figure 70 is the nucleotide frame-shift that occurs to allow the same nucleotide sequence to be read as an entirely different three codon code. The codon code of the 'gag' gene reads the nucleotide sequence for the 'gag' gene. The 'pol' gene utilizes the same nucleotide sequence but reads the 3-nucleotide codon code with a shift of one nucleotide to the left. Shown in the figure the codon code 'aat' read as a 'gag' codon code, the 't' becomes incorporated into a 'ttt' codon code for the first codon of the 'pol' gene.

HIV gene= "gag" CDS: 336-1838. ———

HIV gene= "pol" CDS: 1631-4642. —————·

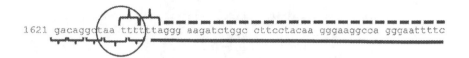

1621 gacaggctaa ttttttaggg aagatctggc cttcctacaa gggaaggcca gggaattttc

Figure 70 Frame-shift allowing 'gag' gene
to share sequencing with 'pol' gene

Figure 70 is a clear example of a base-three code embedded in a base-four code for the purpose of data compression.

Figure 71 illustrates the latter portion of HIV's 'vif' gene. The 'vif' gene extends from nucleotide 4487 to 5165. Figure 71 shows the 'vif' gene from nucleotides 5041 to 5165.

Gene= vif 4487-5165   —————

```
5041  cattaataac accaaaaaag ataaagccac ctttgcctag tgttacgaaa ctgacagagg

5101  atagatggaa caagccccag aagaccaagg gccacagagg gagccacaca atgaatggac

5161  actagagctt ttagaggagc ttaagaatga agctgttaga cattttccta ggatttggct

5221  ccatggctta gggcaacata tctatgaaac ttatggggat acttgggcag gagtggaagc

5281  cataataaga attctgcaac aactgctgtt tatccatttt cagaattggg tgtcgacata

5341  gcagaatagg cgttactcga cagaggagag caagaaatgg agccagtaga tcctagacta

5401  gagccctgga agcatccagg aagtcagcct aaaactgctt gtaccaattg ctattgtaaa

5461  aagtgttgct ttcattgcca agtttgtttc ataacaaaag ccttaggcat ctcctatggc

5521  aggaagaagc ggagacagcg acgaagagct catcagaaca gtcagactca tcaagcttct

5581  ctatcaaagc agtaagtagt acatgtaatg caacctatac caatagtagc aatagtagca

5641  ttagtagtag caataataat agcaatagtt gtgtggtcca tagtaatcat agaatatagg

5701  aaaatattaa gacaaagaaa aatagacagg ttaattgata gactaataga aagagcagaa

5761  gacagtggca atgagagtga aggagaaata tcagcacttg tggagatggg ggtggagatg

5821  gggcaccatg ctccttggga tgttgatgat ctgtagtgct acagaaaaat tgtgggtcac
```

Figure 71 HIV 'vif' gene from 5041 to 5165

The 'vpr' gene extends from nucleotide 5105 to nucleotide 5341. The 'vif' gene overlaps the 'vpr' gene from nucleotide 5105 to nucleotide 5165. Figure 72 demonstrates the location of both the 'vif' and the 'vpr' genes.

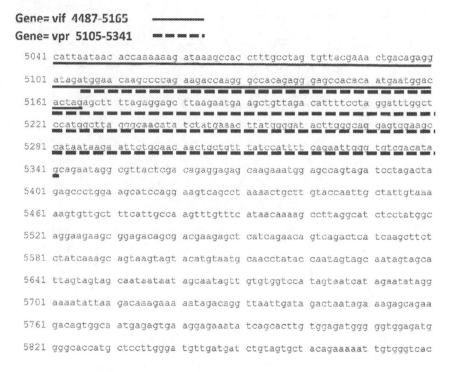

Figure 72 HIV 'vif' gene and 'vpr' gene

Figure 73 illustrates the 'vif' gene, the 'vpr' gene and the 'tat' gene.

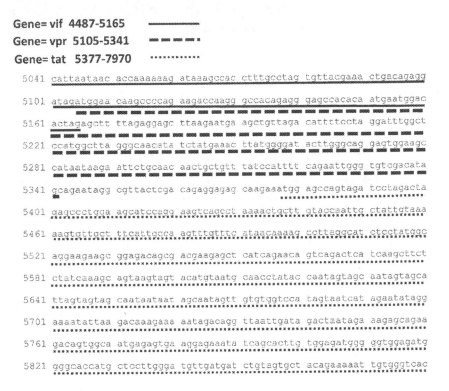

Figure 73 HIV 'vif' gene, 'vpr' gene and 'tat' gene

Figure 74 illustrates the 'vif' gene, the 'vpr' gene, the 'tat' gene and the 'rev' gene. Note the 'rev' gene rests within the boundaries of the 'tat' gene.

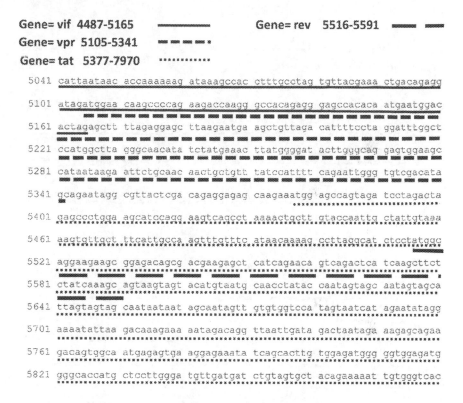

Figure 74 HIV 'vif' gene, 'vpr' gene, 'tat' gene and 'rev' gene

Figure 75 illustrates the 'vif' gene, the 'vpr' gene, the 'tat' gene, the 'rev' gene and the 'vpu' gene. Note the genetic coding for both the 'rev' gene and the 'vpu' gene rest within the boundaries of the 'tat' gene.

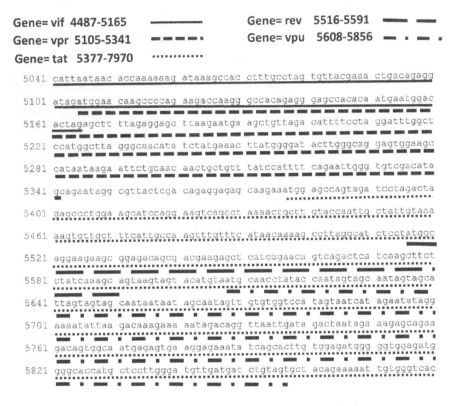

Figure 75 HIV 'vif' gene, 'vpr' gene, 'tat' gene, 'rev' gene, and 'vpu' gene

Figure 76 illustrates the 'vif' gene, the 'vpr' gene, the 'tat' gene, the 'rev' gene, the 'vpu' gene and the 'env' gene. Both the 'rev' gene and the 'vpu' gene rest within the boundaries of the 'tat' gene. Astonishingly, from nucleotide 5771 to nucleotide 5856 of the 'tat' gene, the 'vpu' gene and the 'env' gene there is an overlap of the codon code generated by frame-shifting of the codon code.

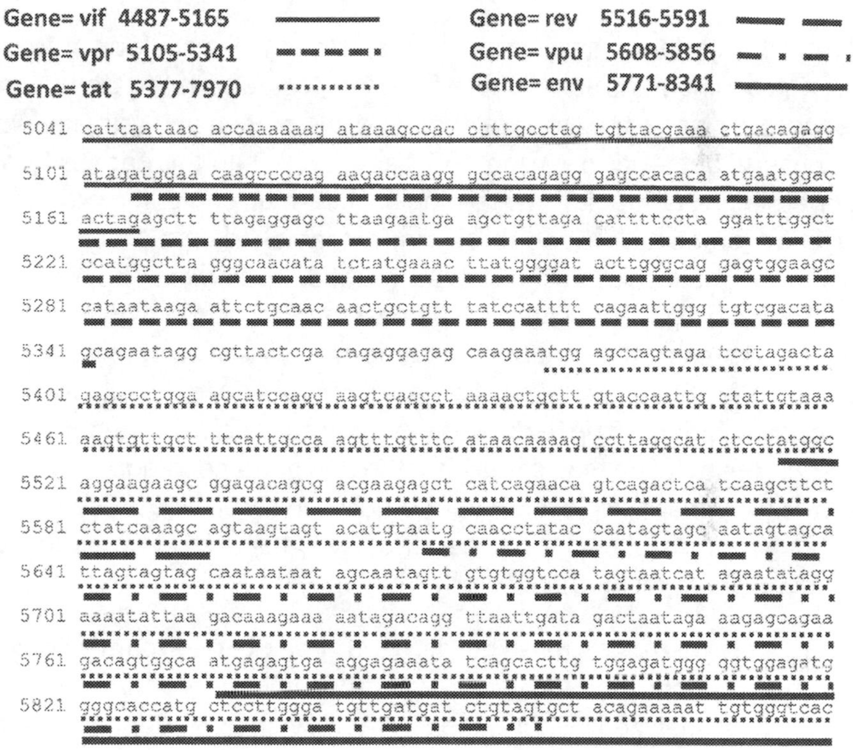

Gene= vif 4487-5165 ——————   Gene= rev 5516-5591 ━━ ━━
Gene= vpr 5105-5341 ▬ ▬ ▬ ▬ ▪   Gene= vpu 5608-5856 ▬ ▪ ▬ ▪
Gene= tat 5377-7970 ············   Gene= env 5771-8341 ═══════════

```
5041  cattaataac accaaaaaag ataaagccac ctttgcctag tgttacgaaa ctgacagagg
5101  atagatggaa caagccccag aagaccaagg gccacagagg gagccacaca atgaatggac
5161  actagagctt ttagaggagc ttaagaatga agctgttaga cattttccta ggatttggct
5221  ccatggctta gggcaacata tctatgaaac ttatggggat acttgggcag gagtggaagc
5281  cataataaga attctgcaac aactgctgtt tatccatttt cagaattggg tgtcgacata
5341  gcagaatagg cgttactcga cagaggagag caagaaatgg agccagtaga tcctagacta
5401  gagccctgga agcatccagg aagtcagcct aaaactgctt gtaccaattg ctattgtaaa
5461  aagtgttgct ttcattgcca agtttgtttc ataacaaaag ccttaggcat ctcctatggc
5521  aggaagaagc ggagacagcg acgaagagct catcagaaca gtcagactca tcaagcttct
5581  ctatcaaagc agtaagtagt acatgtaatg caacctatac caatagtagc aatagtagca
5641  ttagtagtag caataataat agcaatagtt gtgtggtcca tagtaatcat agaatatagg
5701  aaaatattaa gacaaagaaa aatagacagg ttaattgata gactaataga aagagcagaa
5761  gacagtggca atgagagtga aggagaaata tcagcacttg tggagatggg ggtggagatg
5821  gggcaccatg ctccttggga tgttgatgat ctgtagtgct acagaaaaat tgtgggtcac
```

Figure 76 HIV 'vif' gene, 'vpr' gene, 'tat' gene, 'rev' gene, 'vpu' gene and 'env' gene

The presence of Figure 76, demonstrates an incredible intelligence where the tat gene coding is frame-shifted to create the vpu gene, then frame-shifted again to code for the env gene.

HIV genome is able have genes share segments of the genome by frame-shifting the base three codon code by one or two codons to create a new segment of codon code. This high-level command of the codon code exhibits evidence of a bio programming design created by an extraordinary intelligence. Such a sophisticated, extensive frame-shifting of the codon code could not have occurred per random chance of DNA nucleotides having simply been haphazardly jumbled together...no matter how much time was allowed to occur...there are some things that just cannot occur by the hand of random chance and the HIV genome is an example of a physical entity requiring design to make its existence possible.

The HIV genome has been thought to have transferred from primates to humans somewhere from the 1880's to 1929. Computer technology was nonexistent at that time. No person on earth, known to history, before or between 1880 and 1929, had the capability of generating a computer or a biologic base-four computer program with an embedded base-three code that overlapped four gene coding sequences using the same nucleotide sequence. The biologic computer programming and the base-four embedded base-three data compression technique that comprises a virus as sophisticated as HIV's 9618 nucleotide sequence represents quite the intellectual accomplishment. The existence of HIV's genome categorically dispels the notation that, at least for the HIV genome, random events were solely responsible for the genome's construct. The presence of HIV's genome defies the position that Evolution has been principle responsible force for the existence of life.

Viruses often exist as similar, but differing strains of the same genome. As further proof the HIV genome was designed, the strain HIV-1 HXB2 was analyzed. Eight genes in the HIV-1 HXB2 genome were found to be compressed. The frame-shifting compression technique shortened the genome by 825 nucleotides, most likely allowing the HIV-1 HXB2 genome to fit inside the HIV virion. Remarkably, there is a triple frame-shift at nucleotide 8380 to include the genes: env, tat2 and rev2. See the last figures of this text for details regarding the HIV-1 HXB2 analysis.

POST SCRIPT 4

NEW PARADIGM IN RHEUMATOID ARTHRITIS: TREATING WITH A NORMAL RHEUMATOID FACTOR

Rheumatoid arthritis (RA) is a systemic disease that usually results in a bilateral and generally symmetrical inflammatory arthritis. The cause of rheumatoid arthritis has yet to be clearly defined. It has been long thought that a person who develops rheumatoid arthritis is in fact a body harboring a genetic predisposition to inflammatory arthritis, which encounters an environmental stimulant, which vigorously triggers a cascade of immune responses. The up-regulated inflammatory changes generate cytokines and other proteins that have destructive effects on cartilage and bone. Left unchecked, the end result of an inflammatory arthritis is a crippling joint disease.

There are factors to suggest that the current cause and effect theory to rationalize the inflammatory changes that accompany rheumatoid arthritis may need to be modified. The current commonly used method for testing for rheumatoid arthritis invokes the rate nephlometry method. The original method utilized to test for RA was the latex agglutination method. The latex agglutination method suggested that the object of the test, the Rheumatoid Factor (RF), was a normal protein in the body that had somehow undergone a transformation into an abnormal protein and demonstrated abnormal functions. The latex agglutination test method was a test to detect the presence of a RF in the blood of patients with RA. The latex agglutination test method detected the presence of a RF by the introduction of latex particles into a sample of serum obtained from a patient with RA and when the RF molecule was present, the RF would attach to the latex particles causing the latex particles to coalesce together. The coalescence of latex particles could be seen by the naked eye, resulting in a visual confirmation of the presence of a RF in the patient's sera. Approximately 75-80% of patients with RA demonstrated the presence of a RF by the latex agglutination method.

The first factor to challenge the current cause-and-effect theory for RA is therefore the previous notion that the rheumatoid factor seen in patients with rheumatoid arthritis represented a previously normal protein that somehow transformed into an abnormal protein. This has been seen in patients, where by the RF started out negative or normal at the beginning of the disease, and the RF titer became positive later in the course of the disease.

The second factor to challenge the current cause-and-effect theory for RA is the perspective that the previous management strategy for rheumatoid arthritis was to rest the joints. In the 1960's, patients were hospitalized for in some cases months to manage RA. During such hospitalizations patients were provided regular physical therapy, but for the most part, patients were treated with bed rest as the mainstay for managing the inflammatory arthritis.

The third factor to challenge the current cause-and-effect theory for RA is the treatment with intravenous gammaglobulins (IVIG) appears to be beneficial to patients with rheumatoid arthritis. Intravenous immunoglobulin is a blood product administered intravenously. It contains the pooled, polyvalent, IgG antibodies extracted from the plasma of over one thousand blood donors.

Published studies document that IVIG therapy is beneficial. One study involving ten patients reports that serial measurement of cytokines revealed a rapid and persistent decrease in serum TNF alpha and a late and significant reduction in sIL-2R concentrations.[1,2]

The three factors of the RF representing a normal protein that turned abnormal, rest being a treatment of RA and the treatment of IVIG being beneficial to RA patients suggest a different theory to explain rheumatoid arthritis might be possible. Taking the observation that IVIG is effective therapy and that the RF is a protein that was once normal, but transformed into an abnormal form suggests that RA may be the result of a lack of a normal RF protein.

The normal use of the joints may cause inflammation. A routine analogy is that the normal use of a car engine causes heat. Heat damages functional mechanical parts. Excess heat must be extracted from a car engine by the use of external airflow and internal coolant, otherwise the car engine fails due to excessive fatigue caused by an intolerant rise in temperature.

There is the chance that simple use of the joints causes a similar set of circumstances. That like heat to an engine, inflammation to the joints needs to be kept under control and maintained at a tolerant level for the internal parts of a joint to operate properly and not wear out excessively. The RF may be the governor of the control mechanism that manages joint inflammation. The lack of a proper amount of 'normal' RF in the body may lead to joint inflammation and damage. In the case of active RA, the RF may become abnormal, thus not being able to properly perform its role as a natural anti-inflammatory protein to control naturally occurring joint inflammation. Thus, in patients with an abnormal noneffective RF protein, the inflammation proceeds unchecked and eventually destroys the joints.

The lack of a normal RF dampening protein would help to explain why the disease is symmetrical and also why the disease tends to be more destructive on the dominant side of the body.

1. Long term treatment of rheumatoid arthritis with high doses of intravenous immunoglobulins: effects on disease activity and serum cytokines. C Muscat, A Bertotto, R Ercolani, Ann Rheum Dis. 1995 May; 54(5): 382–385.

2. Intravenous immunoglobulin in the treatment of polyarticular juvenile rheumatoid arthritis: a phase I/II study. Pediatric Rheumatology Collaborative Study Group. Giannini EH, Lovell DJ, Silverman ED, Sundel RP, J Rheumatol. 1996 May;23(5):919-24.

POST SCRIPT 5

THEORY OF LIGHT

'Light Representing the Presence of a Physical Medium'

It has long been observed that light exhibits at least two competing and somewhat incompatible behaviors. Light sometimes acts as a wave, and then sometimes light acts as a ball. These two behaviors of light remain a mystery.

Light has been considered its own entity. The equation $E=MC^2$, the famous equation derived by Dr. Albert Einstein, has suggested that light is a stand alone entity; leading us to believe that light flows through the universe uninterrupted, independent of all other factors and features comprising the universe. It is a simple concept to accept, since on any clear night, an observer can gaze up at the stars in the night sky and accept the fact that the only way light traveled billions of light years from distant galaxies to the eyes in one's head, is if light were its own independent entity.

But then the controversy occurs, when one ponders why Dr. Albert Einstein was awarded the 1921 Nobel Prize for physics for his law of the photoelectric effect. Dr. Einstein calculated that as light passed by an object in space exhibiting a large gravitational field, light would bend toward the gravitational field. 1919 saw the first successful attempt to measure the gravitational deflection of light. Two British expeditions were organized and sponsored by the Royal Astronomical Society and the Royal Society. Each of the two groups took photographs of a region of the sky centered on the Sun during the May 1919 total solar eclipse and compared the positions of the photographed stars with those of the same stars photographed from the same locations in July 1919 when the Sun was far from that region of the sky. The results showed that light was deflected, and also that this deflection was consistent with general relativity but not with "Newtonian" physics.

So, despite the brain observing that light may travel unimpeded billions of light years from a distant galaxy to reach our eyes as we observe starry bodies in a night sky, Dr. Einstein suggested that the path of light can be influenced by celestial bodies that exhibit intense gravitational fields.

There is also the thought that a black hole can trap light due to an intense gravitational field. The gravity at the center of a black hole is so strong, that light traversing the vicinity of a black hole gets absorbed into the black hole, never to exit the black hole.

Similar to the world populace considering the Earth was flat until Christopher Columbus sailed west across the Atlantic Ocean and discovered the Americas, maybe light is not its own independent entity, but instead, representative of a medium that exits that fills the universe. This medium might be considered an ether. Over a hundred years ago, to classical science, the universe was not considered to consist of a void, but instead, the territory between stars and planets was considered to be comprised of a medium referred to as ether.

The age old mystery of light is that in certain circumstances light behaves in a concentrated form like a 'ball', while in other instances light appears to behave like a 'wave'. The simplest analogy would be to compare 'light' to 'water'. It is well known that when water is undisturbed and void of sediment, that viewing through water can be rather clear; as if the water did not exist. The term 'crystal clear' is often used in terms of description if viewing an object through a body of water, and the object is exceptionally clear visually.

Water can act as a medium. Water has the capacity to act like a 'wave' when within a certain temperature range, water exists as a liquid. Water may also act as a 'ball' when the temperature of water drops below freezing, and water takes on the form of a solid. Like many physical substances, 'temperature' tends to be the primary factor influencing whether 'water' exists as a gas, a liquid or as a solid.

Water can be stationary. We can hold water in our hand. Light is an entity that we can see, but we cannot hold it in our hand. Light does not appear to be affected by temperature, that we know of, but light is supposedly affected by gravity. Theoretically, a black hole exhibits enough gravity to trap light. If light is truly affected by gravity, then theoretically if one could hold a black hole in their hand, they could also hold light trapped by such a black hole in their hand.

If light is not affected by temperature but instead gravity, then this would reflect that light represents a medium that is smaller than atoms, and therefore is not influenced by the vibrational changes in the atomic structures of molecules. It is these sub-sub atomic particles that are affected by gravity.

Light is representative of that an 'ether' exists at a level that is sub-sub atomic. The behavior of light demonstrates that there is a particle that is smaller to an electron, a proton, or a neutron. This particle acting as the ether of the universe are 'quadsitrons'. Quadsitrons are the most elemental particle comprised of four separate poles: (1) a positive pole, (2) a negative pole, (3) a neutral pole and (4) a true absolute zero pole. The description of a quadsitron suggests that the state of 'neutral' is a separate state of energy equal to the charged states of 'positive' and 'negative' and does not represent zero, as has been described in the past. 'Neutral' representing its own physical 'state' is suggested by the fact that 'neutrons' do not represent a void, but exist in atoms and serve a purpose to complement protons and electrons in providing stability to the structure of an atom. Further, the Beta decay of a neutron produces not only a proton and an electron, but also a neutrino and additional energy.

If such an ether exists, then like water, light could behave like a ball or a wave, depending upon the physical nature of the ether. The energy of light could be temporarily trapped by this ether to produce electrons, protons and neutrons. The ether could conduct the travel of light. A black hole then represents light traveling into a vortex of swirling ether, similar to the swirling winds of a tornado, waterspout or hurricane that might be seen in the lower denser atmosphere on earth. The physical phenomenon of a black hole is that of light following the path of quadsitrons being sucked into the vortex of the galactic tornado, while a quasar represents light compressed as it passes through the vortex and emitted out the opposite side of the black hole (like a laser beam) as the quadsitrons stream out the opposite side of the black hole.

Light, like other energy described in the electromagnetic spectrum travels in a wave as described above. The presence of a medium such as an ether would conveniently explain the behavior of light and other energies moving through space or on planet earth as a wave.

Galaxies with a black hole for a center, in fact may be the universe's hurricanes, one of the many visible means of appreciating the immense unbridled energy that ebbs and flows through the universe. The Earth circling Sol, one of thousands of stars in the Orion Spur carried along by the galactic winds as collectively the star studded spiral arms swirl around the central vortex of the Milky Way galaxy.

The universe may be simply summed up to be comprised of two complimentary entities: energy and an ether comprised of quadsitrons. This ether may be the fabric of the universe, from which all other matter is created.

POST SCRIPT 6

THEORY TO UNIFY GLEAM

'Gravity, Light, Electrons, Atoms and Magnetism'

Several prime fundamental concepts of classical physics dramatically and exceedingly conflict with each other. Light is expected to travel at a constant speed, but it is taught gravity can have such a dominating effect that light cannot escape a black hole. An electron has measureable mass and travels at the speed of light, but an entity achieving the travel velocity of the speed of light is not expected to have mass.

It is taught that a positively charged proton and a negatively charged electron equal a neutron. Often the concept of a neutron has been synonymous with the concept of zero. Yet, the study of the subject of beta decay demonstrates that it requires not only the combination of a proton and electron, but the addition of an anti-neutrino to create a neutron. An anti-neutrino represents a measure of both energy and mass. The study of beta decay also demonstrates that when a neutron decays to a proton the resultant mass is not sufficient to generate either a solid spherical mass the size of an electron nor sufficient to generate a hollow spherical shell the size of an electron.

The advent of quantum physics overshadowed and disavowed the previously commonly accepted concept that the universe was comprised of an ether. In 1887, the concept of an ether was nullified when the speed of light traveling in one axis and at an axis ninety degrees to the first axis were found to be the same; The Michelson-Morley experiment proposed that if there was a luminiferous ether there would exist a cosmic wind as the earth moved forward in the planet's orbit around the sun and this cosmic wind would disrupt one of the two beams of light causing a measurable difference in the speed of the two beams of light. Current physics theory struggles to concretely explain the existence of several basic concepts including how gravity exerts a force on an object, the conflicting behaviors of light, the presence of the electron (traveling at the speed of light) and how magnetism exists.

The theory presented here founded on a unifying theory to explain gravity, light, electrons, atoms and magnetism is the concept that the universe is comprised solely of two nonreducible, nondestructible, wholly conserved elements, and only two elements. These two primary elements include 'quadsitrons' and 'energy'. From the combination of quadsitrons and energy all other matter in the universe is created.

Quadsitrons singly represent the most elemental particle of the universe. All quadsitrons are physically identical, including size, shape, weight, and charges. Quadsitrons contain four charge states including: positive, negative, neutral and absolute zero. Figure 77. A key innovative concept is that neutral represents its own state of physical properties of matter and does not represent the entity of 'zero'.

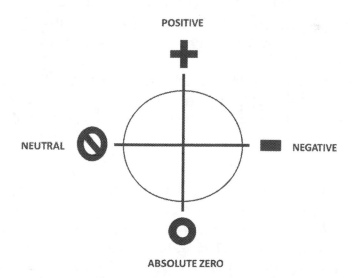

Figure 77 Four distinct charge states of matter including Positive, Negative, Neutral and Absolute Zero

A quadsitron contains four poles each representing one of positive, negative, neutral and absolute neutral. Each of the four poles of a quadsitron project 120 degrees from the neighboring poles. Various differing configurations of quadsitrons result in the existence of protons, neutrons, electrons and dark matter. See Figure 78.

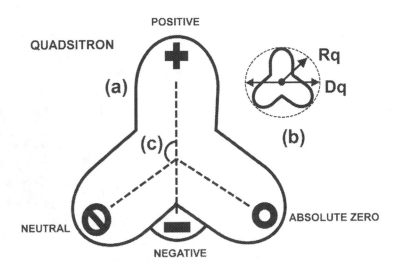

Figure 78 Illustration of a quadsitron with differing four poles each at 120 degrees apart

Energy represents the force that drives all action in the universe. Energy is a nonreducible entity and exists either in a state of flow or energy is trapped by some configuration of quadsitrons, either by quadsitrons themselves or macro structures, from protons to atoms to molecular objects, all comprised of quadsitrons.

Free energy exists such as waves or photons with energy levels depending upon the frequency and wavelength as represented as the electromagnetic spectrum. Energy that flows at low frequencies, such as sound, vibrate molecules of the transfer medium. Energy that flows at high frequencies vibrate quadsitrons as the means of energy transfer. At the speed of light, quadsitrons are the medium by which energy moves from one position to the next. Quadsitrons are a nonreducible entity, therefore quadsitrons transfer energy from one location to another or trap emery.

Trapped energy may exist captured between two quadsitrons to form a neutrino, trapped in a proton, neutron or electron, trapped within the structure of a molecule, trapped in a macromolecule and trapped as potential energy as dictated by gravity or a magnetic field. Various organizations of quadsitrons facilitate the multiple means energy can be captured.

Determining the mass and diameter of a quadsitron is pivotal to unlocking the secrets of the universe. The mass of a quadsitron represented as Qw and the diameter of a quadsitron represented as Qd can be determined by analyzing known quantities and utilizing universal mathematical equations as presented below.

Defining the Radius of a Proton and a Neutron

The proton was theorized in 1815 by William Prout and discovered in 1920 by Ernest Rutherford. The neutron was theorized by Ernest Rutherford in 1920, then discovered by James Chadwick in 1932. There are discrepancies regarding the physical dimensions of both the proton and the neutron.

The exact measurement of the radius of a proton has been so illusive that the term 'proton radius puzzle' has been applied to this phenomenon. The size of a proton has been measured by at least two differing approaches, which include electron-proton scattering and muonic hydrogen Lamb shift experiments. Electron-proton scattering experiments where a proton is bombarded by electrons estimates the proton root mean square charge radius to be 0.8751(61) fm which is listed in 2014 CODATA.[8] The muonic hydrogen Lamb shift experiments, where proton is engaged by a muonon, 200 times the weight of an electron, estimates the proton radius to be 0.8409(4) fm.[10] The Baryon Summary Table in the Review of Particle Physics[12] by Nakamura lists the charge radius of a proton as 0.877 fm. There is obvious disagreement in the proton radius between these two approaches.

Arriving at a determination of the radius of the neutron is equally perplexing. 2014 CODATA does not list a radius for a neutron. The Baryon Summary Table in the Review of Particle Physics[12] by

Nakamura lists the mean square charge radius of a neutron as $<r^2_n>$ = -0.1161 fm^2, or by deriving the square root the r_n might calculate to be 0.3407345 fm.

Attempting to determine the radius of a neutron, the neutron charge radius might be derived by calculating the radius from neutron transmission of liquid ^{208}Pb and ^{209}Bi.[13] Pb symbol for the element lead and Bi symbol for the element bismuth. The neutron-electron scattering length b_{ne} is related to the charge radius $<r^2_n>$ by the equation:

$$<r^2_n> = \frac{3 * me * a0}{mn} * bne$$

Where me is electron mass, mn is neutron mass, a0 is Bohr radius, bne is neutron-electron scattering length.

The b_{ne} for ^{208}Pb determined to be -1.33 x 10^{-3} fm and the b_{ne} for ^{209}Bi -1.44 x 10^{-3} fm. The charge radius of the neutron $<r^2_n>$ is the mean squared radius. Positive and negative values for the charge radius are possible due to distribution of valence quarks and negative meson cloud of the neutron. The meson cloud can lead to a negative value for $<r^2_n>$.[13]

Taking the above b_{ne} for both liquid ^{208}Pb and ^{209}Bi and solving for an approximation for the radius of a neutron or r_n leads to:

^{208}Pb b_{ne} determined to be -1.33 x 10^{-3} fm

$$<r^2_n> = \frac{3 * me * a0}{mn} * bne$$

$$<r^2_n> = \frac{3*(9.10938356 \, x10-31kg)*(5.2917721067 \, x10-11m)}{(16,749.27471 x10-31kg)} * -1.33 x10-3fm$$

$<r^2_n>$ = 0.1148325097 x 10^{-30} m^2

r_n = 0.3388694582 x 10^{-15} m

The approximation of a neutron radius using b_{ne} of ^{208}Pb is 0.3388694582 fm.

^{209}Bi b_{ne} determined to be -1.44 x 10^{-3} fm

$$< r^2_n >= \frac{3 * me * a0}{mn} * bne$$

$$< r^2_n >= \frac{3*(9.10938356 \times 10-31kg)*(5.2917721067 \times 10-11m)}{(16,749.2747 \times 10-31kg)} * -1.44 \times 10-3fm$$

$<r^2_n> = 0.124330552$ x 10^{-30} m^2

$r_n = 0.352605378$ x 10^{-15} m

The approximation of a neutron radius using b_{ne} of ^{209}Bi is 0.352605378 fm.

The approximation of the neutron radius per ^{208}Pb and ^{209}Bi do not agree. In addition, the approximation of neutron radius per both ^{208}Pb and ^{209}Bi is much does not correlate with that of the proton root mean square charge radius to be 0.8751(61) fm which is listed in 2014 CODATA. In the results of the reference it is stated 'Results were obtained for both liquid samples of ^{208}Pb and ^{209}Bi applying the evaluation procedure in Sec IVB. The given statistical uncertainties include the additional uncertainty introduced by the uncertainty of the free normalization parameter.'[13] Attempting to determine the radius of a neutron per means performed above may not be acceptable or practical.

Some presentations of the root mean square charge radius of the proton and neutron place the size of the proton being larger than the size of the neutron. Such an example is free proton root mean charge square radius being 0.8305 fm, while the free neutron root mean charge square radius is 0.8269 x 10^{-15} m.[5] This may be accurate depending upon the behavior of the exterior layers or cloud of the proton and the neutron. The interaction of the positive and negative charges may cause a neutron to become more compact in the process of the transformation of a proton to a neutron. Conceptually, since the neutron is known to possess more mass than a proton, and a neutron harbors within its volume a proton, an electron and a neutrino, it would be logical for a neutron to be larger in size than a proton.

Sha Yin Yue, in the study *On the Radius of the Neutron, Proton, Electron and the Atomic Nucleus*, uses math to calculate the radius of the proton and the neurton.[2] Yue calculates the proton radius to be $1.112772961016 \times 10^{-15}$ m and the neutron radius to be $1.113284057367 \times 10^{-15}$ m. Sha Yin Yue utilizes the following equations and defines the following constants as presented below:

'x' signifies the mathematical multiplication function.

Rn = radius of a neutron = K x Qp x Qe/ ((Mn-Mp) x C ^2)

Rp = radius of proton = (Mp/Mn) ^(1/3) x Rn

Re = (Me/Mn) ^(1/3) x Rn

K is the electromagnetic constant.

Qp is electric charge of a proton.

Qe is the electric charge of an electron.

Mn represents the mass of a neutron.

Mp represents the mass of a proton.

Me represents the mass of an electron.

C is light velocity.

Physically, these calculations are in harmony with what one would expect and that is the size of the neutron, having more mass than a proton, being larger than the size of the proton. Since this study utilizes math to define the physical characteristics of a quadsitron, Sha Yin Yue's calculations will be utilized for the radius of the proton and the neutron, given the measured physical dimensions of both the proton and neutron remain controversial to date.

References:

1. R. Pohl, Antognini A, Nez F...et al, Nature, 213-216, 8 July 2010.

2. Antognini A...et al, Science 339, 417 (2013)

3. Mohr PJ, Newel DB, and Taylor BN,(2015), arXiv: 1507.07956

4. Bernauer JC, Distler MO, Avoiding common pitfalls and misconceptions in extraction of the proton radius, http://arxiv.org/pdf/1606.02159.pdf

5. Nakamura K...et al, Review of Particle Physics, The Baryon Summary Table, Journal of Physics G: Nuclear and Particle Physics, Volume 37, article 075021.

6. Kopecky S, Harvey JA, Hill NW...et al, Neutron charge radius determined from the energy dependence of the neutron transmission of liquid ^{208}Pb and ^{209}Bi, Physical Review C, Vol 56, No.4, 2229-2237, October 1997.

Solving for Weight of an Individual Quadsitron (Qw) and Diameter for an Individual Quadsitron (Qd)

List of Common Variables Utilized in this Text

N = neutron.

P = proton.

E = electron.

Q = quadsitron.

Ve = neutrino

Nw = neutron weight (mass).

Pw = proton weight (mass).

Ew = electron weight (mass).

Vew = anti-neutrino weight (mass).

Qw = quadsitron weight (mass).

a = number of quadsitrons comprising a neutron by weight and volume.

b = number of quadsitrons comprising a proton by weight and volume.

g = number of quadsitrons comprising an electron by weight and volume.

h = number of quadsitrons comprising an anti-neutrino.

Nd = diameter of a neutron.

Nr = radius of a neutron.

Pd = diameter of a proton.

Pr = radius of a proton.

Ed = diameter of an electron.

Er = radius of an electron.

Ved = diameter of an anti-neutrino.

Ver = radius of an anti-neutrino.

Qd = diameter of a quadsitron.

Qr = radius of a quadsitron.

m = number of quadsitrons comprising the diameter of a neutron.

s = number of quadsitrons comprising the diameter of a proton.

t = number of quadsitrons comprising the radius of a proton.

u = number of quadsitrons comprising the diameter of an electron.

U = theoretical number of quadsitrons that would be present in an electron, if an electron were a solid sphere, and if quadsitrons could be packed tightly together with no separation of space.

U' = theoretical number of quadsitrons that would be present in an electron, if an electron were a hollow sphere, and if quadsitrons could be packed tightly together with no intervening space on the surface of the sphere.

U# = theoretical number of quadsitrons that would be present comprising an electron, if an electron were one hollow ring or series of consecutive hallow rings (or spirals).

y = number of quadsitrons comprising the change from neutron to proton.

z = number of quadsitrons comprising the change of neutron to proton minus electron.

Nvol = volume of neutron.

Pvol = volume of a proton.

Evol = volume of an electron.

Qvol = volume of a quadsitron.

Esur = surface area of an electron.

Ecir = circumference of an electron.

Qarea = area taken at the center of a quadsitron

List of Equations

'*' represents the function of multiplication of the two quantities surrounding the symbol.

Neutron weight = Nw = a * Qw

Proton weight = Pw = b * Qw

Electron weight = Ew = g * Qw

Anti-Neutrino weight = Vew = h * Qw

Nw = Pw + Ew + Vew = b * Qw + g * Qw + h * Qw

Change Nw to Pw = Nw − (Pw + Ew + Vew)

Volume sphere = 4/3 * π * r^3

Neutron volume = Nvol = 4/3 * π*(Nd/2)^3

Proton volume = Pvol = 4/3 * π*(Pd/2)^3

Quadsitron volume = 4/3 * π*(Qr) ^{3}

Qr = Qd/2

Quadsitron volume = 4/3 * π*(Qd/2) ^{3}

Change Nd to Pd = m * Qd − s * Qd

Change Nd to Pd = u * Qd + w * Qd

Surface area of a sphere = 4 * π * r^2

Circumference of a circle = 2 * π * r

Area of a circle = π * r^2

Beta Decay of a Neutron = P + E + Ve

List of Known Constants/Quantities

Neutron weight = Nw = 16,749.27471 x 10^{-31} kg (ref 1)

Proton weight = Pw = 16,726.21898 x 10^{-31} kg (ref 1)

Electron weight = Ew = 9.10938356 x 10^{-31} kg (ref 1)

Neutron-Proton mass difference is 1.29 MeV (ref 1)

Kinetic energy of an electron = 0.51 MeV (ref 1)

Maximum kinetic energy Beta Decay of free Neutron = 1.29 MeV- 0.51 MeV = 0.78 Mev (ref 7)

Neutron radius = Nr = $1.113284057367 \times 10^{-15}$ m (ref 2)

Proton radius = Pr = $1.112772961016 \times 10^{-15}$ m (ref 2)

Free neutron root mean square radius = 0.8269×10^{-15} m (ref 5)

Proton root mean square radius = Mainz electron scattering = 0.8775×10^{-15} m (ref 3)

Proton root mean square radius = hydrogen 2S-2P lamb shift = 0.84087×10^{-15} m (ref 3)

Free proton root mean charge square radius = 0.8305 fm (ref 5)

Change in the radius of Nr to Pr = $5.11096351 \times 10^{-19}$ m (ref 2)

Change in the diameter of Nd to Pd = $10.22186352 \times 10^{-19}$ m (ref 2)

Electron radius = Er = $2.8179403227 \times 10^{-15}$ m (ref 1)

Electron radius = $9.087345835484 \times 10^{-17}$ m (ref 2)

Free electron root mean square charge radius = 0.0118 fm (ref 5)

Electron diameter = Ed = 5.63588×10^{-15} m (ref 1)

a0 = Bohr radius = $5.2917721067 \times 10^{-11}$ m (ref 1)

c = speed of light = 2.99792458×10^{8} m/s (ref 1)

π = 3.141592653 (ref 4)

fm = fentimeter = 10^{-15} m

1 electron volt = 1 eV = $1.6021766208 \times 10^{-19}$ joules (ref 1)

1 electron volt divided by the speed of light squared = $1\ eV/C^2$

$1\ eV/c^2 = 1.6021766208 \times 10^{-19}$ joules/$(2.99792458 \times 10^{8}$ m/s$)^2$

$1\ eV/c^2 = 1.782661907 \times 10^{-36}$ kg (ref 1)

Energy = mass multiplied by speed of light squared = m * c^2

Mass of three neutrinos = 0.32 ± 0.081 eV/c^2 (ref 6)

References:

1. CODATA Internationally recommended 2014 values of the Fundamental Physical Constants, Physical Measurement Laboratory of National Institute of Standards and Technology, http://physics.nist.gov/cuu/Constants/index.html

2. On the Radius of the Neutron, Proton, Electron and the Atomic Nucleus, Sha Yin Yue, the General Science Journal, http://www.gsjournal.net/old/physics/yue.pdf

3. Carlson CE, The Proton Radius Puzzle, Physics Department, College of William and Mary, Williamsburg, VA 23187, USA, February 19, 2015 https://arxiv.org/pdf/1502.05314.pdf

4. Wilson D, The History of Pi https://www.math.rutgers. edu/~cherlin/History/Papers2000/wilson.html

5. Storti RC, Desiato TJ, Derivation of Fundamental Particle Radii: Electron, Proton, and Neutron, April 10, 2015. http://documents.mx/documents/derivation-of-fundamental-particle-radii-electron-proton-neutron.html

6. Battye RA, Moss A, Evidence for Massive Neutrinos from Cosmic Microwave Background and Lensing Observations, Phys. Rev. Lett. 112, 051303, 6 February 2014, http://journals.aps.org/prl/abstract/10.1103/PhysRevLett.112.051303

7. Nuclear Physics, PHY303, Solution 2, http://physics-database.group.shef.ac.uk/phy303/303soltn2.html

STEP #1 Solve for Weight of One Neutrino:

It is deduced that a neutrino represents two quadsitrons. The two quadsitrons are configured to trap energy between three of the poles of the two quadsitrons. The weight of a single quadsitron is half of the weight of a neutrino.

Energy = mass multiplied by speed of light squared = $m * c^2$

Mass of three neutrinos = 0.32 ± 0.081 eV/c^2

Approximate mass of one neutrino = 0.1066 eV/c^2

1 eV/c^2 = 1.782661907 x 10^{-36} kg (ref 1)

Mass (kilograms) of 3 neutrinos = (0.32 eV/c^2 * 1.782661907 x 10^{-36} kg/ eV/c^2)

Mass (kilograms) of 3 neutrinos = 0.57045181024 x 10^{-36} kg

Mass (kilograms) of 1 neutrinos or 1 anti-neutrino = 0.57045181024 x 10^{-36} kg / 3

Mass (kilograms) of 1 neutrino or 1 anti-neutrino = 1.90150603413 x 10^{-37} kg.

STEP #2 Solve for Weight of Quadsitron (Qw):

Antineutrino weight (kg) = Vew = 1.90150603413 x 10^{-37} kg

It is theorized that two quadsitrons combine to trap energy. Two quadsitrons make up a neutrino or anti-neutrino.

Qw is ½ the size of an anti-neutrino = 1.90150603413 x 10^{-37} kg / 2

The weight of a quadsitron is 9.507530170666 x 10^{-38} kg.

STEP #3 Solve for Number of Quadsitrons Comprising a Neutron designated variable 'a':

Knowing the weight of a single quadsitron, and utilizing the weight of a known neutron, the number of quadsitrons present in a neutron can be calculated.

Neutron weight = Nw = 16,749.27471 x 10^{-31} kg

Neutron weight = Nw = 1.674927471 x 10^{-27} kg

Weight of a quadsitron = Qw = 9.5075301706 x 10^{-38} kg

Nw = a * Qw

a = Nw / Qw

a = 1.674927471 x 10^{-27} kg / 9.5075301706 x 10^{-38} kg

a = 1.7616851495 x 10^{10}

Number of Quadsitrons comprising a Neutron using Nw and Qw is 1.7616851495 x 10^{10}.

STEP #4 Solve for Number of Quadsitrons Comprising a Proton designated variable 'b':

Knowing the weight of a single quadsitron, and utilizing the known weight of a proton, the number of quadsitrons present in a proton can be calculated.

Proton weight = Pw = 16,726.21898 x 10^{-31} kg

Proton weight = Pw = 1.672621898 x 10^{-27} kg

Weight of a quadsitron = Qw = 9.5075301706 x 10^{-38} kg

Pw = b * Qw

b = Pw / Qw

b = 1.672621898 x 10^{-27} kg / 9.5075301706 x 10^{-38} kg

b = 1.7592601527 x 10^{10}

Number of Quadsitrons comprising a Proton using Pw and Qw is 1.7592601527 x 10^{10}.

STEP #5 Solve for Neutron Volume:

The radius of a neutron is taken from the calculated value from reference 2 as Nr = 1.113284057367 x 10^{-15} m. Approximating that a neutron is in the shape of a sphere, utilizing the radius of a neutron, the volume of a neutron can be calculated.

Neutron volume = Nvol = a * Qvol = 4/3 * π * (Nr)^3

Radius of a neutron = Nr = 1.113284057367 x 10^{-15} m

Neutron Volume = 4.18879020 * (1.113284057367 x 10^{-15} m)^3

Neutron Volume = 4.18879020 * 1.379805810823 x 10^{-45} m^3

Neutron Volume = 5.779717058280 x 10^{-45} m^3.

STEP #6 Solve for Proton Volume:

The radius of a proton is from the calculated value from reference 2 as Pr = 1.112772961016 x 10^{-15} m. Approximating that a proton is in the shape of a sphere, utilizing the radius of a proton, the volume of a proton can be calculated.

Proton volume = Pvol = b * Qvol = 4/3 * π * (Pr)^3

Radius of a proton = Pr = 1.112772961016 x 10^{-15} m

Proton Volume = 4.18879020 * (1.112772961016 x 10^{-15} m)^3

Proton Volume = 4.18879020 * 1.377906322537 x 10^{-45} m^3

Proton Volume = 5.771760500361 x 10^{-45} m^3.

STEP #7 Solve for Change in Neutron Volume to Proton Volume:

If a neutron is approximated to be a sphere and a proton is a sphere, and if the neutron is larger by volume than a proton, the change in volume of a neutron during a Beta decay to a proton can be calculated.

Change in Neutron Volume to Proton Volume = Nvol - Pvol

Neutron Volume to Proton Volume = $5.779717058280 \times 10^{-45}$ m³ - $5.771760500361 \times 10^{-45}$ m³

Change in Neutron Volume to Proton Volume = $7.956557919 \times 10^{-48}$ m³.

Change in volume when a free neutron decays to a proton is $7.956557919 \times 10^{-48}$ m³ *.

*Using the radius of a neutron = Nr = $1.113284057367 \times 10^{-15}$ m and radius of a proton = Pr = $1.112772961016 \times 10^{-15}$ m.

STEP #8 Solve for Diameter of a Quadsitron (Qd) by Means of Nvol:

A neutron is approximated to be in the shape of a sphere. A quadsitron, has four poles with each pole separated by 120 degrees and equiradius from the center of the quadsitron. Given the four poles are equiradius from the center of the quadsitron, the diameter of a quadsitron can be approximated by treating the quadsitron as if it were a sphere. In fact, a quadsitron may be likened to a sphere with four poles. Treating the quadsitron as a sphere allows for the calculation of the gross approximate volume of a quadsitron. Knowing the number of quadsitrons present in a neutron as calculated by weight allows to solve for the diameter of a quadsitron.

Nvol = a * Qvol

a = Nvol / Qvol = Nw / Qw = $1.7616851495 \times 10^{10}$

$Qvol = Nvol / a$

$Qvol = 4/3 * \pi * (Qr)^3$

$Qvol = 4/3 * \pi * (Qd/2)^3$

$Qd = (\sqrt[3]{\left(Qvol * \dfrac{3}{4}\right) / \pi}) * 2$

$Qd = (\sqrt[3]{\left(\left(\dfrac{Nvol}{a}\right) * \dfrac{3}{4}\right) / \pi}) * 2$

$Qd = (\sqrt[3]{\dfrac{\dfrac{4}{3} * \pi * (Nr)\char94 3 * \dfrac{3}{4}}{\pi * a}}) * 2$

$Qd = (\sqrt[3]{(Nr)\char94 3 / a}) * 2$

$a = 1.7616851495 \times 10^{10} = 1.7616851495 \times 10\char94 10$

$Nr = 1.113284057367 \times 10^{-15}$ m $= 1.113284057367 \times 10\char94 \text{-}15$ m (ref 2)

$(Nr)^3 = (Nr)\char94 3 = 1.379805810823 \times 10^{-45}$ m^3

$Qd = (\sqrt[3]{(Nr)\char94 3 / 1.7616851495 \times 10\char94 10}) * 2$

$Qd = (\sqrt[3]{(1.113284057367 \times 10\char94{-15} \text{ m})\char94 3 / 1.7616851495 \times 10\char94 10}) * 2$

$Qd = (\sqrt[3]{1.379805810823 \times 10\char94{-45} \text{ m}\char94 3 / 1.7616851495 \times 10\char94 10}) * 2$

$Qd = (\sqrt[3]{78.323065345394 \times 10\char94{-57} \text{ m}\char94 3}) * 2$

$Qd = 4.278549479083791 \times 10^{-19}$ m $* 2$

$Qd = 8.557098958167 \times 10^{-19}$ m

Diameter of a quadsitron using Nvol is $8.557098958167 \times 10^{-19}$ m

$Qr = 4.278549479083791 \times 10^{-19}$ m

Radius of a quadsitron using Nvol is $4.278549479083791 \times 10^{-19}$ m

STEP #9 Solve for Diameter of a Quadsitron (Qd) by Means of Pvol:

A proton is approximated to be in the shape of a sphere. A quadsitron, has four poles with each pole separated by 120 degrees and equiradius from the center of the quadsitron. Given the four poles are equiradius from the center of the quadsitron, the diameter of a quadsitron can be approximated by treating the quadsitron as if it were a sphere. Treating the quadsitron as a sphere allows for the calculation of the gross approximate volume of a quadsitron. Knowing the number of quadsitrons present in a proton as calculated by weight allows to solve for the diameter of a quadsitron.

$Pvol = b * Qvol$

$b = Pvol / Qvol = Pw / Qw = b = 1.7592601527 \times 10^{10}$

$Qvol = 4/3 * \pi * (Qr)^3$

$Qvol = 4/3 * \pi * (Qd/2)^3$

$$Qd = (\sqrt[3]{\left(Qvol * \frac{3}{4}\right) / \pi}) * 2$$

$$Qd = (\sqrt[3]{\left(\left(\frac{Pvol}{b}\right) * \frac{3}{4}\right) / \pi}) * 2$$

$$Qd = (\sqrt[3]{\frac{\frac{4}{3} * \pi * (Pr)^{\wedge}3 * \frac{3}{4}}{\pi * b}}) * 2$$

$$Qd = (\sqrt[3]{(Pr)^{\wedge}3 / b}) * 2$$

$b = 1.7592601527 \times 10^{10} = 1.7592601527 \times 10^{\wedge}10$

$Pr = 1.112772961016 \times 10^{-15}$ m $= 1.112772961016 \times 10^{\wedge}-15$ m (ref 2)

$(Pr)^3 = 1.377906322537 \times 10^{-45}$ m³ $= 1.377906322537 \times 10^{\wedge}-45$ m³

$$Qd = (\sqrt[3]{(Pr)3 / 1.7592601527 \times 10^{\wedge}10}) * 2$$

Qd $= (\sqrt[3]{(1.112772961016 \times 10^{-15}\ m)3}\ /\ 1.7592601527 \times 10^{10})*\ 2$

Qd $= (\sqrt[3]{1.377906322537 \times 10^{-45}\ m3}\ /\ 1.7592601527 \times 10^{10})*\ 2$

Qd $= (\sqrt[3]{78.323056452013 \times 10^{-57}\ m3})*\ 2$

Qd = 4.278549317144 x 10^{-19} m * 2

Qd = 8.557098634288 x 10^{-19} m

Diameter of a quadsitron using Pvol is 8.557098634288 x 10^{-19} m

Qr = 4.278549317144 x 10^{-19} m

Radius of a quadsitron using Pvol is 4.278549317144 x 10^{-19} m

Calculated radius of a quadsitron per Nvol and Pvol are equal to 4.278549 x 10^{-19} m.

Calculated diameter of a quadsitron per Nvol and Pvol equal to 8.557098 x 10^{-19} m.

STEP #10 Solving for Energy Anti-Neutrino (Ve) in Beta Decay of Free Neutron using Qw:

The known resultant kinetic energy of an electron in the Beta decay of a free neutron is 0.51 MeV. The known kinetic energy of an anti-neutrino in the Beta decay of a free neutron is 1.29 MeV - 0.51 MeV to equal 0.78 MeV Utilizing the weight of a quadsitron, the kinetic energy associated with an anti-neutrino should be calculable. To do this, first the number of quadsitrons associated with an electron is determined by taking the weight of the electron and dividing by the weight of a single quadsitron. Then the number of quadsitrons associated with the change in weight of a neutron decaying to a proton is determined by taking the weight associated with the change in weight of a neutron to a proton and dividing this number by the weight of a single quadsitron. Taking the number of quadsitrons associated with the change in weight of a neutron to a proton and subtracting the number of quadsitrons associated with an electron results in the number of quadsitrons associated with the energy of the anti-neutrino in the Beta decay of a free neutron.

Known energy of a electron = 0.51 MeV

Known quantity is Beta decay of a free neutron is = 1.29 MeV = 0.51 MeV + 0.78 MeV

$E_w = g * Q_w$, where g is the number of quadsitrons comprising an electron

$Q_w = 9.5075301706 \times 10^{-38}$ kg

$E_w = 9.10938356 \times 10^{-31}$ kg (ref 1)

$g = E_w / Q_w$

$g = 9.10938356 \times 10^{-31}$ kg $/ 9.50753017 \times 10^{-38}$ kg

$g = 9.581230 \times 10^{6}$

Change in weight N_w to $P_w = 23.05573 \times 10^{-31}$ kg

y = Number quadsitrons N_w to $P_w / Q_w = 23.05573 \times 10^{-31}$ kg $/ 9.5075301706 \times 10^{-38}$ kg

y = Number quadsitrons in N_w to $P_w = 2.4249967 \times 10^{7}$

z = Number of quadsitrons following removal of electron = $y - g$

z = Number of quadsitrons removal of electron = $2.4249967 \times 10^{7} - 9.581230 \times 10^{6}$

z = Number of quadsitrons following removal of electron = 1.4668737×10^{7}

Energy of antineutrino in Beta Decay = $V_e = z * Q_w$

$V_e = z * Q_w$

$V_e = 1.4668737 \times 10^{7} * 9.5075301706 \times 10^{-38}$ kg

Ve = 13.946345959 x 10^{-31} kg

mass = 1.782661907 x 10^{-36} kg / 1 eV/c^2

Energy result of Beta Decay = Ve / mass conversion

Energy of Beta Decay = 13.946345959 x 10^{-31} kg / 1.782661907 x 10^{-36} kg / 1 eV/c^2

Energy result of Beta Decay = 0.78233263999 x 10^6 eV/c^2

Energy result of Beta Decay by using Qw is 0.78233263999 MeV/c^2.

Energy result of Beta Decay by using Qw is 0.782533263999 MeV/c^2, which is similar to the published measured value assigned to the anti-neutrino of the Beta decay of a free neutron, which is 0.78 MeV/c^2.

STEP #11 Solve for Number of Quadsitrons Comprising a Neutron designated variable 'a':

Neutron Volume = 5.77971705828 x 10^{-45} m^3

Quadsitron volume = Qvol = 4/3 * π * $(Qd/2)^3$

Qvol = 4/3 * π * $(8.557098958167$ x 10^{-19} m/2$)^3$

Qvol = 4/3 * π * $(4.278549479083$ x 10^{-19} m$)^3$

Qvol = 3.280788888658 x 10^{-55} m^3

a = Nvol / Qvol

a = 5.77971705828 x 10^{-45} m^3 / 3.280788888658 x 10^{-55} m^3

a = 1.7616851478 x 10^{10}

Number of quadsitrons present in volume of Neutron = 1.7616851478 x 10^{10}.

Neutron weight = Nw = 16,749.27471 x 10^{-31} kg

Quadsitron weight = Qw = 9.507530170666 x 10^{-38} kg

Nw = a * Qw

a = Nw / Qw

a = 1.674927471 x 10^{-27} kg / 9.507530170666 x 10^{-38} kg

a = 1.7616851494 x 10^{10}

Number of Quadsitrons comprising a Neutron using Nw and Qw is 1.7616851494 x 10^{10}

The number of quadsitrons calculated by volume and calculated by weight for a neutron are both equal at 1.76168514 x 10^{10}.

STEP #12 Solve for Number of Quadsitrons Comprising a Proton designated variable 'b':

Proton Volume = 5.771760500361 x 10^{-45} m^3

Qvol = 3.280788888658 x 10^{-55} m^3

Proton Volume = Pvol = b * Qvol

b = Pvol / Qvol

b = 5.771760500361 x 10^{-45} m^3 / 3.280788888658 x 10^{-55} m^3

b = 1.7592599513 x 10^{10}

Number of quadsitrons present in volume of Proton = 1.7592599513 x 10^{10}.

Proton weight = Pw = 16,726.21898 x 10^{-31} kg

Quadsitron weight = Qw = 9.507530170666 x 10^{-38} kg

$Pw = b * Qw$

$b = Pw / Qw$

$b = 1.672621898 \times 10^{-27}$ kg $/ 9.507530170666 \times 10^{-38}$ kg

$b = 1.7592601527 \times 10^{10}$

Number of Quadsitrons comprising a Proton using Pw and Qw is $1.7592601527 \times 10^{10}$.

The number of quadsitrons calculated by volume and calculated by weight for a proton are both equal at 1.75926×10^{10}.

STEP #13 Solve for Number Quadsitrons in Change in Neutron Volume to Proton Volume:

The number of quadsitrons associated with the change in weight when a free neutron undergoes Beta decay to a proton was calculated previously. Here the number of quadsitrons associated with the change in volume when a free neutron undergoes Beta decay to a proton is calculated using the derived diameter of a quadsitron. The number of quadsitrons associated with change of a free neutron to a proton during Beta decay calculated by change in weight should equal the number of quadsitrons associated with change of a free neutron to a proton during Beta decay calculated by volume. First quadsitron volume is calculated using the derived diameter of a quadsitron.

Neutron Volume $= 5.77971705828 \times 10^{-45}$ m^3

Proton Volume $= 5.771760500361 \times 10^{-45}$ m^3

Qvol $= 3.280788888658 \times 10^{-55}$ m^3

Change in Neutron Volume to Proton Volume = Nvol - Pvol

Neutron Volume to Proton Volume = $5.77971693 \times 10^{-45}$ m^3 - $5.77176048 \times 10^{-45}$ m^3

Change in Neutron Volume to Proton Volume = $7.956557919 \times 10^{-48}$ m^3

Number of quadsitrons present in change in volume of Neutron Volume to Proton Volume = (Nvol − Pvol) / Qvol

Number of quadsitrons present in change in volume of Neutron Volume to Proton Volume = $7.956557919 \times 10^{-48}$ m^3 / $3.280788888658 \times 10^{-55}$ m^3.

Number of quadsitrons present in change in volume of Neutron Volume to Proton Volume = y = 2.4251966×10^7.

Neutron weight = Nw = $16,749.27471 \times 10^{-31}$ kg

Proton weight = Pw = $16,726.21898 \times 10^{-31}$ kg

Quadsitron weight = Qw = $9.507530170666 \times 10^{-38}$ kg

Change in Neutron weight to Proton Weight = Nw − Pw = y * Qw

y = (Nw − Pw) / Qw

y = ($1.674927471 \times 10^{-27}$ kg − $1.672621898 \times 10^{-27}$ kg) / $9.507530170666 \times 10^{-38}$ kg

y = (23.05573×10^{-31} kg) / $9.507530170666 \times 10^{-38}$ kg

y = 2.4249968×10^7

The number of quadsitrons calculated by volume and calculated by weight for the change of a neutron to a proton are both approximately equal to 2.425×10^7.

STEP #14 Solve for Change in Radius of a Neutron to Proton

During Beta decay of a neutron, the neutron transforms into a proton.

Change in Radius of a Neutron to Proton = Nr – Pr

Nr – Pr = 11,132.84057367 x 10^{-19} m – 11,127.72960 x 10^{-19} m

Nr – Pr = 5.11096351 x 10^{-19} m

Change in the radius of a Neutron to a Proton is 5.11096351 x 10^{-19} m.

STEP #15 Solve for Number of Quadsitrons in the Radius of a Proton

Proton radius = t * Qd

Pr = t * Qd

Number quadsitrons in radius of proton = t = Pr/Qd

t = Pr/Qd = 11,127.72926 x 10^{-19} m/8.557098 x 10^{-19} m

t = Pr/Qd = 1,300.40923

Number of Quadsitrons comprising the radius of a Proton is 1,300.31626 or simplified 1,300.

STEP #16 Solve for Number of Neutrinos in the Radius of a Proton

Two quadsitrons comprise a neutrino.

Neutrinos comprising the radius of a proton = t/2

t/2 = 1300/2

Number of neutrinos in the radius of a proton is 650.

STEP #17 Solve for the Number of Quadsitrons Available to Comprise an Electron

$Ew = 9.10938356 \times 10^{-31}$ kg

The weight of a quadsitron is $9.5075301706 \times 10^{-38}$ kg

$Ew = g \times Qw$

$g = Ew / Qw$

$g = 9.10938356 \times 10^{-31}$ kg $/ 9.5075301706 \times 10^{-38}$ kg

$g = 9.581230 \times 10^{6}$

The number of quadsitrons available by weight to comprise an electron is 9.581230×10^{6}.

STEP #18 Solve for the Number of Quadsitrons That Would Comprise Electron Volume if an Electron Were a Solid Sphere

Electron radius $= Er = 2.81794 \times 10^{-15}$ m

$Evol = U * Qvol$

where U is the theoretical number of quadsitrons that would be present in an electron, if an electron were a solid sphere, and if quadsitrons could be packed tightly together with no separation of space.

Volume of an electron $= Evol = 4/3 * \pi * (Er)^3$

$Evol = 4/3 * \pi * (2.81794 \times 10^{-15}$ m$)^3$

$Evol = 93.731126080 \times 10^{-45}$ m^3

$Qr = 4.2785494790 \times 10^{-19}$ m

Volume of a quadsitron = Qvol = $4/3 * \pi * (Qr)^3$

Qvol = $4/3 * \pi * (Qr = 4.278549479 \times 10^{-19}$ m$)^3$

Qvol = $3.280788888658 \times 10^{-55}$ m^3

U = Evol / Qvol

U = $93.731126080 \times 10^{-45}$ m^3 / $3.280788888658 \times 10^{-55}$ m^3

U = $28.56969139466 \times 10^{10}$ quadsitrons

The number of quadsitrons by weight calculated to comprise an electron is 9.581230×10^6. To create a solid sphere the number of quadsitrons needed would be $28.56969139466 \times 10^{10}$, Therefore, an electron cannot be a solid sphere comprised of quadsitron derived from the resultant mass change of the neutron decaying to a proton. There is an insufficient number of quadsitrons generated by a neutron decaying to a proton to create a solid sphere the size of an electron.

STEP #19 Solve for the Number of Quadsitrons That Would Comprise Electron Volume if an Electron Were the Surface Shell of a Sphere

Electron radius = Er = 2.81794×10^{-15} m

Surface area of an electron = Esur = U' * Qarea

where U' is the theoretical number of quadsitrons that would be present in an electron, if an electron were a hollow sphere, and if quadsitrons could be packed tightly together with no intervening space on the surface of the sphere.

Surface of an electron = Esur= $4 * \pi * (Er)^2$

Esur = $4 * \pi * (Er)^2$

Esur = 4 * π * (2.81794 x 10⁻¹⁵ m)²

$Esur = 4 * \pi * (2.81794 \times 10^{-15} \text{ m})^2$

$Esur = 9.978685786 \times 10^{-29} \text{ m}^2$

$Qr = 4.2785494790 \times 10^{-19} \text{ m}$

Area taken at center of a quadsitron = $Qarea = \pi * (Qr)^2$

$Qarea = \pi * (4.2785494790 \times 10^{-19} \text{ m})^2$

$Qarea = 5.75099500059 \times 10^{-37} \text{ m}^2$

$U' = Esur / Qarea$

$U' = 9.978685786 \times 10^{-29} \text{ m}^2 / 5.75099500059 \times 10^{-37} \text{ m}^2$

$U' = 1.735123362996 \times 10^8$ quadsitrons

The number of quadsitrons by weight calculated to comprise an electron is 9.581230×10^6. To create a hollow sphere the number of quadsitrons needed would be $1.735123362996 \times 10^8$, Therefore, an electron cannot be a hollow sphere comprised of quadsitrons derived from the resultant mass change of the neutron decaying to a proton. There is an insufficient number of quadsitrons generated by a neutron decaying to a proton to create a hollow sphere the size of an electron.

STEP #20 Solve for the Number of Quadsitrons That Would Comprise Electron Volume if an Electron Were a Series of Hollow Rings

Electron radius = $Er = 2.81794 \times 10^{-15}$ m

Circumference of an electron = $Ecir = 2 * \pi * Er$

where $U^\#$ is the theoretical number of quadsitrons that would be present comprising an electron, if an electron were one hollow ring:

$Ecir = 2 * \pi * (2.81794 \times 10^{-15} \text{ m})$

$Ecir = 17.7056392011 \times 10^{-15} \text{ m}$

$Ecir = 1.77056392011 \times 10^{-14} \text{ m}$

$Qd = 8.557098 \times 10^{-19} \text{ m}$

$U^{\#} = Ecir / Qd$

$U^{\#} = 1.77056392011 \times 10^{-14} \text{ m} / 8.557098 \times 10^{-19} \text{ m}$

$U^{\#} = 20,690$ quadsitrons

The number of quadsitrons by weight calculated to comprise an electron is 9.581230×10^{6}. To create a single hollow ring, the number of quadsitrons needed would be 20,690 quadsitrons, Therefore, an electron cannot be one hollow ring.

Number of hollow rings = 9,581,230 / 20,690

Number of hollow rings = 463.085 hollow rings

An electron could be comprised of 463 hollow rings.

If an electron is comprised of 463 hollow rings (or spiral rings similar to a coil), then an electron is 463 * diameter of a quadsitron = 463 * 8.557098×10^{-19} m = $3.96193637 \times 10^{-16}$ m in length while having a circular radius of 2.81794×10^{-15} m.

Discussion

With regards to the above calculations the weight of a quadsitron is $9.5075301706 \times 10^{-38}$ kg, and the diameter of a quadsitron is 8.557098×10^{-19} m per the above calculations. As a note, alternatively, if Sha Yin Yue's calculations for the diameter of a neutron and proton are adjusted specifically to the constants used in the above calculations, then the diameter of a single quadsitron would be calculated per both volume of a neutron and volume of a proton means to be $8.557941465 \times 10^{\wedge}{-19}$ m.

A neutrino is theorized to be composed of two quadsitrons. One quadsitron on the left side projects a negative pole toward the left sided end of the neutrino, with its positive, neutral and absolute zero poles pointed toward the inside of the neutrino. The second quadsitron on the right projects its positive pole at the opposite end of the neutrino, with its negative, neutral and absolute zero poles pointed toward the inside of the neutrino. Inside the neutrino, the positive pole of the left neutrino attaches to the negative pole of the right neutrino, while the neutral pole and absolute zero poles of each quadsitron attach to each other. See Figure 79. Cradled inside the inside of the two quadsitrons that comprise a neutrino is a quantity of energy. The amount of energy trapped inside the core of the neutrino equal to 0.1066 eV/c². The amount of weight of the two quadsitrons, which combine to create a neutrino, is 1.90150603413 x 10⁻³⁷ kg.

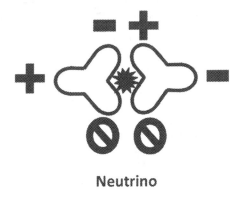

Neutrino

Figure 79 Illustration of a neutrino

A proton is theorized to be a sphere comprised of a volume of 1.75926 x 10¹⁰ quadsitrons. The radius of the proton is comprised of 1300 quadsitrons. A proton is theorized to be comprised of a sphere of neutrinos. At the center of a proton is Dark Matter. The entity of Dark Matter is comprised of two neutrons oriented with the absolute zero pole pointed outward and a quanta of energy trapped in-between the two quadsitrons. See Figure 80.

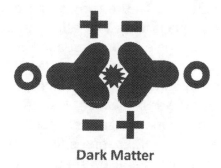

Dark Matter

Figure 80 Illustration of a Dark Matter

The radius of a proton would be 650 neutrinos. Within a proton, the neutrinos would have their negative pole directed toward the center of the proton and their positive pole pointed toward the exterior of the proton.

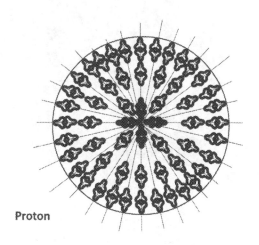

Proton

Figure 81 Concept drawing of a proton comprised
of quadsitrons (configured as neutrinos)

A neutron is comprised of a volume of $1.76168514 \times 10^{10}$ quadsitrons. A neutron is theorized to be a sphere with a radius of 1301 quadsitrons. The difference is the radius of a neutron and the radius of a proton is only $5.11096351 \times 10^{-19}$ m. This difference in the radius of a neutron and the radius of a proton is smaller than the diameter of a quadsitron, which is 8.557098×10^{-19} m by sixty percent of the diameter of a quadsitron. The reason of the discrepancy is that the exterior layer of quadsitrons that attach to the exterior of the proton are a shell of single layer of quadsitrons that fit onto the exposed positive end of the neutrinos on the surface of the proton. The neutrinos on the surface of the proton project their positive pole into space. The layer of quadsitrons that cover the layer of neutrinos to make a proton a neutron project their neutral pole into space. Due to the angle of 120 degrees that separates each of the four poles of a quadsitron, this allows a quadsitron to sit on top of another quadsitron, with a forty percent by volume overlap of the two quadsitrons. See Figure 82.

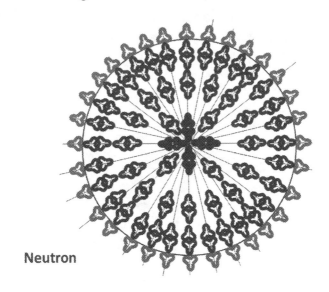

Neutron

Figure 82 Concept of a neutron as a proton with
a layer of quadsitrons covering the surface

In Figure 83, the concept of Beta Decay is illustrated with the most exterior layer of quadsitrons separating from the body of the underlying proton.

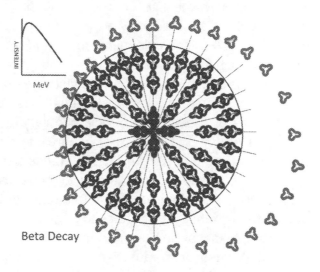

Figure 83 Exterior layer of quadsitrons separating
from the neutron to produce a proton

Note, the graph of Beta decay of a Neutron included in Figure 83 demonstrates an initial up rise of energy to a peak, then a gradual decline in energy as the process completes the transformation from neutron to proton. If the neutron exists as a three dimensional ball, then the process of Beta decay can be thought of similar to removing the outer skin of an orange. As the orange peel is peeled away from the surface of the fruit, by hand with an instrument such as a spoon, generally the process of removing the skin starts at a point, then spreads across the surface till a peak amount of the peel is removed, then the process is continued until the remainder of the peel has been separated from the orange. The process of Beta decay of a neutron may start a one point on the surface of the neutron and progress across the three dimensional surface of the neutron until the single outer layer of quadsitrons is shed and the resulting proton emerges from inside the neutron.

Conclusion

The Michelson-Morley experiment of 1887, may have been flawed in its approach to disavow the existence of an ether. The overall observation is that objects are solid. Instead, all atoms are comprised mostly of space, therefore most molecules are comprised mostly of space. To an object such as a quadsitron measuring Qd = 8.557098 x 10^{-19} m, Bohr's radius 5.291772 x 10^{-11} m, the distance between the nucleus and the electron of a hydrogen atoms is quite substantial compared to the size of a quadsitron. As a corollary, the Earth's diameter is 6,378.1 km or 6.3781x 10^6 m, where the distance of the Earth to the Sun is 1.49 x 10^{11} m. The difference between the diameter of a quadsitron and the radius of a hydrogen atom is in the magnitude of 10^8. The difference in the diameter of the Earth and the distance to the sun is in the magnitude of 10^5. Most would believe there is a substantial amount of open space between the Earth and the Sun. A gross macro assessment of the existence of a cosmic wind would be inaccurate. Therefore, to accurately disavow the presence of an ether, one must be prepared to measure the presence of a cosmic wind as such a wind interacts with the surface of a proton or the surface of a neutron comprising the nucleus of an atom.

The universe is fundamentally about energy flow and the trapping of energy. Gravity and magnetism are simply the physical results of energy flow through quadsitrons and energy trapping by quadsitrons. Quadsitrons make up the fabric of the universe. We believe sound waves occur because air molecules or water molecules are caused to vibrate at various frequencies in the sound spectrum. We believe air or water act as the medium to propagate sound waves. But then consider the Planck constant. The Planck constant (6.62607004 x 10^-34 m^2 kg/s), the physical constant that is the quantum of action, remains the same across the electromagnetic spectrum, whether considering low energy waves or high energy waves. Sound, a lower energy wave, is considered to be propagated due to air or water and light, a higher energy wave, is considered to have no medium that causes it to transfer from one location to another. The obvious question is, how does the Planck constant adequately describe both low energy waves such as sound and high-energy waves such as light and microwaves when there is an obvious change in the medium that transfers the waves from one location to another. The clear answer is that there is a consistent medium, that being quadsitrons, which is responsible for the propagation of energy from one location in the universe to another location in the universe. Being neither created nor destroyed, energy waves travel through the fabric of quadsitrons in the universe and through all objects unless the energy is reflected or trapped by either the quadsitrons, the atoms, the molecules or the macrostructure of the object. Breaking down of the macrostructure or the molecule or the atom or a neutrino into separate quadsitrons releases trapped energy.

The concept of a ubiquitous underlying fabric of the universe comprised of quadsitrons as the building block of all matter, creates the pathway to design anti-gravity engines to replace combustion engines, create engines for speed of light space travel and design means of portable magnetic fields powerful enough to protect humans and other organic matter during the course of space travel.

POST SCRIPT 7

NEW FRONTIERS IN MEDICAL MANAGEMENT OF OSTEOARTHRITIS

Osteoarthritis is generally associated with the degenerative wear of the cartilage surface of joints. Cartilage acts to protect the ends of the bone and the rounded polished-like surface of the cartilage results in smooth movement of joints. Chondrocytes embedded under the surface of cartilage generate a protein matrix that comprises the cartilage. Degenerative changes involving the joints is most often assumed to be related to aging processes that occur as the body grows older. Joints that incur serious injury can accelerate the process of degenerative changes to the cartilage and lead to premature osteoarthritis involving an injured joint.

Osteoarthritis or degenerative arthritis is a chronic debilitating condition involving the joints. Approximately 46 million people in the United States,[1] or 10 to 12% of the adult population, have symptomatic osteoarthritis.[2-4] Recent estimates suggest that knee osteoarthritis affects approximately 250 million people worldwide.[5]

Osteoarthritis is generally considered the result of the articular cartilage of the joints wearing out. The prevailing opinion has been that the 1.6 mm of cartilage covering the distal surface of bones of the knee including the femur, the posterior surface of the patella and the tibia plateau in essence remains the same over a person's lifetime. Degenerative arthritis is generally presumed to occur when the 1.6 mm of cartilage covering the ends of the bone eventually succumbs to the mechanical stresses generated by ambulation and deteriorates, frays, breaks down, and wears off.

If a person lives to 90 years of age, in their lifetime they will walk an estimated 110,000 miles. The circumference of the earth is 24,901 miles, which implies a person who reaches 90 years old would have walked the equivalent of more than four times around the earth in their lifetime. In contrast to presuming the same 1.6 mm of cartilage exists over the lifetime of an individual, an automotive car tire wears from 8 mm thickness to 1.6 mm thickness over the course of approximately 30,000 miles of travel; a car tire is generally considered unsafe at a thickness of 1.6 mm or less and is usually replaced.

An emerging consciousness is that the articular surface of cartilage is not a static process, but represents a dynamic or active process. Chondrocytes most likely sense the utilization and degradation of the cartilage across the articular surface and replace cartilage as appropriate. At certain points due to injury or other stressor, the chondrocytes are not able to maintain an appropriate supply of cartilage production, and breakdown of the cartilage covering the surface of the bone occurs in one or more joints. It has been shown that presence of osteoarthritis is associated with the up-regulation of pro-inflammatory cytokines and chemokines.[6] Pro-inflammatory cytokines and chemokines result in cell death of chondrocytes and degradation of cartilage. It is theorized that if the pro-inflammatory cytokines and chemokines could be neutralized then chondrocytes might be able to generate enough cartilage to repair and rejuvenate the articular surface of a joint that had suffered osteoarthritis.

To maintain a thickness of 1.6 mm of cartilage over the course of 110,000 miles of ambulation, it would seem that the cartilage would need to be slowly and precisely replaced over the lifetime of an individual. By necessity, it would seem that chondrocytes residing in the periarticular region of the knee would need to slowly generate replacement cartilage to replace the cartilage surface damaged by the combined stresses of compressive forces and tangential friction forces that occur across the surface of the knee with ambulation. As an approximation, if an automotive tire loses 6.4 mm of cartilage over 30,000 miles, then a human could generate and wear of 23.47 mm of cartilage over the 110,000 miles of ambulation in a patient's lifetime. During the course of 89 years of time at 365 days/year this results in 32,485 days, which translates into an average loss of 7.2249×10^{-3} mm cartilage a day. In other words, collectively for each articular surface in the knee joint, the chondrocytes associated with the articular surface of each bone would need to generate 7.2249 x 10^{-3} mm of cartilage per day in some locations of the knee in order to prevent excessive wear, if the wear pattern of the articular cartilage is similar to the wear pattern of a vehicle tire. Therefore, it would take an interval of 1385 days (or 3.79 years) of repair in order to replace 1.0 mm of cartilage on the surface of the bones in the knee.

The mean difference between cartilage per MRI study versus histologic comparison has been shown to be 10%. If cartilage is 1.6 mm in thickness, then MRI difference would be 0.16 mm change. In order to appropriately measure a true change in cartilage, the tissues would have to grow to more than 0.16 mm, which by the above-mentioned analogy would take approximately 222 days. Thus for a 0.25 ± 0.025 mm change in cartilage due to repair of the cartilage it would take 346.25 days; for a 0.50 ± 0.05 mm change in cartilage it would take 692.5 days; for a 0.75 ± 0.075 mm change in cartilage it would take an estimated 1,038.75 days.

Thus any prospective study of the cartilage where MRI technology is utilized to define measureable improvement in cartilage may need to be almost four years in duration regarding patient follow up in order to appreciate a true repair of the cartilage surface of the knee.

Study of the biochemistry of human joints demonstrates that compressive forces generate TNF-alpha and interleukin-1beta (IL-1β). The synovitis in OA is quantitatively milder but qualitatively very similar to synovitis in rheumatoid arthritis.[7] The presence of pro-inflammatory cytokines and chemokines including TNF-alpha, IL-1β, IL-6, IL-8 and IL-17 have been implicated in OA and appear to activate transcription of nuclear factor kB (NF-kB). NF-kB regulates the expression of many cytokines, chemokines, adhesion molecules, inflammatory mediators and several matrix-degrading enzymes, including metalloproteinases.[8] TNF-alpha becomes a potential therapeutic target in the medical management of OA.

TNF-alpha appears to generate several affects that are deleterious to cartilage including causing an increase in the death rate of chondrocytes and up-regulating production of metalloproteinases. Molecules such as metalloproteinases serve to breakdown cartilage.

TNF alpha is expressed not only in aging cartilage, but also in joints that have incurred injury. It has been long recognized that in the adult years, if a joint is seriously injured, there is a high likelihood the joint will undergo premature degenerative changes. Inhibiting TNF alpha activity when a joint shows signs of aging and/or at the time of injury to a joint, may reduce the risk of the occurrence of degenerative changes.

Studies of the use of a TNF-alpha blocking agent as a means of suppressing inflammation and repairing cartilage damage associated with osteoarthritis have been pursued. In an open labeled study, 20 patients with osteoarthritis of the knee received six biweekly subcutaneous injections of adalimumab, NCT00686439. Seventeen patients completed the study with withdrawals unrelated to lack of efficacy or adverse events. At 12 weeks, 14 (70%) patients achieved an OARSI/OMERACT response by intent-to-treat analysis.[9] In a randomized, double-blind, placebo-controlled, parallel group patients randomized to receive adalimumab 40 mg two subcutaneous injections at a 15-day interval or placebo and monitored for six months. The conclusion was that adalimumab was not superior to placebo.[10]

The commonly used TNF-alpha blocking agents include infliximab, etanercept, adalimumab, golimumab, certolizumab pegol. Infliximab is a chimeric monoclonal antibody, with human constant and murine variable regions with molecular mass 149 kilodaltons (kDa). Etanercept recombinant human protein, ligand-binding portion of 75 kDa TNFR fused to Fc portion of IgG1 with an overall molecular mass of 150 kDa. Adalimumab is a recombinant human IgG1 monoclonal antibody specific for human tumor necrosis factor with molecular mass 148 kDa. Golimumab is a human IgG1k monoclonal antibody exhibits multiple glycoforms with molecular mass 150-151 kDa. Certolizumab pegol is a pegylated human tumor necrosis factor alpha inhibitor with molecular mass 91 kDa formed by combing antigen-binding fragment 50 kDa with a 40 kDa polyethylene glycol (PEG) moiety.

The results of studies regarding the use of TNF-alpha blocking agents to manage cartilage damage associated with osteoarthritis have generally been less than conclusive. Studies investigating the benefit of TNF-alpha blocking agents are generally limited due to: (1) studies being conducted over short interval; (2) Intra-articular studies using TNF-alpha blocking molecules that are possibly too large to penetrate cartilage and therefore possibly unable to optimally generate a therapeutic response to benefit chondrocytes; and (3) the prime end point of the investigations being the subjective reduction in 'pain' over a short study period, rather than demonstrating an objective end point such as a measurable cartilage repair (by MRI) over a treatment interval that might need to last over a span of several years rather than weeks or months.

The currently existing TNF alpha inhibitors, which generally exist in the size range of 91 kDa to 150 kDa, may not be small enough to adequately diffuse into the deeper tissues of the cartilage. The larger the molecule, the more difficult it may be for the therapeutic medication to penetrate the surface of the cartilage and then diffuse through the cartilage to the deeper tissues of the cartilage. The currently existing TNF alpha inhibitors may be too large to penetrate the cartilage and therefore may not be able to provide an optimal benefit to chondrocytes that exist deep in the cartilage tissues. A small molecule tumor necrosis factor alpha (smTNF$_\alpha$) inhibitor might be fashioned to be injected directly into a joint space. Being a small molecule, such a smTNF$_\alpha$ inhibitor may effectively penetrate the cartilage and deliver to the tissues surrounding the chondrocytes the positive effects of blocking the action of tumor necrosis factor alpha. Blocking TNF alpha should reduce the rate of cell death of chondrocytes and decrease the release of metalloproteinases, molecules that act to degrade cartilage.

An IgG molecule typically functions as an antibody coded to attach to and neutralize a particular target molecule. An IgG is generally comprised of four smaller proteins connected together. The typical IgG molecule is constructed with two heavy chains connected together, acting as the backbone of the molecule. A single light chain protein is connected to the same end of each heavy chain protein. The tip of the heavy chain and tip of the light chain are variable regions and act to attach to a molecular target the variable region is coded to attach to, and functionally engage.

Single-chain variable fragment (scFv) antibody represents only the functional end of a larger IgG molecule. Single-chain variable fragment (scFv) antibody technology takes the variable end of the heavy chain and light chain of an IgG molecule and connects the two subset protein molecules with a small protein chain. Theoretically, a scFv antibody would perform similarly to the larger IgG molecule, but by being much smaller, the scFv antibody would be able to more easily diffuse into denser tissues than a larger IgG molecule.

Single-chain variable fragment antibody with inhibitory activity against tumor necrosis factor alpha shows promise for being small enough to effectively diffuse through articular cartilage.[6] A scFv antibody has been shown to have comparable efficacy to neutralizing tumor necrosis factor alpha as the full length IgG TNF alpha inhibitor molecule infliximab, which has a size of 150 kDa. The molecular mass of the studied scFv is 26 kDa,[6] which makes it much smaller in size than full length IgG TNF alpha inhibitor molecules which typically have a size of approximately 148-150 kDa. Penetration of cartilage by proteins is dependent upon molecular weight and the charge of the protein. Study of bovine cartilage penetration of the scFv versus infliximab demonstrated the small molecule TNF alpha inhibitor had the appropriate size and charge for therapeutic intra-articular use, and infliximab might be to be too large to optimally penetrate cartilage.[6]

CONCLUSION:

A small molecule with inhibitory activity against tumor necrosis factor alpha may have intra-articular therapeutic efficacy for managing knee osteoarthritis by neutralizing the up-regulated production of TNF alpha seen in degenerative cartilage and following serious injury to a joint. Injecting such a small molecule TNF alpha inhibitory molecule into a joint may mitigate systemic side effects the molecule might generate. An advantage of injecting a medical therapy into a joint space is that the joint space acts as a natural reservoir to temporarily store such a medication. Constructing the small molecule TNF alpha inhibitor molecule to have a variable degradation strategy, such that the configuration of the molecule utilized the environment (such as naturally occurring enzymes) inside the joint space to act to variably degrade the small molecule TNF alpha inhibitor molecule, creating a timed release of the molecule facilitating a variation in diffusion of the small molecule TNF alpha inhibitor molecule into the cartilage could generate a treatment program that exhibited immediate as well as extended beneficial effects to the cartilage.

Such a treatment strategy may assist anyone with elevated TNF alpha levels. Science suggests TNF alpha levels are elevated in progressive osteoarthritis, the setting of a joint injury, obesity and inflammatory joint diseases such as rheumatoid arthritis. Elevated levels of TNF alpha in the region of the joint space, results in increased death of chondrocytes and degradation of cartilage, which leads to the progression of osteoarthritis. Delivering small molecule TNF alpha inhibitor molecules to the cartilage of patients with osteoarthritis, injury, obesity and rheumatoid arthritis may act as a medical treatment to prevent and/or treat, possibly reverse osteoarthritis.

References:

1. Helmick CG, Felson DT, Lawrence RC, et al. Estimates of the prevalence of arthritis and other rheumatic conditions in the United States: part I. Arthritis Rheum 2008; 58: 15-25.

2. Prevalence and impact of chronic joint symptoms — seven states, 1996. MMWR Morb Mortal Wkly Rep 1998; 47: 345-51.

3. Dunlop DD, Manheim LM, Song J, Chang RW. Arthritis prevalence and activity limitations in older adults. Arthritis Rheum 2001; 44: 212-21.

4. Lawrence RC, Helmick CG, Arnett FC, et al. Estimates of the prevalence of arthritis and selected musculoskeletal disorders in the United States. Arthritis Rheum 1998; 41: 778-99.

5. Murray CJ, Vos T, Lozano R, et al. Disability-adjusted life years (DALYs) for 291 diseases and injuries in 21 regions, 1990-2010: a systematic analysis for the Global Burden of Disease Study 2010. Lancet 2012; 380: 2197-223.

6. Urech DM, Feige U, et al. Anti-inflammatory and cartilage-protecting effects of an intra-articularly injected anti-TNF-alpha single-chain Fv antibody (ESBA105) designed for local therapeutic use, Ann Rheum Dis 2010; 69:443-449.

7. Farahat MN, Yanni G, et al. Cytokine expression in synovial membranes of patients with rheumatoid arthritis and osteoarthritis, Ann Rheum Dis 1993; 52:870-5.

8. Mobasheri A. The future of osteoarthritis therapeutics: emerging biologic therapy, Curr Rheum Rep, 2013, 15:385.

9. Maksymowych WP, Russell AS, et al. Targeting tumor necrosis factor alleviates signs and symptoms of inflammatory osteoarthritis of the knee, Arthritis Res Ther. 2012; 14(5): R206, published online 2012 Oct 4.

10. Chevalier C, Ravaud P, Maheu E, et al, Adalimumab in patients with hand osteoarthritis refractory to analgesics and NSAIDs: a randomized, multicentre, double-blinded, placebo-controlled trial, Ann Rheum Dis 2015 Sep; 74(9):1697-705.

COMRIONS: MICRO RNA
INTRACELLULAR COMMUNICATION

Like the term 'virion' generally refers to a vessel that transports a viral genome for a host cell to a target cell, the term 'comrion' refers to a vessel that transports microRNA from a host cell to target cells for cellular cell-to-cell communication purposes.

Hormones are proteins or chemicals that are generally recognized as means of conveying communication to cells in a body. Male and female hormones generally guide sexual development in target tissues. Thyroid hormone acts as a master hormone guiding the health of numerous tissues. Many differing types of hormones provide the necessary communication throughout the body needed to orchestrate a healthy state in a body.

The genome has been considered comprised of functional DNA referred to as genes and nonfunctional DNA referred to as 'noncoding DNA'. Genes, when transcribed, produce messenger RNA (mRNA) molecules, which in the cytoplasm of the cell mRNAs are used as templates to produce proteins. There have been thought to be approximately 30,000 genes in the human genome, because there have been identified 30,000 differing proteins present in the human body. The coding portion of the human genome is approximately five percent of the 3 billion base pairs that comprise human DNA. Noncoding DNA does not generate messenger RNAs and therefore does not generate proteins. Noncoding DNA is thought to comprise ninety-five percent of the human genome and is often considered to be 'genetic junk'.

MicroRNAs have recently been identified being generated inside the nucleus of a cell. The term 'microRNA' generally refers to small RNAs, often approximately 25 nucleotides in length, that may act to modify cell function. MicroRNAs are noncoding RNAs and some are thought to up-regulate or down-regulate transcription of certain specific target genes.

Emerging science is suggesting that some microRNAs are being expressed by some cells in order to communicate with other cells. To accomplish this task, a cell produces a microRNA, packages the microRNAs into a vessel comprised of a budding portion of the cell membrane and releases the vessel. Such a vessel that carries a microRNA in an extracellular environment may be referred to as a 'comrion' or 'communication transport vessel', likened to the term 'virion' used to identify a transport vessel that carries a viral genome in the extracellular environment from a host cell to a target cell.

Current theory is that an originator cell produces a microRNA that the cell wishes to utilize to communicate with another cell. The originator cell packages the microRNAs into a vessel comprised of a budding portion of the cell membrane and releases the vessel, a comrion, into the extracellular environment. The comrion traverses the extracellular environment to seek out and engage a target cell. When the comrion encounters a target cell, the comrion inserts the microRNA that the vessel carries into the target cell. Once inside the target cell, the microRNA acts to modify a cell function either in the cytoplasm of the target cell, or in the nucleus of the target cell.

Observing and understanding the function of comrions will all usher in an entirely new pharmaceutical technology. Constructing medical therapeutic comrions to carry microRNAs to cancer cells to activate apoptosis in cancer cells may provide an entirely new approach to targeted cancer therapy. Understanding the programming code utilized by these microRNAs may facilitate an abundance of other therapies designed to up-regulate the metabolism in injured or aging cells or down-regulate the internal metabolism of overactive cells that are harmful to the body. Deciphering microRNA cell-to-cell communication may lead to the discovery of an entirely new network of cell function that can be utilized to benefit patients and advance the quality and effectiveness of healthcare.

The concept of microRNAs also suggests that a portion of the DNA considered to be junk, which has been estimated to be 95% of the nuclear DNA, may in fact be genes that are comprised not of genes that produce messenger RNAs intended to produce proteins, but instead microRNAs that are designed to deliver commands inside and outside of a cell. It is well recognized that numerous functions inside and outside cells must occur in a very precise and coordinated manner. Genes comprising the 'junk' DNA may in fact code for series of microRNAs, these microRNAs meant to coordinate biologic functions inside the cell as well as coordinate actions or development amongst sister cells in a body. Once the language comprising the biologic code that has been used to program the DNA has been deciphered, very little, if any, of the DNA will be found to be junk. There are at least 240 different cell types comprising the human body, and each cell type requires its own set of instructions to properly regulate initial development, maturity and management.

PROPOSALS TO DEVELOP DNA VACCINES UTILIZING A VIRTUAL LAB

PART A

PROPOSAL TO DEVELOP AN EMBEDDED DNA VACCINE TO SILENCE HUMAN IMMUNODEFICIENCY VIRUS

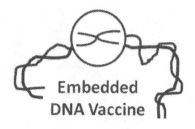

Copyright 2015

Phase 1: Identify the 3D biochemical molecular structure of the HIV.

Phase 2: Computer model the 3D biochemical molecular structure of HIV.

Phase 3: Derive a Transcription Factor to intercept and neutralize the HIV genome.

Phase 4: Computer model the 3D molecular structure of the TFIIIA to silence HIV.

Phase 5: Computer model the internal environment of the cell to test HIV RNA and TFIIIA.

Phase 6: Design the messenger RNA molecule to generate a therapeutic TFIIIA.

Phase 7: Computer model the molecular structure of the mRNA intended to produce TFIIIA.

Phase 8: Design an embeddable segment of DNA to generate an mRNA to produce TFIIIA.

Phase 9: Computer model the molecular structure of the DNA segment to produce mRNA.

Phase 10: Computer model the environment inside the nucleus of a cell to test DNA vaccine.

Phase 11: Work with a bio-lab to construct TFIIIA and DNA vaccine, and test both molecules.

White Paper Proposal

PHASE 1

DECIPHER BASE-FOUR PROGRAMMING
INSTRUCITON CODES COMPRISING HIV GENOME

Lane B. Scheiber II, MD
Osteoporosis & Arthritis Center, Inc.

Objective: Decipher the base-four biologic instruction code programming language comprising the HIV genome.

Description of Effort: Similar to the DNA, the HIV DNA sequence represents a base-four biologic computer program. Dissection of each nucleotide comprising the HIV DNA sequence to cross-correlate segments of the HIV genome with known functions of the segments; then analyzing subsegments of the HIV genome that are not accounted for with known processes required to construct the complete HIV virion and cross-correlate with cell organelles and known function of cell organelles and cross-correlate with known function of enzymes and other proteins present in the cytoplasm of the cell. Convert nucleotides to a 0-3 numbering system to enhance study of the HIV genome, similar to how a binary computer code would be studied to decipher the programming instructions.

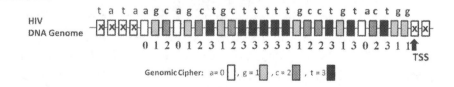

Figure 85

Benefits of Proposed Technology: By establishing knowledge of the instruction codes comprising the HIV genome that dictate how the proteins and ultimately the virus's virion is assembled allows for expanded means to predict, interdict and halt lethal viral infections such as HIV. Deciphering the base-four language of HIV leads to the opportunity to unlock the programming instructions that control biologic cell functions.

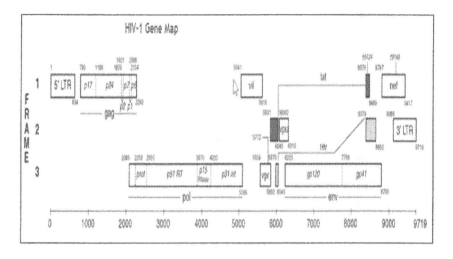

Figure 86

Challenges: Currently, only the subsections of the DNA sequence that act as templates to manufacture proteins are recognized, there is no knowledge of the instruction codes required to construct complex proteins or structures inside the boundaries of a cell. Of rather challenging complexity is discerning the base four programming language comprising the DNA sequence. Arriving at the proper cipher to be used to correctly assign a numerical system to the letter system, that was arbitrarily assigned to the DNA/RNA nucleotides in the late 1800's, is a sophisticated puzzle to decode. The genomic cipher A0G1C2T3 utilized in the figure below was published in an abstract accepted to the 2014 annual meeting of the European Society of Human Genetics. It is understood that the HIV genome remains an RNA molecule, not represented as a DNA genome, during the life-cycle of the HIV and therefore each thymine nucleotide (DNA) actually represents a uracil nucleotide (RNA). By convention, HIV's DNA sequence represents the virus's DNA.

<u>Major Goals/Milestones</u>: Identify the instruction codes comprising the HIV genome that direct how the viral virion is assembled. Decipher the means by which the HIV virion is constructed in order to identify vulnerabilities that can be exploited to halt the infectious nature of the virus. Gain knowledge of a base-four programming language utilized to generate viral genomes. This project would represent the first effort to convert the individual nucleotides comprising the viral genome to numbers for the purposes of trying to decipher the base-four programming language that comprises the HIV genome.

<u>Approximate Period of Performance</u>: 36 months

<u>References</u>: 1. *Fourth Generation Biologics: Molecular Virus Killers*, L. B. Scheiber II, Lane B. Scheiber, iUniverse, 2014.

2. ScheiberL, ScheiberL, Presenting the genomic cipher adenine = 0, guanine =1, cytosine = 2, thymine = 3 derived directly from the DNA to convert nucleotide names/letters to numbers to study patterns of unique identifiers to detect command genes in the human genome, Control No. 2014-A-616-ESHG, European Conference of Human Genetics 2014.

White Paper Proposal

PHASE 2

GENERATE AN INTERACTIVE THREE DIMENSIONAL
COMPUTER MODEL OF THE HIV DNA SEQUENCE

Lane B. Scheiber II, MD
Osteoporosis & Arthritis Center, Inc.

Objective: Establish a prototype three dimensional interactive computer model of the HIV single stranded DNA sequence as it appears in the cell, this three dimensional interactive computer model of the HIV to act as a target for therapeutic molecules such a modified TFIIIA molecules and to be interactive within a computer model of the human cell.

Description of Effort: The occurrence of the HIV outbreak demonstrates that a future critical battlefield will be security of the human cell. To effectively design therapies to combat HIV, a three dimensional interactive model of the HIV DNA sequence is to be designed and generated. Such a three dimensional model of the HIV DNA sequence to be designed to be compatible with a three dimensional model of the human cell. Such a computer simulation of the HIV to act as a virtual laboratory specimen to study viral threats as they reside inside the host cell where viral genomes are copied and ejected from host as viral virions.

Benefits of Proposed Technology: A three dimensional interactive model of the HIV DNA sequence facilitates the means to design and study neutralizing therapeutic molecules such as a modified TFIIIA in real time to determine an optimal design of therapeutic molecules to combat RNA viral genomes in the cytoplasm. A detailed 3D computer graphics representation of the current HIV threats and future variations of the HIV (See Second Figure). A 3D computer graphics representation of the HIV DNA sequence allows for simulations to be performed to study the biochemistry and behavior of the HIV DNA sequence as it interacts with a 3D graphics representation of potential neutralizing therapeutic molecules that might be utilized to seek out HIV DNA sequence as the viral genome resides inside the cytoplasm.

Challenges: Constructing a computer model with precise detail of the HIV genome at the molecular level and accounting for the three dimensional behavior of the nucleotides that comprise the viral genome. The complexity rises sharply when accounting for the factors of how the individual nucleotides of the viral genome interact with the cytoplasm medium, and organelles and the wide variety of proteins naturally suspended in the cytoplasm of the host cell. Such a project requires a very high level of computer processing power, extensive memory storage capacity and sophisticated state-of-the-art software programming. There is limited knowledge of subprograms comprising HIV DNA sequence.

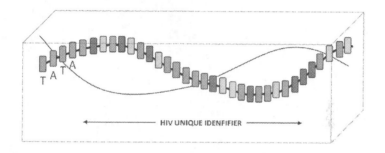

HIV UNIQUE IDENFIFIER

Figure 87

Major Goals/Milestones: Identify design parameters of 3D model of HIV RNA. Design 3D physical representation of Wild Type HIV DNA sequence. Design 3D computer representation of HIV DNA sequence to be interactive with 3D computer TFIIIA molecule. If 3D computer model of the cell is completed, design 3D computer representation of HIV DNA sequence to be interactive with a 3D computer model of the cell. Test and improve 3D computer representation of HIV DNA sequence to simulate real time, life-like interaction of HIV DNA sequence with neutralizing therapeutic molecules such as a modified TFIIIA hunter-killer molecule which would seek out and bind to 3D simulation of wild type HIV RNA in the cytoplasm of the cell inside 3D model of the cell. Final goal is to simulate by computer assisted design the HIV DNA sequence to act as a target to facilitate the development of effective means to neutralize the threat of the HIV DNA sequence and future variations of the virus, which the computer assisted design of a neutralizing therapeutic molecule once perfected can then be sent to the lab for production of actual biologic therapeutic molecules to be tested and used in humans as a treatment against an HIV infection.

Approximate Period of Performance: 60 months

WHITE PAPER PROPOSAL

PHASE 3

DEVELOP MEANS TO COMBAT HIV GENOME WITH A NOVEL MODIFIED TFIIIA MOLECULE

Lane B. Scheiber II, MD
Osteoporosis & Arthritis Center, Inc.

Objective: Develop a means to rapidly and efficiently seek out and neutralize the Human Immunodeficiency Virus (HIV) DNA sequence in the host cells of an infected individual utilizing a modified Transcription Factor IIIA (TFIIIA) molecule to bind to and silence HIV DNA sequence.

Description of Effort: Utilize a modified TFIIIA molecule, target the HIV genome directly as it resides in the host cell. Prevent translation of the viral genome by binding the modified TFIIIA molecule to a unique identifier in the viral genome upstream from the NP gene. Halting translation of the HIV genome arrests the viral infection and the lethal effects of the virus.

Recent events regarding the HIV outbreak in West Africa suggest two undeniable concerns: (1) a viral pathogen is capable of efficiently killing large numbers of individuals and (2) current capability to combat viral infections including isolation, vaccines, and infusions of antibodies are not necessarily sufficient to arrest virulent viral infections and insure survival of an infected patient. Given viruses mutate, a third concern is emergence of an airborne strain of HIV.

Currently HIV consists of 6 known strains. Human Immunodeficiency Virus (HIV) was the first strain recorded in 1976, and is responsible for the two most recent 2014 epidemics. HIV is an RNA negative sense virus, activating and replicating in the cytoplasm of a host cell. The HIV genome is approximately 19,000 nucleotides and comprised of 7 genes including 3'-NP-VP35-VP40-GP/sGP-VP30-VP24-L-5'. VP40 protein assists with forming the exterior viral coat. Respiratory Syncytial Virus (RSV) is an RNA negative sense virus with a genome comprised of approximately 15,277 nucleotides. The RSV genome is comprised of ten genes including 3'-N1-N2-N-M-P-G-F-SH-M2-L-5'. The genes G-F-SH code for RSV's external coat.

THREAT OF HIV MUTATION TO MORE VIRULENT VIRUS

HIV genome, NCBI Reference Sequence: AY354458 has a 25 nucleotide sequence 5'-tcttttgtgtgcgaataactatgag-3' positioned at 34 to 58, which serves as a unique identifier for HIV's NP gene. NP gene's product is vital for virus replication. The human genome was studied and this unique identifier is not found as a complete sequence in the human genome. This unique identifier can be used as an inimitable target.

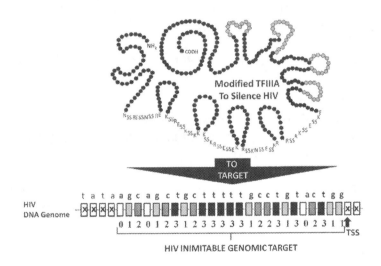

Figure 88

MODIFIED TFIIIA MOLECULE

This effort utilizes HIV's NP gene's unique identifier as an inimitable therapeutic target. TFIIIA molecules initiate decoding of viral genomes. The first 5 zinc fingers of a TFIIIA molecule are modified to seek out and attach to NP's unique identifier. The algorithm responsible for replacing the amino acids of zinc fingers 1-5 is derived from a novel biochemical analysis of the bonding characteristics of nucleotides-to-amino acids, detailed in the listed reference. Zinc fingers 6-9 are modified to prevent binding of other transcription factors. The COOH tail is modified to maintain the TFIIIA in the cytoplasm. This novel approach provides a modified TFIIIA designed to seek out and bind to NP gene's unique identifier to avert translation of the NP gene to arrest construction of copies of the HIV virion. Halting HIV virion construction neutralizes the threat.

Benefits of Proposed Technology: The modified TFIIIA technology is versatile and allows expansion of the technology to treat various versions of HIV as well as the means to target most DNA/RNA viral pathogens that might be encountered on the battlefield.

Challenges: Insuring the modified TFIIIA molecule does not interact with other structures inside the human cell. Accounting for genetic variation in HIV genome. Insuring modified TFIIIA neutralizing effect is permanent enough to restrict HIV genome from being translated.

Major Goals/Milestones: Identify design parameters of modified TFIIIA molecule. Explore computer modeling of amino acid bonding to nucleotides. Versatile system to treat viral threats.

Approximate Period of Performance: 24 months.

Reference: *Fourth Generation Biologics: Molecular Virus Killers*, L Scheiber, iUniverse, 2014.

WHITE PAPER PROPOSAL

PHASE 4

REPRESENT BY INTERACTIVE 3D COMPUTER MODEL A MODIFIED TFIIIA MOLECULE TO NEUTRALIZE HIV

Lane B. Scheiber II, MD
Osteoporosis & Arthritis Center, Inc.

Objective: Develop three dimensional computer graphics model of a modified Transcription Factor IIIA (TFIIIA) molecule to seek out Human Immunodeficiency Virus (HIV) genome in a host cell and silence the virus's genome in order to neutralize the effects of the virus and halt viral replication.

Description of Effort: Utilize a modified TFIIIA molecule, target the HIV genome directly as it resides in the host cell. Prevent translation of the viral genome by binding the modified TFIIIA molecule to a unique identifier in the viral genome upstream from the NP gene. Halting translation of the HIV genome arrests the viral infection and the lethal effects of the virus.

Recent events regarding the HIV outbreak in West Africa suggest two undeniable concerns: (1) a viral pathogen is capable of efficiently killing large numbers of individuals and (2) current capability to combat viral infections including isolation, vaccines, and infusions of antibodies are not necessarily sufficient to arrest virulent viral infections and insure survival of an infected patient. Given viruses mutate, a third concern is emergence of an airborne strain of HIV.

HIV genome, NCBI Reference Sequence: AY354458 has a 25 nucleotide sequence 5'-tcttttgtgtgcgaataactatgag-3' positioned at 34 to 58, which serves as a unique identifier for HIV's NP gene. NP gene's product is vital for virus replication. The human genome was studied and this unique identifier is not found as a complete sequence in the uninfected human genome. Thus, this unique identifier in the HIV genome can be used as an inimitable target (See Figure 89).

The 3D model for the HIV genome is already expected to have been generated as a part of a prior software development effort.

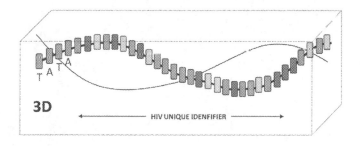

Figure 89

Modified TFIIIA Molecule This effort utilizes HIV's NP gene's unique identifier as an inimitable therapeutic target. In nature TFIIIA molecules initiate decoding of viral genomes. The first 5 zinc fingers of a TFIIIA molecule are modified to seek out and attach to NP's unique identifier. The algorithm responsible for replacing the amino acids of zinc fingers 1-5 is derived from a novel biochemical analysis of the bonding characteristics of nucleotides-to-amino acids detailed in the listed reference. Zinc fingers 6-9 are modified to prevent binding of other transcription factors. The COOH tail is modified to maintain the TFIIIA in the cytoplasm. This novel approach provides a modified TFIIIA designed to seek out and bind to NP gene's unique identifier to avert translation of the NP gene to arrest construction of copies of the HIV virion in the cytoplasm of the cell. Halting HIV virion construction would neutralize the HIV threat.

Design and construct a physical model of the modified TFIIIA molecule intended to seek out and neutralize Human Immunodeficiency Virus, to be utilized as the source to generate a computer graphics representation of the TFIIIA molecule. Construct a 3D computer graphics model of the modified TFIIIA molecule (See Figure 90).

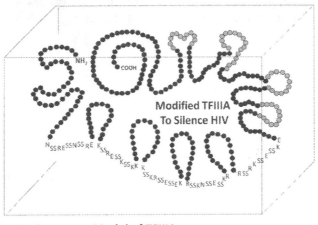

3D Computer Model of TFIIIA

Figure 90

Construct a 3D software model of the DNA target sequence in order to study the proper bonding of the three dimensional TFIIIA molecule to the three dimensional twisting DNA sequence. See Figure 91.

Benefits of Proposed Technology: The modified TFIIIA technology is versatile and allows expansion of the technology to treat variations of HIV as well as most DNA/RNA viral pathogens that might be encountered on the battlefield. A detailed 3D computer graphics representation of the TFIIIA molecule allows for study of the biochemistry and bonding of the TFIIIA molecule to current HIV threats and future variations of HIV.

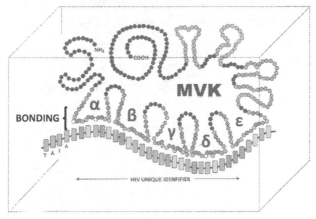

3D Computer Model of TFIIIA and HIV Genome

Figure 91

Challenges: Insuring the modified TFIIIA molecule does not interact with other structures inside the human cell. Complexity rises sharply when accounting for how the individual amino acids comprising the TFIIIA molecule will interact with the cytoplasm and organelles of the host cell. Insuring a modified TFIIIA bonds to the HIV genome in a permanent enough manner to sufficiently restrict the HIV genome from being translated or copied. Such a project requires a very high level of computer processing power, extensive memory storage capacity and sophisticated state-of-the-art software programming technology.

Major Goals/Milestones: Design 3D physical representation of TFIIIA molecule. Design 3D computer representation of TFIIIA molecule to be interactive with 3D computer model of HIV RNA. If 3D computer model of the cell is available, design 3D computer representation of TFIIIA to be interactive with a 3D computer model of the cell. Test and improve 3D computer representation of TFIIIA to simulate real time, life-like interaction of TFIIIA hunter-killer molecule to seek out and bind to 3D simulation of wild type HIV RNA in the cytoplasm inside 3D model of the cell. Once computer TFIIIA simulation perfected, information to be sent to lab for production of biologic therapeutic molecules to be tested for use in humans to treat HIV.

<u>Approximate Period of Performance</u>: 60 months

<u>Reference</u>: *Fourth Generation Biologics: Molecular Virus Killers*, L Scheiber, iUniverse, 2014.

White Paper Proposal

PHASE 5

GENERATE INTERACTIVE THREE DIMENSIONAL COMPUTER MODEL OF THE HUMAN CELL WITH INANIMATE NUCLEUS

Lane B. Scheiber II, MD
Osteoporosis & Arthritis Center, Inc.

Objective: Establish a prototype three dimensional interactive computer model of a human cell with functional cytoplasm, organelles, microtubule architecture and an inanimate nucleus.

Description of Effort: The occurrence of the HIV outbreak demonstrates that the next critical medical research frontier will be the security of the human cell. Develop a three dimensional interactive model of the human cell with functional cytoplasm. See Figure 92. Model the specifics of the interior of the cell including characteristics of the cytoplasm, external characteristics of organelles including the nucleus, Golgi apparatus, vacuoles, mitochondria and molecules including ribosomes and proteins.

Benefits of Proposed Technology: A three dimensional interactive model of the human cell facilitates the means to design and study molecules such as a modified TFIIIA in real time to determine an optimal design of therapeutic molecules to combat the genomes of viral pathogens including HIV. Development of a virtual laboratory to act as a means to study the behavior of viral pathogens and therapeutic molecules without placing human laboratory personnel at risk, with such a laboratory being capable of running numerous scenarios in order to arrive at an optimal design of a therapeutic molecule to combat the HIV genome.

Challenges: Constructing a realistic computer representation of the precise detail of a human cell's three dimensional exterior membrane. Constructing a computer representation of the precise detail of the organelles and proteins comprising the interior structures of a human cell. Correctly modeling the fluid dynamics of the cell cytoplasm and the effects of the cell's internal microtubule architecture. The complexity of the project rises sharply when such a three dimensional computer representation is then required to be interactive with the insertion of both molecular structures that might attack the cell such a viral genome, as well as the insertion of molecular structures of therapeutic molecules that might be used to benefit the cell by neutralizing a threatening viral genome. Such a project requires a very high level of computer processing power, extensive memory storage capacity and sophisticated state-of-the-art software programming. There is limited knowledge of the molecular architecture of the organelles and behavior of the organelles as they are suspended in the cell cytoplasm. Fluid dynamics of the cytoplasm is affected by numerous factors including fluid channels in the exterior membrane, fluid channels present in the nuclear membrane, numerous complex shaped free-floating structures, the microtubule architecture, the attractive and repulsive forces inherent to the electrical charges present on molecular surfaces.

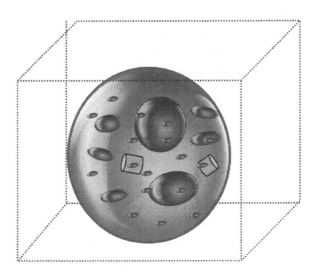

3D COMPUTER MODEL OF THE CELL

Figure 92

<u>Major Goals/Milestones</u>: Identify design parameters of a three dimensional (3D) model of a cell. Design 3D physical representation

of the cell membrane and internal cytoplasm and microtubule architecture. Design 3D physical representation of organelles and proteins. Consolidate 3D physical representations of outer cell membrane and 3D physical representation of organelles and proteins into a 3D physical model of the cell that can be used as a reference to design a 3D computer model of a cell. Design 3D computer model representation of the cell membrane and internal cytoplasm and microtubule architecture. Design 3D computer representation of organelles. Design 3D computer representation of proteins. Consolidate 3D computer representations of cell membrane, cell's internal cytoplasm, microtubule architecture organelles and 3D computer representations of proteins into 3D computer model of a human cell. Assimilate the software programming into 3D Computer Model of the Cell capable of to interactions with 3D computer model of the HIV and 3D computer model of a modified TFIIIA molecule or 3D computer model of equivalent therapeutic molecule. Establish a virtual laboratory to act as a means to study the behavior of viral pathogens and therapeutic molecules capable of running numerous scenarios in order to arrive at an optimal design of a therapeutic molecule to combat the current HIV genomes and future variations to the HIV genome.

Approximate Period of Performance: 60 months

WHITE PAPER PROPOSAL

PHASE 6

INTRACELLULAR mRNA VACCINE TO GENERATE TFIIIAs
INSIDE HOST CELL TO NEUTRALIZE HIV

Lane B. Scheiber II, MD
Osteoporosis & Arthritis Center, Inc.

Objective: Develop an intracellular vaccine consisting of a messenger ribonucleic acid (mRNA) to be translated to generate therapeutic Transcription Factor IIIA (TFIIIA) molecules coded to seek out the Human Immunodeficiency Virus (HIV) genome in host cells and to engage and silence the virus's genome to halt viral replication and arrest the viral infection. See Figure 93.

Description of Effort: The goal is to produce a vaccine that consists of a mRNA that produces TFIIIA molecules designed to silence the HIV DNA sequence if the HIV genome breaches the cell's membrane and enters the cytoplasm. The life-cycle of the Hepatitis C virus demonstrates it is possible to embed functional mRNA into specific target cells.

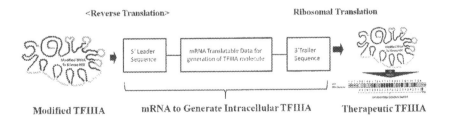

Figure 93

HIV genome, NCBI Reference Sequence: AY354458, has a 25 nucleotide sequence 5'-tcttttgtgtgcgaataactatgag-3' positioned at 34 to 58, which serves as a unique identifier for HIV's NP gene. NP gene's product is vital for virus replication. The human genome was studied and this unique identifier is not found as a complete sequence in the uninfected human genome. Thus, this unique identifier in the HIV genome can be used as an inimitable target.

This effort utilizes HIV's NP gene's unique identifier as an inimitable therapeutic target. Once the design parameters of the TFIIIA molecule are established, a reverse translation process is undergone to design the translatable portion of a mRNA molecule that when translated by ribosomes in the cytoplasm of a host cell will produce the TFIIIA molecule, this TFIIIA molecule capable of hunting down and engaging the HIV DNA sequence. See Figure 94.

Prevention of translation of the viral genome by binding the therapeutic TFIIIA molecule to a unique identifier in the viral genome upstream from the NP gene halts translation of the HIV genome and arrests the viral infection.

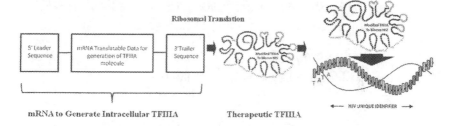

Figure 94

Benefits of Proposed Technology: The mRNA intracellular vaccine technology designed to produce therapeutic TFIIIA molecules is versatile and allows expansion of the mRNA vaccine technology to provide protection for US troops against numerous high risk endemic DNA/RNA viral pathogens that might be encountered on battlefields around the globe. The mRNA technology is the frontrunner effort which provides the necessary technical information regarding mRNA design in order to develop an embedded DNA vaccine.

Challenges: Establishing a reverse translation process that will generate the translatable segment of an mRNA; this effort includes deciphering the quaternary computer aspects of human genetics.

Design of a complete functional mRNA molecule to be inserted into the human cell. Design of the complete mRNA molecule so as to be recognized and translated by a ribosomal complex in the cytoplasm of a host cell to generate functional TFIIIA molecules. Design the 3' trailer sequence of the mRNA to modulate the life of the mRNA's presence in the cytoplasm.

Major Goals/Milestones: Design an intercellular vaccine utilizing a mRNA molecule that will generate therapeutic TFIIIA molecules that will engage the HIV DNA sequence if it enters the protected cell. Describe how a ribosomal complex effects translation of a specific therapeutic intracellular mRNA vaccine. Design functional 5' trailer sequence of mRNA molecule. Design functional 3' trailer sequence of the mRNA molecule to extend the life of the mRNA.

Approximate Period of Performance: 48 months

References: 1. *Fourth Generation Biologics: Molecular Virus Killers*, L. B. Scheiber II, Lane B. Scheiber, iUniverse, 2014.

2.*Changing Global Approach to Medicine, Medical Vector Therapy*, L. B. Scheiber II, Lane B. Scheiber, iUniverse, 2011.

WHITE PAPER PROPOSAL

PHASE 7

COMPUTER MODEL 'INTRACELLULAR' mRNA VACCINE TO GENERATE TFIIIAs TO NEUTRALIZE HIV

Lane B. Scheiber II, MD
Osteoporosis & Arthritis Center, Inc.

Objective: Develop three dimensional computer graphics model of a messenger RNA designed to be translated by the ribosomes of the host cell to generate modified Transcription Factor IIIA (TFIIIA) molecules coded to seek out Human Immunodeficiency Virus (HIV) genome in the host cell to engage and silence the virus's genome in order to arrest viral replication.

Description of Effort: Utilize computer graphics to represent the messenger ribonucleic acid (mRNA) designed to be translated to generate modified TFIIIA molecules, to target the HIV genome directly if the HIV DNA sequence breaches the host cell membrane and enters the host cell. Utilizing computer graphics demonstrate that the therapeutic mRNA can be engaged and decoded by a ribosomal complex to produce the intended TFIIIA molecules. See Figure 95.

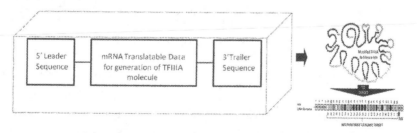

3D Computer Model of mRNA to Generate Intracellular TFIIIA   TFIIIA to Target HIV

Figure 95

This effort utilizes HIV's NP gene's unique identifier as an inimitable therapeutic target. Once the design parameters of the TFIIIA molecule are established, a reverse translation process is undergone to design the translatable portion of a mRNA molecule that when translated by ribosomes in the cytoplasm of a host cell will produce the TFIIIA molecule.

Design and construct a physical model of the proposed mRNA sequence intended to generate mRNA molecules intended to be translated to produce TFIIIAs capable of seeking out and neutralizing Human Immunodeficiency Virus, to be utilized as the source to generate a computer graphics representation of the TFIIIA molecule. The goal is to produce a realistic 3D graphics representation of an intracellular vaccine that consists of a mRNA that produces TFIIIA molecules designed to silence the HIV DNA sequence if the HIV genome breaches the outer membrane of a host cell and enters the cell's cytoplasm. See Figure 96.

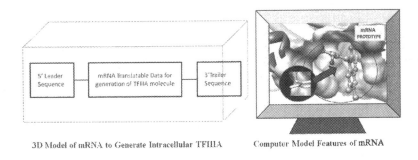

3D Model of mRNA to Generate Intracellular TFIIIA   Computer Model Features of mRNA

Figure 96

Benefits of Proposed Technology: Computer modeling of the mRNA intracellular vaccine technology designed to produce therapeutic TFIIIA molecules provides expansion of the mRNA vaccine technology to make available protection for US troops against high risk endemic DNA/RNA viral pathogens that might be encountered on battlefields around the globe.

Challenges: Computer modeling the design of a complete functional sequence of mRNA. Defining how the ribosomal complex engages the mRNA molecule. Discern in the 5' leader segment of the mRNA the signal required to initiate assembly of a ribosomal complex and subsequent engagement of the therapeutic mRNA molecule. Model representations of the ribosome molecules to interface with the mRNA model to run simulations to show the mRNA will be translated when present in a biologic cell's cytoplasm. Such a project requires a very high level of computer processing power, extensive memory storage capacity and sophisticated state-of-the-art software programming technology.

Major Goals/Milestones: Design 3D physical representation of mRNA sequence to produce therapeutic TFIIIA molecules. Develop a 3D computer representation of the mRNA sequence to be interactive with 3D computer model of a ribosomal complex. Establish definition of the signaling of mRNA to initiate translation of an mRNA molecule. Establish design parameters of the 3' tail segment of the mRNA molecule that will dictate the functional life of a mRNA molecule in cytoplasm of the host cell.

Once computer mRNA simulation is perfected, information to be sent to lab for production of biologic therapeutic molecules to be tested for use in humans to prevent HIV infections from occurring in individuals at risk of infection due to exposure to HIV.

Approximate Period of Performance: 60 months

Reference Fourth Generation Biologics: Molecular Virus Killers, L. B. Scheiber II, Lane B. Scheiber, iUniverse, 2014.

WHITE PAPER PROPOSAL

PHASE 8

DEVELOP EMBEDDED DNA INTRACELLULAR VACCINE TO GENERATE TFIIIAs TO NEUTRALIZE HIV

Lane B. Scheiber II, MD
Osteoporosis & Arthritis Center, Inc.

Objective: Develop an intracellular vaccine consisting of a deoxyribonucleic acid (DNA) segment designed to be transcribed by the host cell's RNA Polymerase II to generate messenger RNA (mRNA) to be translated to generate therapeutic Transcription Factor IIIA (TFIIIA) molecules coded to seek out Human Immunodeficiency Virus (HIV) genome in host cells to engage and silence the virus's genome to halt viral replication and arrest the viral infection.

Description of Effort: The goal is to produce a vaccine that consists of a segment of DNA (See Figure 97) that once embedded in the human genome perpetually produces TFIIIA molecules designed to silence the HIV DNA sequence if the HIV genome breaches the cell. The life-cycle of the Human Immunodeficiency Virus demonstrates that it is possible to embed functional segments of DNA into a specific target cell's genome.

HIV genome, NCBI Reference Sequence: AY354458, has a 25 nucleotide sequence 5'-tcttttgtgtgcgaataactatgag-3' positioned at 34 to 58, which serves as a unique identifier for HIV's NP gene. NP gene's product is vital for virus replication. The human genome was studied and this unique identifier is not found as a complete sequence in the uninfected human genome. Thus, this unique identifier in the HIV genome can be used as an inimitable target.

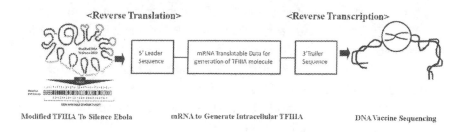

<Reverse Translation>   <Reverse Transcription>

| 5' Leader Sequence | mRNA Translatable Data for generation of TFIIIA molecule | 3' Trailer Sequence |

Modified TFIIIA To Silence Ebola   mRNA to Generate Intracellular TFIIIA   DNA Vaccine Sequencing

Figure 97

This effort utilizes HIV's NP gene's unique identifier as an inimitable therapeutic target. Once the design parameters of the TFIIIA molecule are established, a reverse translation process is undergone to design the translatable portion of a mRNA molecule that when translated by ribosomes in the cytoplasm of a host cell will produce the TFIIIA molecule. Once the design parameters of the mRNA molecule is established, a reverse transcription process is utilized to design an embeddable therapeutic segment of DNA.

Design a segment of DNA to be embedded in the human genome that when transcribed would generate mRNA molecules designed to be translated in the cytoplasm of the host cell to generate therapeutic TFIIIA molecules to target the HIV genome directly if the HIV DNA sequence breaches the host cell membrane and enters the host cell. Prevent translation of the viral genome by binding the therapeutic TFIIIA molecule to a unique identifier in the viral genome upstream from the NP gene. Halting translation of the HIV genome arrests the viral infection.

Benefits of Proposed Technology: The DNA embedded intracellular vaccine technology designed to produce therapeutic TFIIIA molecules is versatile and allows expansion of the DNA vaccine technology to provide permanent protection for US troops against numerous high risk endemic DNA/RNA viral pathogens that might be encountered on battlefields around the globe.

Challenges: Establishing a reverse transcription process that will generate the transcribable segment; this effort includes deciphering the quaternary computer aspects of the human gene utilized by the gene to locate and transcribe genetic information as needed by the cell. Design of a complete functional sequence of DNA to be seamlessly embedded into the human genome; avoiding undue influence of the sex cells. Design of the complete DNA sequence so as to be recognized and transcribed by a transcription complex to generate a functionally mature mRNA molecule.

Major Goals/Milestones: Design an intercellular vaccine utilizing a DNA sequence that will generate mRNA molecules to produce therapeutic TFIIIA molecules that will engage the HIV DNA sequence if the virus's genome enters the protected cell. Describe how RNA Polymerase II would engage reverse transcribed DNA to effect transcription of therapeutic DNA to mRNA. Design functional 5' upstream sequence of DNA. Design functional 3' downstream sequence of DNA.

Approximate Period of Performance: 60 months

References: 1. *Fourth Generation Biologics: Molecular Virus Killers*, L. B. Scheiber II, Lane B. Scheiber, iUniverse, 2014.

2.*Changing Global Approach to Medicine, Medical Vector Therapy*, L. B. Scheiber II, Lane B. Scheiber, iUniverse, 2011.

WHITE PAPER PROPOSAL

PHASE 9

COMPUTER MODEL DNA 'INTRACELLULAR' VACCINE TO GENERATE TFIIIAs TO NEUTRALIZE HIV

Lane B. Scheiber II, MD
Osteoporosis & Arthritis Center, Inc.

Objective: Develop a three dimensional computer graphics model representative of a segment of deoxyribonucleic acid (DNA) designed to be embedded in the human genome to be transcribed by the host cell to generate messenger RNA molecules to be translated to generate modified Transcription Factor IIIA (TFIIIA) molecules coded to seek out Human Immunodeficiency Virus (HIV) genome in host cell and engage, then silence the virus's genome to arrest a viral infection.

Description of Effort: Utilize computer assisted design technology to generate a model of an embeddable segment of DNA that when transcribed would produce messenger RNA (mRNA) designed to be translated to generate modified TFIIIA molecules to target and neutralize the HIV genome directly if the HIV genome breaches the host cell membrane and enters the cell. Utilizing computer graphics demonstrate that the DNA segment can be inserted into the human genome. Further, demonstrate through computer modeling that a transcription complex is able to engage and decode the DNA sequence to produce the intended mRNA.

HIV genome, NCBI Reference Sequence: AY354458, has a 25 nucleotide sequence 5'-tcttttgtgtgcgaataactatgag-3' positioned at 34 to 58, which serves as a unique identifier for HIV's NP gene. NP gene's product is vital for virus replication. The human genome was studied and this unique identifier is not found as a complete sequence in the uninfected human genome. Thus, this unique identifier in the HIV genome can be used as an inimitable target.

This effort utilizes HIV's NP gene's unique identifier as an inimitable therapeutic target. Once the design parameters of the TFIIIA molecule are established, a reverse translation process is undergone to design the translatable portion of a mRNA molecule that when translated by ribosomes in the cytoplasm of a host cell will produce the TFIIIA molecule. Once the design parameters of the mRNA molecule is established, a reverse transcription process is utilized to design a segment of DNA that will generate mRNA when transcribed by a transcription complex.

The goal is to produce an embeddable intracellular vaccine that consists of a segment of DNA that inserted into the human genome that perpetually produces TFIIIA molecules designed to silence the HIV DNA sequence if the HIV genome breaches the cell. The life-cycle of the Human Immunodeficiency Virus demonstrates that it is distinctly possible to embed functional segments of DNA into a specific target cell's genome.

Design and construct a physical model of the proposed DNA sequence intended to generate mRNA molecules intended to be translated to produce TFIIIAs capable of seeking out and neutralizing Human Immunodeficiency Virus, to be utilized as the source to generate a computer graphics representation of the embeddable DNA Vaccine sequence. Construct a 3D computer graphics model of the proposed DNA sequence. See Figure 98.

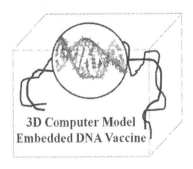

3D Computer Model
Embedded DNA Vaccine

Figure 98

Benefits of Proposed Technology: Computer modeling of the DNA intracellular vaccine technology designed to produce therapeutic TFIIIA molecules provides expansion of the DNA vaccine technology to make available permanent protection for US troops against high risk endemic DNA/RNA viral pathogens that might be encountered on battlefields across the globe.

Challenges: Modeling the design of a complete functional sequence of DNA to be seamlessly embedded into the human genome. Detailing the quaternary computer programming of the DNA. Computer modeling the basic construct of the forty proteins comprising an interactive transcription complex. Such a project requires a very high level of computer processing power, extensive memory capacity and sophisticated state-of-the-art software programming technology.

Major Goals/Milestones: Design 3D physical representation of DNA sequence to produce mRNA that when translated will produce therapeutic TFIIIA molecules. Design 3D computer representation of the DNA sequence to be interactive with 3D computer model of the human genome. Once computer DNA sequence simulation perfected, information to be sent to lab for production of biologic therapeutic molecules to be tested for use in humans to prevent HIV infections from occurring in individuals at risk of infection due to exposure to HIV.

Approximate Period of Performance: 48 months

References: 1. *Fourth Generation Biologics: Molecular Virus Killers*, L. B. Scheiber II, Lane B. Scheiber, iUniverse, 2014.

2.*Changing Global Approach to Medicine, Medical Vector Therapy*, L. B. Scheiber II, Lane B. Scheiber, iUniverse, 2011.

White Paper Proposal

PHASE 10

GENERATE AN INTERACTIVE THREE DIMENSIONAL COMPUTER MODEL OF THE HUMAN CELL NUCLEUS

Lane B. Scheiber II, MD
Osteoporosis & Arthritis Center, Inc.

Objective: Establish a prototype three dimensional interactive computer model of a human cell nucleus.

Description of Effort: The occurrence of the HIV outbreak demonstrates in the future it will be critical to make human cell secure against pathologic viruses. To effectively design rapidly deployable therapies to combat DNA viral genomes utilizing a three dimensional interactive model of the human cell nucleus as a platform for study of the behavior of a viral genome as well as study of the behavior of therapeutic molecules that can be utilized to neutralize an embedded viral threat. Model the specifics of the interior of the cell nucleus including fluid characteristics of the nuclear cytoplasm and molecular characteristics of structures including the DNA, histones, nucleosomes, spliceosomes, RNAs and proteins. See Figure 99.

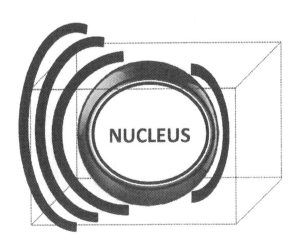

Figure 99

Benefits of Proposed Technology: By modeling the nucleus of the cell, a virtual laboratory can be established to study the strategy to efficiently embed a sequence of therapeutic DNA into the human genome to act as a vaccine. Once the embedding process has been established the computer model can be used to study the process of transcription where a transcription complex assembles and decodes the genetic information in the embedded sequence of therapeutic DNA.

A secondary benefit is that by computer modeling the nucleus of the human cell is that a substantial number of viruses exhibit a DNA phase where the viral genome is represented as DNA nucleotide code and is embedded in the nuclear DNA of the host cell. A viral genome that is capable of being represented as a segment of DNA and becomes inserted in the nuclear DNA of a host cell may lay dormant until a trigger is activated that generates transcription of the viral DNA genome. The DNA genome of the human immunodeficiency virus is known to lay dormant, termed proviral latency, for years. It is known that viral DNA genomes once transcribed are capable of overriding the normal command and control mechanisms of a cell and redirect the operations of the host cell to generate copies of the virus. A three dimensional interactive model of the nucleus of the human cell facilitates the means to design and study molecules such as a modified TFIIIA in real time to determine an optimal design of therapeutic molecules to combat viral DNA genomes that may be embedded in the DNA of human cells. See Figure 100.

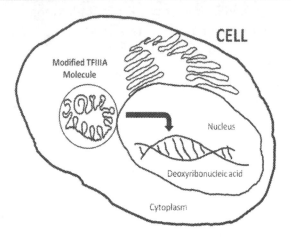

Figure 100

Challenges: Constructing computer model with precise detail of nuclear structures including inclusion of electrical charges emanating from structures comprising nucleus. Such a project requires a very high level of computer processing power, extensive memory storage capacity and sophisticated state-of-the-art software programming. There is limited detailed knowledge of molecular architecture of the individual nuclear structures, and even less knowledge of precisely how the nuclear structures actually function.

Major Goals/Milestones: Design 3D physical representation of nuclear structures. Design 3D physical representation of nuclear proteins. Design 3D computer representation of nuclear structures. Design 3D computer representation of nuclear proteins. Consolidate 3D representations into computer model. Construct and interactive three dimensional model of a cell's base-four biologic computer memory and processing components to be utilized as a platform to study the behavior of embedded DNA viral genomes and learn how to best neutralize the threat of DNA viral genomes which target and become embedded in the human genome.

Approximate Period of Performance: 60 months

References: 1. *Fourth Generation Biologics: Molecular Virus Killers*, L. B. Scheiber II, Lane B. Scheiber, iUniverse, 2014.

2.*Changing Global Approach to Medicine, Medical Vector Therapy*, L. B. Scheiber II, Lane B. Scheiber, iUniverse, 2011.

PART B

PROPOSAL TO DEVELOP AN EMBEDDED DNA VACCINE TO SILENCE EBOLAVIRUS
(and other viral pathogens)

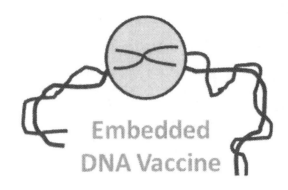

Copyright 2015

Phase 1: Decode and identify the 3D biochemical molecular structure of Ebolavirus.

Phase 2: Computer model the 3D biochemical molecular structure of EBOV.

Phase 3: Derive a Transcription Factor to intercept and neutralize the EBOV genome.

Phase 4: Computer model the 3D molecular structure of the TFIIIA to silence EBOV.

Phase 5: Computer model the internal environment of the cell to test EBOV RNA and TFIIIA.

Phase 6: Design the messenger RNA molecule to generate a therapeutic TFIIIA.

Phase 7: Computer model the molecular structure of the mRNA intended to produce TFIIIA.

Phase 8: Design an embeddable segment of DNA to generate an mRNA to produce TFIIIA.

Phase 9. Computer model the molecular structure of the DNA segment to produce mRNA.

Phase 10: Computer model the environment inside the nucleus of a cell to test DNA vaccine.

Phase 11: Work with a bio-lab to construct TFIIIA and DNA vaccine, and test both molecules.

White Paper Proposal

PHASE 1B

DECIPHER BASE-FOUR PROGRAMMING INSTRUCITON CODES COMPRISING EBOLAVIRUS GENOME

Lane B. Scheiber II, MD
Osteoporosis & Arthritis Center, Inc.

Objective: Decipher the base-four biologic instruction code programming language comprising the Ebola genome. See Figure 102.

Description of Effort: Similar to the DNA, the Ebolavirus RNA genome represents a base-four biologic computer program. Dissection of each nucleotide comprising the Ebolavirus RNA genome to cross-correlate segments of the Ebolavirus genome with known functions of the segments; then analyzing subsegments of the Ebolavirus genome that are not accounted for with known processes required to construct the complete Ebolavirus virion and cross-correlate with cell organelles and known function of cell organelles and cross-correlate with known function of enzymes and other proteins present in the cytoplasm of the cell. Convert nucleotides to a 0-3 numbering system to enhance study of the Ebola genome, similar to how a binary computer code would be studied to decipher the programming instructions.

Zaire Ebolavirus Genome (EBOV)
Genus Ebolavirus
Family Filoviridae

Single stranded RNA virus (-)

≈19,000 bps

7 Genes
7 encoded viral proteins and
3'leader and 5'trailer sequences

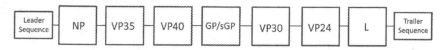

Figure 102

Benefits of Proposed Technology: By establishing knowledge of the instruction codes comprising the Ebolavirus genome that dictate how the proteins and ultimately the virus's virion is assembled allows for expanded means to predict, interdict and halt lethal viral infections such as Ebola. Deciphering the base-four language of Ebolavirus leads to the opportunity to unlock the programming instructions that control biologic cell functions.

Challenges: Currently, only the subsections of the RNA genome that act as templates to manufacture proteins are recognized, there is no knowledge of the instruction codes required to construct complex proteins or structures inside the boundaries of a cell. Of rather challenging complexity is discerning the base four programming language comprising the RNA genome. Arriving at the proper cipher to be used to correctly assign a numerical system to the letter system, that was arbitrarily assigned to the DNA/RNA nucleotides in the late 1800's, is a sophisticated puzzle to decode. The genomic cipher A0G1C2T3 utilized in Figure 103, below, was published in an abstract accepted to the 2014 annual meeting of the European Society of Human Genetics. It is understood that the Ebolavirus genome remains an RNA molecule, not represented as a DNA genome, during the life-cycle of the Ebolavirus and therefore each thymine nucleotide (DNA) actually represents a uracil nucleotide

(RNA). By convention, Ebola virus's RNA genome represents the virus's DNA.

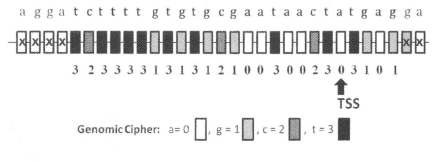

Figure 103

Major Goals/Milestones: Identify the instruction codes comprising the Ebolavirus genome that direct how the viral virion is assembled. Decipher the means by which the Ebolavirus virion is constructed in order to identify vulnerabilities that can be exploited to halt the infectious nature of the virus. Gain knowledge of a base-four programming language utilized to generate viral genomes. This project would represent the first effort to convert the individual nucleotides comprising the viral genome to numbers for the purposes of trying to decipher the base-four programming language that comprises the Ebolavirus genome.

Approximate Period of Performance: 36 months

References: 1. *Fourth Generation Biologics: Molecular Virus Killers*, L Scheiber, iUniverse, 2014.

2. ScheiberL, ScheiberL, Presenting the genomic cipher adenine = 0, guanine =1, cytosine = 2, thymine = 3 derived directly from the DNA to convert nucleotide names/letters to numbers to study patterns of unique identifiers to detect command genes in the human genome, Control No. 2014-A-616-ESHG, European Conference of Human Genetics 2014.

White Paper Proposal

PHASE 2B

GENERATE AN INTERACTIVE THREE DIMENSIONAL COMPUTER MODEL OF THE EBOLAVIRUS RNA

Lane B. Scheiber II, MD
Osteoporosis & Arthritis Center, Inc.

Objective: Establish a prototype three dimensional interactive computer model of the Ebolavirus single stranded RNA genome as it appears in the cell, this three dimensional interactive computer model of the Ebolavirus to act as a target for therapeutic molecules such a modified TFIIIA molecules and to be interactive within a computer model of the human cell. See Figure 104.

Description of Effort: The occurrence of the 2014 West Africa Ebolavirus outbreak demonstrated that the future security of the human cell is critical. To effectively design therapies to combat Ebolavirus, a three dimensional interactive model of the Ebolavirus RNA genome is to be designed and generated. Such a three dimensional model of the Ebolavirus RNA genome to be designed to be compatible with a three dimensional model of the human cell. Such a computer simulation of the Ebolavirus to act as a virtual laboratory specimen to study viral threats as they reside inside the host cell where viral genomes are copied and ejected from host as viral virions.

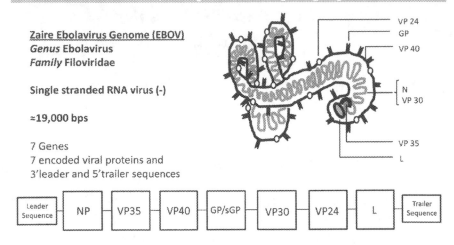

Figure 104

Benefits of Proposed Technology: A three dimensional interactive model of the Ebolavirus RNA genome facilitates the means to design and study neutralizing therapeutic molecules such as a modified TFIIIA in real time to determine an optimal design of therapeutic molecules to combat RNA viral genomes in the cytoplasm. A detailed 3D computer graphics representation of the current Ebolavirus threats and future variations of the Ebolavirus (See Second Figure). A 3D computer graphics representation of the Ebolavirus RNA genome allows for simulations to be performed to study the biochemistry and behavior of the Ebolavirus RNA genome as it interacts with a 3D graphics representation of potential neutralizing therapeutic molecules that might be utilized to seek out Ebolavirus RNA genome as the viral genome resides inside the cytoplasm. See Figure 105.

Challenges: Constructing a computer model with precise detail of the Ebolavirus genome at the molecular level and accounting for the three dimensional behavior of the nucleotides that comprise the viral genome. The complexity rises sharply when accounting for the factors of how the individual nucleotides of the viral genome interact with the cytoplasm medium, and organelles and the wide variety of proteins naturally suspended in the cytoplasm of the host cell. Such a project requires a very high level of computer processing power, extensive memory storage capacity and sophisticated state-of-the-art software programming. There is limited knowledge of subprograms comprising Ebolavirus RNA genome.

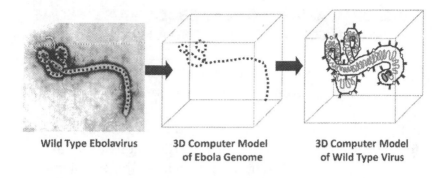

Wild Type Ebolavirus   3D Computer Model   3D Computer Model
of Ebola Genome   of Wild Type Virus

Figure 105

<u>Major Goals/Milestones</u>: Identify design parameters of 3D model of Ebolavirus RNA. Design 3D physical representation of Wild Type Ebolavirus RNA genome. Design 3D computer representation of Ebolavirus RNA genome to be interactive with 3D computer TFIIIA molecule. If 3D computer model of the cell is completed, design 3D computer representation of Ebolavirus RNA genome to be interactive with a 3D computer model of the cell. Test and improve 3D computer representation of Ebolavirus RNA genome to simulate real time, life-like interaction of Ebolavirus RNA genome with neutralizing therapeutic molecules such as a modified TFIIIA hunter-killer molecule that would seek out and bind to 3D simulation of wild type Ebolavirus RNA in the cytoplasm of the cell inside 3D model of the cell. Final goal is to simulate by computer assisted design the Ebolavirus RNA genome to act as a target to facilitate the development of effective means to neutralize the threat of the Ebolavirus RNA genome and future variations of the virus, which the computer assisted design of a neutralizing therapeutic molecule once perfected can then be sent to the lab for production of actual biologic therapeutic molecules to be tested and used in humans as a treatment against an Ebolavirus infection.

<u>Approximate Period of Performance</u>: 60 months

WHITE PAPER PROPOSAL

PHASE 3B

DEVELOP MEANS TO COMBAT EBOLAVIRUS GENOME WITH A NOVEL MODIFIED TFIIIA MOLECULE

Lane B. Scheiber II, MD
Osteoporosis & Arthritis Center, Inc.

Objective: Develop a means to rapidly and efficiently seek out and neutralize the Zaire Ebolavirus (EBOV) RNA genome in the host cells of an infected individual utilizing a modified Transcription Factor IIIA (TFIIIA) molecule to bind to and silence EBOV RNA genome.

Description of Effort: Utilize a modified TFIIIA molecule, target the Ebola genome directly as it resides in the host cell. Prevent translation of the viral genome by binding the modified TFIIIA molecule to a unique identifier in the viral genome upstream from the NP gene. Halting translation of the Ebola genome arrests the viral infection and the lethal effects of the virus.

Recent events regarding the 2014 EBOV outbreak in West Africa suggest two undeniable concerns: (1) a viral pathogen is capable of efficiently killing large numbers of individuals and (2) current capability to combat viral infections including isolation, vaccines, and infusions of antibodies are not necessarily sufficient to arrest virulent viral infections and insure survival of an infected patient. Given viruses mutate, a third concern is emergence of an airborne strain of EBOV.

Currently Ebolavirus consists of 6 known strains. Zaire ebolavirus (EBOV) was the first strain recorded in 1976, and is responsible for the two most recent 2014 epidemics. EBOV is an RNA negative sense virus, activating and replicating in the cytoplasm of a host cell. The EBOV genome is approximately 19,000 nucleotides and comprised of 7 genes including 3'-NP-VP35-VP40-GP/sGP-VP30-VP24-L-5'. VP40 protein assists with forming the exterior viral coat. Respiratory Syncytial Virus (RSV) is an RNA negative sense virus with a genome comprised of approximately 15,277 nucleotides. The RSV genome is comprised of ten genes including 3'-N1-N2-N-M-P-G-F-SH-M2-L-5'. The genes G-F-SH code for RSV's external coat.

THREAT OF EBOLAVIRUS MUTATION TO MORE VIRULENT VIRUS

Both EBOV and RSV may utilize a lung cell for virion replication purposes. If EBOV and RSV coexist in the same lung cell, there is the prospect that the EBOV genome may switch VP40 gene with RSV's G-F-SH gene segment. See Figure 106. If the EBOV genome acquires the G-F-SH virion coating genes from RSV it now has the opportunity to act like a respiratory virus. Conversely, RSV might integrate the VP35 and GP genes, utilized by Ebola to circumvent immune responses, into its genome and become a significantly more lethal airborne virus.

EBOV genome, NCBI Reference Sequence: AY354458 has a 25 nucleotide sequence 5'-tcttttgtgtgcgaataactatgag-3' positioned at 34 to 58, which serves as a unique identifier for EBOV's NP gene. NP gene's product is vital for virus replication. The human genome was studied and this unique identifier is not found as a complete sequence in the human genome. This unique identifier can be used as an inimitable target. See Figure 107.

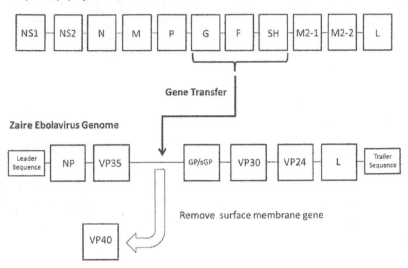

Figure 106

MODIFIED TFIIIA MOLECULE

This effort utilizes EBOV's NP gene's unique identifier as an inimitable therapeutic target. TFIIIA molecules initiate decoding of viral genomes. The first 5 zinc fingers of a TFIIIA molecule are modified to seek out and attach to NP's unique identifier. The algorithm responsible for replacing the amino acids of zinc fingers 1-5 is derived from a novel biochemical analysis of the bonding characteristics of nucleotides-to-amino acids, detailed in the listed reference. Zinc fingers 6-9 are modified to prevent binding of other transcription factors. The COOH tail is modified to maintain the TFIIIA in the cytoplasm. This novel approach provides a modified TFIIIA designed to seek out and bind to NP gene's unique identifier to avert translation of the NP gene to arrest construction of copies of the EBOV virion. Halting EBOV virion construction neutralizes the threat.

Benefits of Proposed Technology: The modified TFIIIA technology is versatile and allows expansion of the technology to treat various versions of Ebolavirus as well as the means to target most DNA/RNA viral pathogens that might be encountered.

Challenges: Insuring the modified TFIIIA molecule does not interact with other structures inside the human cell. Accounting for genetic variation in Ebolavirus genome. Insuring modified TFIIIA neutralizing effect is permanent enough to restrict EBOV genome from being translated.

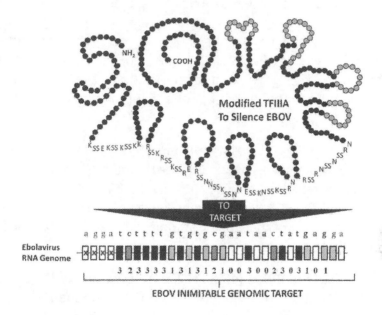

Figure 107

Major Goals/Milestones: Identify design parameters of modified TFIIIA molecule. Explore computer modeling of amino acid bonding to nucleotides. Versatile system to treat viral threats.

Approximate Period of Performance: 24 months.

Reference: *Fourth Generation Biologics: Molecular Virus Killers*, L Scheiber, iUniverse, 2014.

WHITE PAPER PROPOSAL

PHASE 4B

REPRESENT BY INTERACTIVE 3D COMPUTER MODEL A MODIFIED TFIIIA MOLECULE TO NEUTRALIZE EBOLA

Lane B. Scheiber II, MD
Osteoporosis & Arthritis Center, Inc.

Objective: Develop three dimensional computer graphics model of a modified Transcription Factor IIIA (TFIIIA) molecule to seek out Zaire Ebolavirus (EBOV) genome in a host cell and silence the virus's genome in order to neutralize the effects of the virus and halt viral replication.

Description of Effort: Utilize a modified TFIIIA molecule, target the Ebola genome directly as it resides in the host cell. Prevent translation of the viral genome by binding the modified TFIIIA molecule to a unique identifier in the viral genome upstream from the NP gene. Halting translation of the Ebola genome arrests the viral infection and the lethal effects of the virus.

Recent events regarding the 2014 EBOV outbreak in West Africa suggest two undeniable concerns: (1) a viral pathogen is capable of efficiently killing large numbers of individuals and (2) current capability to combat viral infections including isolation, vaccines, and infusions of antibodies are not necessarily sufficient to arrest virulent viral infections and insure survival of an infected patient. Given viruses mutate, a third concern is emergence of an airborne strain of EBOV.

EBOV genome, NCBI Reference Sequence: AY354458 has a 25 nucleotide sequence 5'-tcttttgtgtgcgaataactatgag-3' positioned at 34 to 58, which serves as a unique identifier for EBOV's NP gene. NP gene's product is vital for virus replication. The human genome was studied and this unique identifier is not found as a complete sequence in the uninfected human genome. Thus, this unique identifier in the EBOV genome can be used as an inimitable target. See Figure 108.

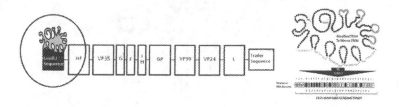

Figure 108

Modified TFIIIA Molecule

This effort utilizes EBOV's NP gene's unique identifier as an inimitable therapeutic target. In nature TFIIIA molecules initiate decoding of viral genomes. The first 5 zinc fingers of a TFIIIA molecule are modified to seek out and attach to NP's unique identifier. The algorithm responsible for replacing the amino acids of zinc fingers 1-5 is derived from a novel biochemical analysis of the bonding characteristics of nucleotides-to-amino acids detailed in the listed reference. Zinc fingers 6-9 are modified to prevent binding of other transcription factors. The COOH tail is modified to maintain the TFIIIA in the cytoplasm. This novel approach provides a modified TFIIIA designed to seek out and bind to NP gene's unique identifier to avert translation of the NP gene to arrest construction of copies of the EBOV virion in the cytoplasm of the cell. Halting EBOV virion construction would neutralize the EBOV threat.

Design and construct a physical model of the modified TFIIIA molecule intended to seek out and neutralize Zaire Ebolavirus, to be utilized as the source to generate a computer graphics representation of the TFIIIA molecule. Construct a 3D computer graphics model of the modified TFIIIA molecule. See Figure 109.

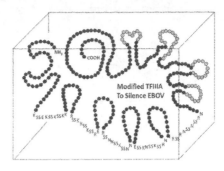

3D Computer Model of TFIIIA

Figure 109

Benefits of Proposed Technology: The modified TFIIIA technology is versatile and allows expansion of the technology to treat variations of EBOV as well as most DNA/RNA viral pathogens that might be encountered on the battlefield. A detailed 3D computer graphics representation of the TFIIIA molecule allows for study of the biochemistry and bonding of the TFIIIA molecule to current EBOV threats and future variations of EBOV.

Challenges: Insuring the modified TFIIIA molecule does not interact with other structures inside the human cell. Complexity rises sharply when accounting for how the individual amino acids comprising the TFIIIA molecule will interact with the cytoplasm and organelles of the host cell. Insuring a modified TFIIIA bonds to the EBOV genome in a permanent enough manner to sufficiently restrict the EBOV genome from being translated or copied. Such a project requires a very high level of computer processing power, extensive memory storage capacity and sophisticated state-of-the-art software programming technology.

Major Goals/Milestones: Design 3D physical representation of TFIIIA molecule. Design 3D computer representation of TFIIIA molecule to be interactive with 3D computer model of EBOV RNA. If 3D computer model of the cell is available, design 3D computer representation of TFIIIA to be interactive with a 3D computer model of the cell. Test and improve 3D computer representation of TFIIIA to simulate real time, life-like interaction of TFIIIA hunter-killer molecule to seek out and bind to 3D simulation of wild type EBOV RNA in the cytoplasm inside 3D model of the cell. Once computer TFIIIA simulation perfected, information to be sent to lab for production of biologic therapeutic molecules to be tested for use in humans to treat EBOV.

Approximate Period of Performance: 60 months

Reference: *Fourth Generation Biologics: Molecular Virus Killers*, L Scheiber, iUniverse, 2014.

White Paper Proposal

PHASE 5B

GENERATE INTERACTIVE THREE DIMENSIONAL COMPUTER MODEL OF THE HUMAN CELL WITH INANIMATE NUCLEUS

Lane B. Scheiber II, MD
Osteoporosis & Arthritis Center, Inc.

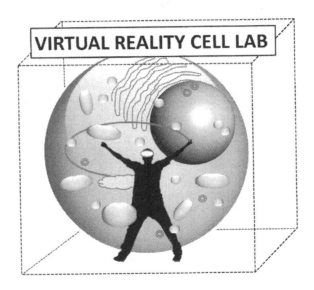

Objective: Establish a prototype three dimensional interactive computer model of a human cell with functional cytoplasm, organelles, microtubule architecture and an inanimate nucleus.

Description of Effort: The occurrence of the 2014 Ebolavirus outbreak in West Africa demonstrates that the next critical thrust in medical research will be bolstering the security of the human cell against lethal viruses. Develop a three dimensional interactive model of the human cell with functional cytoplasm. Model the specifics of the interior of the cell including characteristics of the cytoplasm, external characteristics of organelles including the nucleus, Golgi apparatus, vacuoles, mitochondria and molecules including ribosomes and proteins.

Benefits of Proposed Technology: A three dimensional interactive model of the human cell facilitates the means to design and study molecules such as a modified TFIIIA in real time to determine an optimal design of therapeutic molecules to combat the genomes of viral pathogens including Ebolavirus. Development of a virtual laboratory to act as a means to study the behavior of viral pathogens and therapeutic molecules without placing human laboratory personnel at risk, with such a laboratory being capable of running numerous scenarios in order to arrive at an optimal design of a therapeutic molecule to combat the Ebolavirus genome.

Challenges: Constructing a realistic computer representation of the precise detail of a human cell's three dimensional exterior membrane. Constructing a computer representation of the precise detail of the organelles and proteins comprising the interior structures of a human cell. Correctly modeling the fluid dynamics of the cell cytoplasm and the effects of the cell's internal microtubule architecture. The complexity of the project rises sharply when such a three dimensional computer representation is then required to be interactive with the insertion of both molecular structures that might attack the cell such a viral genome, as well as the insertion of molecular structures of therapeutic molecules that might be used to benefit the cell by neutralizing a threatening viral genome. Such a project requires a very high level of computer processing power, extensive memory storage capacity and sophisticated state-of-the-art software programming. There is limited knowledge of the molecular architecture of the organelles and behavior of the organelles as they are suspended in the cell cytoplasm. Fluid dynamics of the cytoplasm is affected by numerous factors including fluid channels in the exterior membrane, fluid channels present in the nuclear membrane, numerous complex shaped free-floating structures, the microtubule architecture, the attractive and repulsive forces inherent to the electrical charges present on molecular surfaces.

Major Goals/Milestones: Identify design parameters of a three dimensional (3D) model of a cell. Design 3D physical representation of the cell membrane and internal cytoplasm and microtubule architecture. Design 3D physical representation of organelles and proteins. Consolidate 3D physical representations of outer cell membrane and 3D physical representation of organelles and proteins into a 3D physical model of the cell that can be used as a reference to design a 3D computer model of a cell. Design 3D computer model representation of the cell membrane and internal cytoplasm and microtubule architecture. Design 3D computer representation of organelles. Design 3D computer representation of proteins. Consolidate 3D computer representations of cell membrane, cell's internal cytoplasm, microtubule architecture organelles and 3D computer representations of proteins into 3D computer model of a human cell. Assimilate the software programming into 3D Computer Model of the Cell capable of to interactions with 3D computer model of the Ebolavirus and 3D computer model of a modified TFIIIA molecule or 3D computer model of equivalent therapeutic molecule. Establish a virtual laboratory to act as a means to study the behavior of viral pathogens and therapeutic molecules capable of running numerous scenarios in order to arrive at an optimal design of a therapeutic molecule to combat the current Ebolavirus genomes and future variations to the Ebolavirus genome.

Approximate Period of Performance: 60 months

WHITE PAPER PROPOSAL

PHASE 6B

INTRACELLULAR mRNA VACCINE TO GENERATE TFIIIAs INSIDE HOST CELL TO NEUTRALIZE EBOLA

Lane B. Scheiber II, MD
Osteoporosis & Arthritis Center, Inc.

Objective: Develop an intracellular vaccine consisting of a messenger ribonucleic acid (mRNA) to be translated to generate therapeutic Transcription Factor IIIA (TFIIIA) molecules coded to seek out the Zaire Ebolavirus (EBOV) genome in host cells and to engage and silence the virus's genome to halt viral replication and arrest the viral infection.

Description of Effort: The goal is to produce a vaccine that consists of a mRNA (See First Figure) that produces TFIIIA molecules designed to silence the Ebolavirus RNA genome if the Ebolavirus genome breaches the cell's membrane and enters the cytoplasm. The life-cycle of the Hepatitis C virus demonstrates it is possible to embed functional mRNA into specific target cells.

EBOV genome, NCBI Reference Sequence: AY354458, has a 25 nucleotide sequence 5'-tcttttgtgtgcgaataactatgag-3' positioned at 34 to 58, which serves as a unique identifier for EBOV's NP gene. NP gene's product is vital for virus replication. The human genome was studied and this unique identifier is not found as a complete sequence in the uninfected human genome. Thus, this unique identifier in the EBOV genome can be used as an inimitable target.

This effort utilizes EBOV's NP gene's unique identifier as an inimitable therapeutic target. Once the design parameters of the TFIIIA molecule are established, a reverse translation process is undergone to design the translatable portion of a mRNA molecule that when translated by ribosomes in the cytoplasm of a host cell will produce the TFIIIA molecule, this TFIIIA molecule capable of hunting down and engaging the Ebolavirus RNA genome. See Figure 110.

Prevention of translation of the viral genome by binding the therapeutic TFIIIA molecule to a unique identifier in the viral genome upstream from the NP gene halts translation of the Ebolavirus genome and arrests the viral infection. See Figure 111.

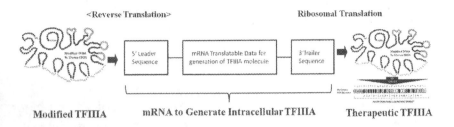

Figure 110

Benefits of Proposed Technology: The mRNA intracellular vaccine technology designed to produce therapeutic TFIIIA molecules is versatile and allows expansion of the mRNA vaccine technology to provide protection for US troops against numerous high risk endemic DNA/RNA viral pathogens that might be encountered on battlefields around the globe. The mRNA technology is the frontrunner effort which provides the necessary technical information regarding mRNA design in order to develop an embedded DNA vaccine.

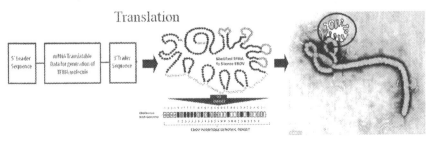

Figure 111

Challenges: Establishing a reverse translation process that will generate the translatable segment of an mRNA; this effort includes deciphering the quaternary computer aspects of human genetics. Design of a complete functional mRNA molecule to be inserted into the human cell. Design of the complete mRNA molecule so as to be recognized and translated by a ribosomal complex in the cytoplasm of a host cell to generate functional TFIIIA molecules. Design the 3' trailer sequence of the mRNA to modulate the life of the mRNA's presence in the cytoplasm.

Major Goals/Milestones: Design an intercellular vaccine utilizing a mRNA molecule that will generate therapeutic TFIIIA molecules that will engage the Ebolavirus RNA genome if it enters the protected cell. Describe how a ribosomal complex effects translation of a specific therapeutic intracellular mRNA vaccine. Design functional 5' trailer sequence of mRNA molecule. Design functional 3' trailer sequence of the mRNA molecule to extend the life of the mRNA.

Approximate Period of Performance: 48 months

References: 1. *Fourth Generation Biologics: Molecular Virus Killers*, LScheiber, iUniverse, 2014.

2.*Changing Global Approach to Medicine, Medical Vector Therapy*, LScheiber, iUniverse,2011.

WHITE PAPER PROPOSAL

PHASE 7B

COMPUTER MODEL 'INTRACELLULAR' mRNA VACCINE TO GENERATE TFIIIAs TO NEUTRALIZE EBOLAVIRUS

Lane B. Scheiber II, MD
Osteoporosis & Arthritis Center, Inc.

Objective: Develop three dimensional computer graphics model of a messenger RNA designed to be translated by the ribosomes of the host cell to generate modified Transcription Factor IIIA (TFIIIA) molecules coded to seek out Zaire Ebolavirus (EBOV) genome in the host cell to engage and silence the virus's genome in order to arrest viral replication.

Description of Effort: Utilize computer graphics to represent the messenger ribonucleic acid (mRNA) designed to be translated to generate modified TFIIIA molecules, to target the Ebola genome directly if the Ebola RNA genome breaches the host cell membrane and enters the host cell. Utilizing computer graphics demonstrate that the therapeutic mRNA can be engage and decoded by a ribosomal complex to produce the intended TFIIIA molecules. See Figure 112.

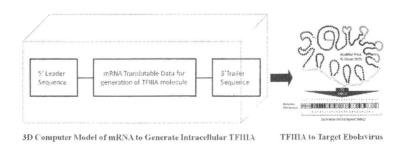

3D Computer Model of mRNA to Generate Intracellular TFIIIA   TFIIIA to Target Ebolavirus

Figure 112

This effort utilizes EBOV's NP gene's unique identifier as an inimitable therapeutic target. Once the design parameters of the

TFIIIA molecule are established, a reverse translation process is undergone to design the translatable portion of a mRNA molecule that when translated by ribosomes in the cytoplasm of a host cell will produce the TFIIIA molecule.

Design and construct a physical model of the proposed mRNA sequence intended to generate mRNA molecules intended to be translated to produce TFIIIAs capable of seeking out and neutralizing Zaire Ebolavirus, to be utilized as the source to generate a computer graphics representation of the TFIIIA molecule. The goal is to produce a realistic 3D graphics representation of an intracellular vaccine that consists of a mRNA that produces TFIIIA molecules designed to silence the Ebolavirus RNA genome if the Ebolavirus genome breaches the outer membrane of a host cell and enters the cell's cytoplasm. See Figure 113.

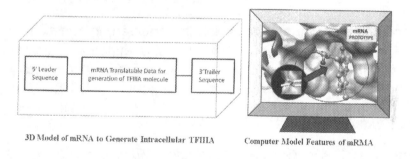

3D Model of mRNA to Generate Intracellular TFIIIA   Computer Model Features of mRMA

Figure 113

Benefits of Proposed Technology: Computer modeling of the mRNA intracellular vaccine technology designed to produce therapeutic TFIIIA molecules provides expansion of the mRNA vaccine technology to make available protection for US troops against high risk endemic DNA/RNA viral pathogens that might be encountered on battlefields around the globe.

Challenges: Computer modeling the design of a complete functional sequence of mRNA. Defining how the ribosomal complex engages the mRNA molecule. Discern in the 5' leader segment of the mRNA the signal required to initiate assembly of a ribosomal complex and subsequent engagement of the therapeutic mRNA molecule. Model representations of the ribosome molecules to interface with the mRNA model to run simulations to show the mRNA will be translated when present in a biologic cell's cytoplasm. Such a project requires a very high level of computer processing power, extensive memory storage capacity and sophisticated state-of-the-art software programming technology.

Major Goals/Milestones: Design 3D physical representation of mRNA sequence to produce be translated will produce therapeutic TFIIIA molecules. Develop a 3D computer representation of the mRNA sequence to be interactive with 3D computer model of a ribosomal complex. Establish definition of the signaling of mRNA to initiate translation of an mRNA molecule. Establish design parameters of the 3' tail segment of the mRNA molecule that will dictate the functional life of a mRNA molecule in cytoplasm of the host cell.

Once computer mRNA simulation is perfected, information to be sent to lab for production of biologic therapeutic molecules to be tested for use in humans to prevent EBOV infections from occurring in individuals at risk of infection due to exposure to EBOV.

Approximate Period of Performance: 60 months

Reference: *Fourth Generation Biologics: Molecular Virus Killers*, L Scheiber, iUniverse, 2014.

WHITE PAPER PROPOSAL

PHASE 8B

DEVELOP EMBEDDED DNA INTRACELLULAR VACCINE TO GENERATE TFIIIAs TO NEUTRALIZE EBOLAVIRUS

Lane B. Scheiber II, MD
Osteoporosis & Arthritis Center, Inc.

Objective: Develop an intracellular vaccine consisting of a deoxyribonucleic acid (DNA) segment designed to be transcribed by the host cell's RNA Polymerase II to generate messenger RNA (mRNA) to be translated to generate therapeutic Transcription Factor IIIA (TFIIIA) molecules coded to seek out Zaire Ebolavirus (EBOV) genome in host cells to engage and silence the virus's genome to halt viral replication and arrest the viral infection.

Description of Effort: The goal is to produce a vaccine that consists of a segment of DNA that is embedded in the human genome that perpetually produces TFIIIA molecules designed to silence the Ebolavirus RNA genome if the Ebolavirus genome breaches the cell. The life-cycle of the Human Immunodeficiency Virus demonstrates that it is possible to embed functional segments of DNA into a specific target cell's genome.

EBOV genome, NCBI Reference Sequence: AY354458, has a 25 nucleotide sequence 5'-tcttttgtgtgcgaataactatgag-3' positioned at 34 to 58, which serves as a unique identifier for EBOV's NP gene. NP gene's product is vital for virus replication. The human genome was studied and this unique identifier is not found as a complete sequence in the uninfected human genome. Thus, this unique identifier in the EBOV genome can be used as an inimitable target.

This effort utilizes EBOV's NP gene's unique identifier as an inimitable therapeutic target. Once the design parameters of the TFIIIA molecule are established, a reverse translation process is undergone to design the translatable portion of a mRNA molecule that when translated by ribosomes in the cytoplasm of a host cell will produce the TFIIIA molecule. Once the design parameters of the mRNA molecule is established, a reverse transcription process is utilized to design a segment of DNA. See Figure 114.

Design a segment of DNA to be embedded in the human genome that when transcribed would generate mRNA molecules designed to be translated in the cytoplasm of the host cell to generate therapeutic TFIIIA molecules to target the Ebolavirus genome directly if the Ebolavirus RNA genome breaches the host cell membrane and enters the host cell. See Figure 115. Prevent translation of the viral genome by binding the therapeutic TFIIIA molecule to a unique identifier in the viral genome upstream from the NP gene. Halting translation of the Ebola genome arrests the viral infection.

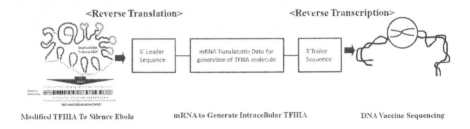

Figure 114

Benefits of Proposed Technology: The DNA embedded intracellular vaccine technology designed to produce therapeutic TFIIIA molecules is versatile and allows expansion of the DNA vaccine technology to provide permanent protection for US troops against numerous high risk endemic DNA/RNA viral pathogens that might be encountered on battlefields around the globe.

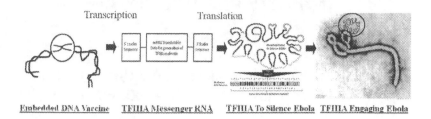

Transcription   Translation

Embedded DNA Vaccine   TFIIIA Messenger RNA   TFIIIA To Silence Ebola   TFIIIA Engaging Ebola

Figure 115

Challenges: Establishing a reverse transcription process that will generate the transcribable segment; this effort includes deciphering the quaternary computer aspects of the human gene utilized by the gene to locate and transcribe genetic information as needed by the cell. Design of a complete functional sequence of DNA to be seamlessly embedded into the human genome; avoiding undue influence of the sex cells. Design of the complete DNA sequence so as to be recognized and transcribed by a transcription complex to generate a functionally mature mRNA molecule.

Major Goals/Milestones: Design an intercellular vaccine utilizing a DNA sequence that will generate mRNA molecules to produce therapeutic TFIIIA molecules that will engage the Ebolavirus RNA genome if the virus's genome enters the protected cell. Describe how RNA Polymerase II would engage reverse transcribed DNA to effect transcription of therapeutic DNA to mRNA. Design functional 5' upstream sequence of DNA. Design functional 3' downstream sequence of DNA.

Approximate Period of Performance: 60 months

Reference1. *Fourth Generation Biologics: Molecular Virus Killers*, LScheiber, iUniverse, 2014.

2.*Changing Global Approach to Medicine, Medical Vector Therapy*, LScheiber, iUniverse, 2011.

WHITE PAPER PROPOSAL

PHASE 9B

COMPUTER MODEL DNA 'INTRACELLULAR' VACCINE TO GENERATE TFIIIAs TO NEUTRALIZE EBOLAVIRUS

Lane B. Scheiber II, MD
Osteoporosis & Arthritis Center, Inc.

Objective: Develop a three dimensional computer graphics model representative of a segment of deoxyribonucleic acid (DNA) designed to be embedded in the human genome to be transcribed by the host cell to generate messenger RNA molecules to be translated to generate modified Transcription Factor IIIA (TFIIIA) molecules coded to seek out Zaire Ebolavirus (EBOV) genome in host cell and engage, then silence the virus's genome to arrest a viral infection.

Description of Effort: Utilize computer assisted design technology to generate a model of an embeddable segment of DNA that when transcribed would produce messenger RNA (mRNA) designed to be translated to generate modified TFIIIA molecules to target and neutralize the Ebola genome directly if the Ebola genome breaches the host cell membrane and enters the cell. Utilizing computer graphics demonstrate that the DNA segment can be inserted into the human genome. Further, demonstrate through computer modeling that a transcription complex is able to engage and decode the DNA sequence to produce the intended mRNA. See Figure 116.

EBOV genome, NCBI Reference Sequence: AY354458, has a 25 nucleotide sequence 5'-tcttttgtgtgcgaataactatgag-3' positioned at 34 to 58, which serves as a unique identifier for EBOV's NP gene. NP gene's product is vital for virus replication. The human genome was studied and this unique identifier is not found as a complete sequence in the uninfected human genome. Thus, this unique identifier in the EBOV genome can be used as an inimitable target.

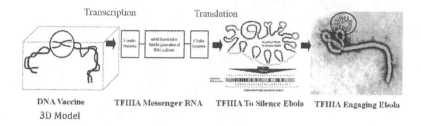

Transcription   Translation

DNA Vaccine   **TFIIIA Messenger RNA**   **TFIIIA To Silence Ebola**   **TFIIIA Engaging Ebola**
3D Model

Figure 116

This effort utilizes EBOV's NP gene's unique identifier as an inimitable therapeutic target. Once the design parameters of the TFIIIA molecule are established, a reverse translation process is undergone to design the translatable portion of a mRNA molecule that when translated by ribosomes in the cytoplasm of a host cell will produce the TFIIIA molecule. Once the design parameters of the mRNA molecule is established, a reverse transcription process is utilized to design a segment of DNA that will generate mRNA when transcribed by a transcription complex.

The goal is to produce an embeddable intracellular vaccine that consists of a segment of DNA that inserted into the human genome that perpetually produces TFIIIA molecules designed to silence the Ebolavirus RNA genome if the Ebolavirus genome breaches the cell. The life-cycle of the Human Immunodeficiency Virus demonstrates that it is distinctly possible to embed functional segments of DNA into a specific target cell's genome.

Design and construct a physical model of the proposed DNA sequence intended to generate mRNA molecules intended to be translated to produce TFIIIAs capable of seeking out and neutralizing Zaire Ebolavirus, to be utilized as the source to generate a computer graphics representation of the embeddable DNA Vaccine sequence. Construct a 3D computer graphics model of the proposed DNA sequence. See Figure 117.

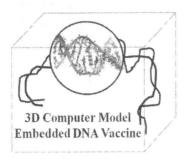

Figure 117

Benefits of Proposed Technology: Computer modeling of the DNA intracellular vaccine technology designed to produce therapeutic TFIIIA molecules provides expansion of the DNA vaccine technology to make available permanent protection for US troops against high risk endemic DNA/RNA viral pathogens that might be encountered on battlefields across the globe.

Challenges: Modeling the design of a complete functional sequence of DNA to be seamlessly embedded into the human genome. Detailing the quaternary computer programming of the DNA. Computer modeling the basic construct of the forty proteins comprising an interactive transcription complex. Such a project requires a very high level of computer processing power, extensive memory capacity and sophisticated state-of-the-art software programming technology.

Major Goals/Milestones: Design 3D physical representation of DNA sequence to produce mRNA that when translated will produce therapeutic TFIIIA molecules. Design 3D computer representation of the DNA sequence to be interactive with 3D computer model of the human genome. Once computer DNA sequence simulation perfected, information to be sent to lab for production of biologic therapeutic molecules to be tested for use in humans to prevent EBOV infections from occurring in individuals at risk of infection due to exposure to EBOV.

<u>Approximate Period of Performance</u>: 48 months

<u>References:</u> 1. *Fourth Generation Biologics: Molecular Virus Killers*, LScheiber, iUniverse, 2014.

2.*Changing Global Approach to Medicine, Medical Vector Therapy*, LScheiber, iUniverse, 2011.

White Paper Proposal

PHASE 10B

GENERATE AN INTERACTIVE THREE DIMENSIONAL
COMPUTER MODEL OF THE HUMAN CELL NUCLEUS

Lane B. Scheiber II, MD
Osteoporosis & Arthritis Center, Inc.

Objective: Establish a prototype three dimensional interactive computer model of a human cell nucleus.

Description of Effort: The occurrence of the Ebolavirus outbreak demonstrates that a future critical battlefield will be security of the human cell. To effectively design rapidly deployable therapies to combat DNA viral genomes utilizing a three dimensional interactive model of the human cell nucleus as a platform for study of the behavior of a viral genome as well as study of the behavior of therapeutic molecules that can be utilized to neutralize an embedded viral threat. Model the specifics of the interior of the cell nucleus including fluid characteristics of the nuclear cytoplasm and molecular characteristics of structures including the DNA, histones, nucleosomes, spliceosomes, RNAs and proteins. See Figure 118.

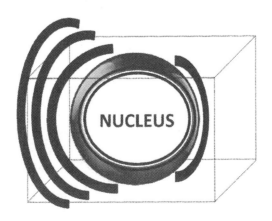

Figure 118

Benefits of Proposed Technology: By modeling the nucleus of the cell, a virtual laboratory can be established to study the strategy to efficiently embed a sequence of therapeutic DNA into the human genome to act as a vaccine. Once the embedding process has been established the computer model can be used to study the process of transcription where a transcription complex assembles and decodes the genetic information in the embedded sequence of therapeutic DNA.

A secondary benefit is that by computer modeling the nucleus of the human cell is that a substantial number of viruses exhibit a DNA phase where the viral genome is represented as DNA nucleotide code and is embedded in the nuclear DNA of the host cell. A viral genome that is capable of being represented as a segment of DNA and becomes inserted in the nuclear DNA of a host cell may lay dormant until a trigger is activated that generates transcription of the viral DNA genome. The DNA genome of the human immunodeficiency virus is known to lay dormant, termed proviral latency, for years. It is known that viral DNA genomes once transcribed are capable of overriding the normal command and control mechanisms of a cell and redirect the operations of the host cell to generate copies of the virus. A three dimensional interactive model of the nucleus of the human cell facilitates the means to design and study molecules such as a modified TFIIIA in real time to determine an optimal design of therapeutic molecules to combat viral DNA genomes that may be embedded in the DNA of human cells. See Figure 119.

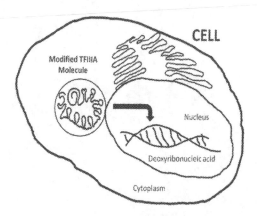

Figure 119

Challenges: Constructing computer model with precise detail of nuclear structures including inclusion of electrical charges emanating from structures comprising nucleus. Such a project requires a very high level of computer processing power, extensive memory storage capacity and sophisticated state-of-the-art software programming. There is limited detailed knowledge of molecular architecture of the individual nuclear structures, and even less knowledge of precisely how the nuclear structures actually function.

Major Goals/Milestones: Design 3D physical representation of nuclear structures. Design 3D physical representation of nuclear proteins. Design 3D computer representation of nuclear structures. Design 3D computer representation of nuclear proteins. Consolidate 3D representations into computer model. Construct and interactive three dimensional model of a cell's base-four biologic computer memory and processing components to be utilized as a platform to study the behavior of embedded DNA viral genomes and learn how to best neutralize the threat of DNA viral genomes which target and become embedded in the human genome.

Approximate Period of Performance: 60 months

Concise summary of composition of human genes

A human gene sequence contains:

5' Upstream segment, transcribable segment, 3' Downstream segment.

In the 5' Upstream segment of a gene, at least ten percent of human genes have a unique identifier that is utilized by the cell to properly direct the transcription complex to assemble in the upstream region of such a gene and transcribe the gene when required.

The transcribable segment contains intron (removed) and exons (much of the information is retained in the mature mRNA).

The final exons when combined must contain the mRNAs 5' nontranslatable region, the translatable region which codes for the protein and includes a START and STOP code, and a 3' nontranslatable region.

There must exist an identifying code in the 5' nontranslatable region of an mRNA to properly signal the ribosomes to attach to the mRNA.

There is a code in the 3' nontranslatable region that dictates how many times the mRNA should be translated. This code is usually represented in eukaryote cells as the number of adenosine amino acids attached to the tail of the mRNA molecule.

Some introns, when transcribed, separate from the maturing mRNA construct and exert command functions in the cell. Certain introns are capable of exerting influence on the mature mRNA in the cytoplasm, that they were associated with during the transcription process in the nucleus.

GLOSSARY & ABBREVIATIONS

BLAST: Basic Local Alignment Search Tool finds regions of local similarity between protein or nucleotide sequences. Reference: NCBI, www.ncbi.nlm.nih.gov/BLAST/.

Chikungunya virus unique identifier: 5'-ctctgcaaagcaagagattaataacccatc-3'.

Dandelion Rift: Concept that life arrived on Earth by a seed and it is the population's responsibility to replicate that seed of life and launch it back out into the universe to cultivate additional planets.

DNA: Deoxyribonucleic acid.

Ecometabolous: the actions of the Prime DNA genome that has resulted in the complete metamorphosis of the ecosystem of the planet and the expected creation of the higher order of organic life known as homo sapiens or 'wise man' based on the combination of (1) a preprogrammed collection of available genetic instructions spanning all organic life and viruses that have occupied the planet since the inception of life on earth and (2) selection based on survival of the fittest given prevailing factors.

ENB: Engineered nuclear biologic, the fourth generation of biologic therapy.

Essential Equation 4 Life: The equation is $3 CO_2 + 8 HN_3 = 4 N_2 + 6 H_2O + 3 CH_4$.

Executable Gene: Executable gene refers to a segment of transcribable DNA that is labeled with a unique identifier. A unique identifier is a sequence of nucleotides used as an identification code which may be comprised of a series of 25 nucleotides. Approximately a quarter of human genes have a segment of 25 nucleotides present in the upstream region of the gene between a TATA box and the transcription start site. A segment of 25 base-four nucleotides could be used to uniquely identify 200,000 different genes for 5 billion different species; and account for a unique genome for all of the species that have ever r existed. Similar to an 'executable statement' in computer science, an 'executable gene' represents (a) a gene by itself or (b) the initial gene of a cluster of genes, and when the unique identifier is targeted by a transcription complex one or more segments of transcribable genetic information are transcribed.

Fourth Generation Biologic: A Fourth Generation Biologic is any man-made molecule that enters into the nucleus to accomplish a medically therapeutic task. Fourth Generation Biologics include synthetic transcription factors, transcription binding proteins, nuclear receptors, nuclear signaling proteins, DNA binding proteins, and control RNA molecules. Fourth Generation Biologics may target nuclear DNA, viral DNA, the transcription complex, the spliceosome, nucleolus, nucleosome, and RNA in the nucleus of a cell. The function of Fourth Generation Biologics include (a) to silence a viral genome by obstructing the viral gene's unique identifier, or (b) activate/deactivate the body's nuclear genes by utilizing a modified transcription factor to locate a gene's unique identifier to turn 'on' or switch 'off' transcription of a specific gene, or (c) engage a specific spliceosome, nucleolus, nucleosome, or RNA in the nucleus of a cell.

Gene: Unit of inheritance that contains transcribable genetic information that will produce a messenger RNA that can be translated to produce a protein.

Genetic Reference Table (GRT): An organized set of genetic material present in nuclear DNA associated with unique identifier comprised of a series of transcribable sequences that when such sequences are transcribed the result is one or more control RNA molecules to activate a specific series of genes.

Genomic Cipher: Genomic Keycode: a=0, g=1, c=2, t=3.

HIV's Unique Identifier: 25 character bp string: 5'-agcagctgcttttttgcctgtactgg-3'.

Holometabolous: Means complete metamorphosis. This is a term that has been applied to the complete metamorphosis observed in some insects. Holometabola refers to a series of ten orders of insects including Coleoptera (beetles), Hymenoptera (bees, wasps, ants), Lepidoptera (moths and butterflies), Diptera (two-winged flies), and Siphonaptera (fleas), which undergo complete metamorphosis.

HSV's Unique Identifier: 25 character bp string 5'-aattccggaaggggacacgggctac-3'.

Medical Vector Therapy: the use of transport devices such as modified viruses to deliver a specific payload to a specific target cell to effect a medical therapy.

NCBI: National Center for Biology Information, www.ncbi.nlm.nih.gov.

Nucleotide bps: Nucleotide base pairs.

Quantum Gene: Genetic material associated with a unique identifier.

RNA: Ribonucleic acid.

TBP: TATA box Binding Protein or Transcription Binding Protein.

TATA_signal: sequence of nucleotides between the TATA box and the transcription start site. This is likely analogous to the unique identifier of the gene. An alternate term for the unique identifier of an executable gene.

TFIIIA: Transcription Factor III A.

Unique Identifier: A sequence of nucleotides used as an identification code for quantum genes, messenger RNAs, ribosomal RNAs and transport RNAs; in the case of the executable gene unique identifier may be comprised of a series of 25 nucleotides.

Universal Dogma of Molecular Biology: 'All protein production is a dynamic process created by a static intelligence stored in the DNA, facilitated by control and command RNAs producing messenger RNA used as templates to generate proteins, the rate of production being controlled by nuclear signaling proteins and control RNAs'.

SYNTHETIC COMPOUNDED HUMAN GENE, REPRESENTING A BIOLOGIC PROGRAM, TO ACT AS AN EMBEDDED DNA VACCINE TO MAKE CELLS DEFENSIBLE AGAINST INFECTION FROM HUMAN IMMUNODEFICIENCY VIRUS

INDIVIDUALS REQUESTING PATENT: Dr. Lane B. Scheiber, ScD and Dr. Lane B. Scheiber II, MD

CITIZENSHIP: Both are United States Citizens

NUMBER OF DRAWINGS: 0

NUMBER OF CLAIMS: 1 Independent Claim

PATENT APPLICATION SPECIFICATION

TITLE OF THE INVENTION:

SYNTHETIC COMPOUNDED HUMAN GENE, REPRESENTING A BIOLOGIC PROGRAM, TO ACT AS AN EMBEDDED DNA VACINE TO MAKE CELLS DEFENSIBLE AGAINST INFECTION FROM HUMAN IMMUNODEFICIENCY VIRUS

CROSS-REFERENCE TO RELATED APPLICATIONS: None.

STATEMENT REGARDING SPONSORED RESEARCH OR DEVELOPEMNT: None.

REFERENCE TO SEQUENCE LISTING, A TABLE, OR COMPUTER LISTING COMPACT DISC APPENDIX: Applicable. Sequence Listing generated by Patent-In 3.5 software and sent separately by US Postal Service as required.

BACKGROUND OF THE INVENTION

1. Field of the Invention

This invention relates to human genes capable of making cells defensible against viral infection.

2. Description of Background Art

[0001] Numerous therapeutic options are available to slow down Human Immunodeficiency Virus (HIV) replication process. A therapeutic means to silence the HIV genome and halt viral replication is necessary. Since HIV's DNA becomes embedded in the human genome of immune cells, it is necessary to produce a means to seek out the HIV genome and neutralize the HIV genome, while the HIV genome resides in the human genome.

[0002] The Tumor Necrosis Factor alpha (TNFalpha) gene is comprised of (1) a 5' Upstream nontranscribable region, (2) a transcription region that codes for an mRNA to act as a template for the TNFalpha protein, and (3) a 3' Downstream nontranscribable region. The TNFalpha gene when transcribed produces a messenger ribonucleic acid (mRNA) that when this template is translated produces tumor necrosis factor alpha protein molecules. The TNFalpha gene is transcribed in response to infections such as an HIV infection.

[0003] Messenger RNA when translated by ribosomes produce proteins. Messenger RNAs are comprised of (1) a 5' nontranslatable region, (2) a translatable region that acts as the template coded to generate a protein when translated by ribosomes, and (3) a 3' nontranslatable region.

[0004] The Transcription Factor IIIA (TFIIIA) gene is comprised of (1) a 5' Upstream nontranscribable region, (2) a transcription region that codes for an mRNA to act as a template for the TFIIIA protein, and (3) a 3' Downstream nontranscribable region. The TNFalpha gene when transcribed produces a messenger ribonucleic acid (mRNA) that when this template is translated produces Transcription Factor IIIA protein molecules.

[0005] TFIIIA molecule is comprised of a sequence of 365 amino acids. The TFIIIA molecule is comprised of (1) a 5' end of the molecule or NH_2 end, (2) nine zinc fingers, (3) amino acid segments that separate each of the zinc fingers, and a 5' end or COOH end of the molecule. The TFIIIA molecule binds to the deoxyribonucleic acid of a genome and acts to facilitate the assembly of a transcription complex. As many as seventy different proteins assemble to form one transcription complex. Once fully assembled, the transcription complex transcribes the gene the transcription complex is attached to downstream from the transcription start site.

[0006] The nine zinc fingers of a TFIIIA molecule each contain a binding loop where amino acids present in the loop bind to either nucleotides or amino acids in other proteins. Of the nine zinc fingers comprising the TFIIIA molecule, zinc fingers 1-5 bid to the nucleotides of the DNA, while zinc fingers 6-9 bind to other transcription factor protein molecules. The sequence of amino acids comprising zinc fingers 1-5 of the TFIIIA molecule dictates which segment of nucleotides along the DNA the TFIIIA molecule binds. Once a TFIIIA molecule has located and bound to a segment of DNA, other transcription factors bind to zinc fingers 6-9 of the bound TFIIIA molecule and assembly of the transcription complex is activated.

BRIEF SUMMARY OF THE INVENTION

[0007] Means to seek out and silence HIV genome a synthetic human gene has been devised. The synthetic gene is 15,636 nucleotides in length. The synthetic human gene is constructed so as when transcribed by a transcription complex is to generate a mRNA, which when this mRNA is translated by cellular ribosomes, the resultant protein is a modified Transcription Factor IIIA (TFIIIA) molecule configured to seek out the unique identifier present in the HIV DNA genome.

DETAILED DESCRIPTION

[0008] TFIIIA molecule gene (NC_000013) produces TFIIIA molecule is comprised of 365 amino acids.

[0009] The synthetic nucleotide sequence presented in this patent application is comprised of: (1) 5' Upstream segment taken from the Tumor Necrosis Factor alpha (TNF alpha) gene (AY214167.1), (2) the transcription region take from the TFIIIA molecule gene (NC_000013), this transcription segment modified to produce a TFIIIA molecule to bind to the HIV genome to prevent replication of the HIV genome, and (3) the 3' segment taken from the Tumor Necrosis Factor alpha (TNF alpha) gene (AY214167.1).

[0010] The nucleotide sequence of the synthetic gene is presented in detail as follows.

[0011] Nucleotides 1 to 1749 of the synthetic gene presented in this text are taken directly from the Tumor Necrosis alpha gene's 5' Upstream Region and represents fully the Tumor Necrosis alpha gene's 5' Upstream Region as it exists in its entirety just prior to the gene's transcription start site.

[0012] Nucleotides 1750 to 1943 represent TFIIIA mRNA 5' untranslatable segment.

[0013] Nucleotides 1944 to 2084 represent TFIIIA protein segment coding for TFIIIA molecule's amino acids 1 to 47.

[0014] Nucleotides 2085 to 2120 represent TFIIIA Binding Loop Number 1 coding for TFIIIA molecules amino acids 48 to 59.

[0015] Nucleotides 2121 to 2144 represent a TFIIIA Intra Loop segment coding for TFIIIA molecule's amino acids 60 to 67.

[0016] Nucleotides 2145 to 4297 represent TFIIIA Intron Number 1.

[0017] Nucleotides 4298 to 4327 represent a TFIIIA Intra Loop segment coding for TFIIIA molecule's amino acids 68 to 77.

[0018] Nucleotides 4328 to 4363 represent TFIIIA Binding Loop Number 2 coding for TFIIIA molecules amino acids 78 to 89.

[0019] Nucleotides 4364 to 4399 represent a TFIIIA Intra Loop segment coding for TFIIIA molecule's amino acids 90 to 101.

[0020] Nucleotides 4400 to 7076 represent TFIIIA Intron Number 2.

[0021] Nucleotides 7077 to 7094 represent a TFIIIA Intra Loop segment coding for TFIIIA molecule's amino acids 102 to 107.

[0022] Nucleotides 7095 to 7130 represent TFIIIA Binding Loop Number 3 coding for TFIIIA molecules amino acids 108 to 119.

[0023] Nucleotides 7131 to 7172 represent a TFIIIA Intra Loop segment coding for TFIIIA molecule's amino acids 120 to 133.

[0024] Nucleotides 7173 to 7738 represent TFIIIA Intron Number 3.

[0025] Nucleotides 7739 to 7756 represent a TFIIIA Intra Loop segment coding for TFIIIA molecule's amino acids 134 to 139.

[0026] Nucleotides 7757 to 7792 represent TFIIIA Binding Loop Number 4 coding for TFIIIA molecules amino acids 140 to 151.

[0027] Nucleotides 7793 to 7828 represent a TFIIIA Intra Loop segment coding for TFIIIA molecule's amino acids 152 to 163.

[0028] Nucleotides 7829 to 9937 represent TFIIIA Intron Number 4.

[0029] Nucleotides 9938 to 9955 represent a TFIIIA Intra Loop segment coding for TFIIIA molecule's amino acids 164 to 169.

[0030] Nucleotides 9956 to 9991 represent TFIIIA Binding Loop Number 5 coding for TFIIIA molecules amino acids 170 to 181.

[0031] Nucleotides 9992 to 10009 represent a TFIIIA Intra Loop segment coding for TFIIIA molecule's amino acids 182 to 187.

[0032] Nucleotides 10010 to 11343 represent TFIIIA Intron Number 5.

[0033] Nucleotides 11344 to 11367 represent a TFIIIA Intra Loop segment coding for TFIIIA molecule's amino acids 188 to 195.

[0034] Nucleotides 11368 to 11404 represent TFIIIA Binding Loop Number 6 coding for TFIIIA molecules amino acids 196 to 207.

[0035] Nucleotides 11405 to 11425 represent a TFIIIA Intra Loop segment coding for TFIIIA molecule's amino acids 208 to 214.

[0036] Nucleotides 11426 to 12009 represent TFIIIA Intron Number 6.

[0037] Nucleotides 12010 to 12033 represent a TFIIIA Intra Loop segment coding for TFIIIA molecule's amino acids 215 to 222.

[0038] Nucleotides 12034 to 12069 represent TFIIIA Binding Loop Number 7 coding for TFIIIA molecules amino acids 223 to 234.

[0039] Nucleotides 12070 to 12126 represent a TFIIIA Intra Loop segment coding for TFIIIA molecule's amino acids 235 to 253.

[0040] Nucleotides 12127 to 12162 represent TFIIIA Binding Loop Number 8 coding for TFIIIA molecules amino acids 254 to 265.

[0041] Nucleotides 12163 to 12219 represent a TFIIIA Intra Loop segment coding for TFIIIA molecule's amino acids 266 to 284.

[0042] Nucleotides 12220 to 12240 represent TFIIIA Binding Loop Number 9A (First half of binding loop 9) coding for TFIIIA molecules amino acids 285 to 291.

[0043] Nucleotides 12241 to 12338 represent TFIIIA Intron Number 7.

[0044] Nucleotides 12339 to 12353 represent TFIIIA Binding Loop Number 9B (Second half of binding loop 9) coding for TFIIIA molecules amino acids 292 to 296.

[0045] Nucleotides 12354 to 12398 represent 3' end of TFIIIA molecule Part A coding for TFIIIA molecules amino acids 297 to 311.

[0046] Nucleotides 12399 to 12638 represent TFIIIA Intron Number 8.

[0047] Nucleotides 12639 to 12803 represent 3' end of TFIIIA molecule Part B coding for TFIIIA molecules amino acids 312 to 365.

[0048] Nucleotides 12804 to 12915 represent TFIIIA mRNA 3' untranslatable segment.

[0049] Nucleotides 12916 to 15636 represent the Tumor Necrosis alpha gene's 3' Downstream Region.

[0050] When the presented synthetic compounded gene is transcribed, the resultant messenger RNA is transcribed from the nucleotides: 1750 to 12915. The introns are removed by cellular mechanisms to generate the mature messenger RNA.

[0051] When the presented synthetic compounded gene is transcribed, and the resultant mature messenger RNA is translated, the resultant protein is a TFIIIA molecule comprised of 365 amino acids. The TFIIIA protein molecule is intended to bind to the HIV genome.

[0052] The molecule of the synthetic compounded gene comprised of nucleotides 1 to 15636 as described above can be easily generated by common production processes offered by any one of a number of manufacturers once the nucleotide sequences is provided.

CONCLUSIONS, RAMIFICATIONS, AND SCOPE

[0053] Accordingly, the reader will see that the synthetic gene represents a new and unique state of the art that has never before been recognized nor appreciated by those skilled in the art.

[0054] Although the description above contains specificities, these should not be construed as limiting the scope of the invention but as merely providing illustrations of some of the presently preferred embodiments of the invention.

NUMBER OF DRAWINGS: 0

CLAIMS

The terms and expressions which are employed here are used as terms of description and are not of limitation and there is no intention, in the use of terms and expressions, of excluding equivalents of the features presented, and described, or portions thereof, it being recognized that various modifications are possible in the scope of the invention or process as claimed.

What is claimed:

1. The following DNA nucleotide sequence:

TNF-TFIIIA Gene Coding

```
   1 ctgctgatag tcccggagct ttcaagaagg attctttcct cccaggggac cacacctccc
  61 tgaatatccc tgatgtctgt ctggctgagg atttcaagcc tgcctaggaa ttcccagccc
 121 aaagctgttg gtctgtccca ccagctaggt ggggcctaga tccacacaca gaggaagagc
 181 aggcacatgg aggagcttgg gggatgacta gaggcaggga ggggactatt tatgaaggca
 241 aaaaaattaa attatttatt tatggaggat ggagagaggg gaataataga agaacatcca
 301 aggagaaaca gagacaggcc caagagatga agagtgagag ggcatgcgca caaggctgac
 361 caagagagaa agaagtaggc atgagggatc acagggcccc agaaggcagg gaaaggctct
 421 gaaagccagc tgccgaccag agccccacac ggaggcatct gcaccctcga tgaagcccaa
 481 taaacctctt ttctctgaaa tgctgtctgc ttgtgtgtgt gtgtctggga gtgagaactt
 541 cccagtctat ctaaggaatg gagggaggga cagagggctc aaagggagca agagctgtgg
 601 ggagaacaaa aggataaggg ctcagagagc ttcagggata tgtgatggac tcaccaggtg
 661 aggccgccag actgctgcag gggaagcaaa ggagaagctg agaagatgaa ggaaaagtca
 721 gggtctggag gggcggggt caggggagctc ctgggagata tggccacatg tagcggctct
 781 gaggaatggg ttacaggaga cctctgggga gatgtgacca cagcaatggg taggagaatg
 841 tccagggcta tggaagtcga gtatggggac ccccccctta acgaagacag ggccatgtag
 901 agggccccag ggagtgaaag agcctccagg acctccaggt atggaataca ggggacgttt
 961 aagaagatat ggccacacac tggggccctg agaagtgaga gcttcatgaa aaaaatcagg
1021 gaccccagag ttccttggaa gccaagactg aaaccagcat tatgagtctc cgggtcagaa
1081 tgaaagaaga aggcctgccc cagtggggtc tgtgaattcc cgggggtgat ttcactcccc
1141 gggggctgtcc caggcttgtc cctgctaccc ccaccagcc tttcctgagg cctcaagcct
1201 gccaccaagc ccccagctcc ttctcccccgc agggacccaa acacaggcct caggactcaa
1261 cacagctttt ccctccaacc ccgttttctc tccctcaagg actcagcttt ctgaagcccc
1321 tcccagttct agttctatct ttttcctgca tcctgtctgg aagttagaag gaaacagacc
1381 acagacctgg tccccaaaag aaatggaggc aataggtttt gaggggcatg gggacggggt
1441 tcagcctcca gggtcctaca cacaaatcag tcagtggccc agaagacccc cctcggaatc
1501 ggagcaggga ggatgggggag tgtgaggggt atccttgatg cttgtgtgtc cccaactttc
1561 caaatccccg cccccgcgat ggagaagaaa ccgagacaga aggtgcaggg cccactaccg
1621 cttcctccag atgagctcat gggtttctcc accaaggaag ttttccgctg gttgaatgat
1681 tctttcccccg ccctcctctc gccccaggga catataaagg cagttgttgg cacacccagc
1741 cagcagacga tgcgcgatct cccggagcat gcgcagcagc ggcgccgacg cggggcggtg
1801 cctggtgacc gcgcgcgctc ccggaagtgt gccggcgtcg cgcgaaggtt cagcagggag
1861 ccgtgggccg ggcgcgccgg ttcccggcac gtgtctcggc acgtggcagc gcgcctggcc
1921 ctgggcttgg aggcgccggc gccctggatc cgccggccgt ggtcgccgag tcggtgtcgt
1981 ccttgaccat cgccgacgcg ttcattgcag ccggcgagag ctcagctccg accccgccgc
2041 gccccgcgct tccccaggagg ttcatctgct ccttccctga ctgcaactcg tcccgtgaat
2101 cgtccacctc gtcccgtgaa cacctgtgca agcacacggg ggaggtgagg ggggcgaggc
2161 tgccaaccct gggcctaggg atggcgcgtg gccccggggt agccactgca gtcgtggcca
2221 ggccgcagg ccccgctgtg cagcgcgttc agctttgaca tccaggactt gggaagggag
2281 ctgaggaagt agacaggaag ttgtaggacc ttcgttctgc gaccttgata tccatggcag
2341 gggctcggga tttactaagc agtcattgat cgtgagtctc ggccagccaa gtgcctcccg
2401 taatctgcaa ataagtgtga ggtttgaggg ggcccaccgc tactagacac ctgccaaaca
2461 ctggcccctg gagctggtac agaaagatgg g ttacatgtac caggggtcgt gaaagcagca
2521 tgtgctcatt tcttcgtaac tccacactgg agagagcagt gagcaaaaca ggcaaacccca
2581 aggtttctgc tgccatggac ctttgttcct gggtcgagcc gaccacagga taggtgggaa
```

— 342 —

```
2641 tgacatgcag tgttgtggtc aggaaaggcc tctctgtgtg agccgtgtaa gaaggaagga
2701 tctagccatg cagacatttg tgctaggtag agagaacaca aagggagcct gtgacccttg
2761 gggtgggagg caggtgggtg tgtttgggtg cggagatcac catatgaggt ctgagaagta
2821 ggcccattag gagttttggat tttattttga gggcaggaga atgtcagata ccatgatatg
2881 acgtggcagc ccatgtcaca cacaagtgag gaaaacgagg gtcatggagg tcaaggaatc
2941 tgcccagctt cccagtttt ggcagagcta ggcttcacac tgcctcagct taaagccctt
3001 aatttcttaa accactgggc tgcagtccat acctttgccc cttgcacctc ctctaattta
3061 tgggccacct tctccaggtg tcctccgggg cctcattcct taacctctcc agcactggaa
3121 ggccgaccgc ttcttccttg agaccttctc tggttctttt cctcttcctc gtctgccctt
3181 ttcgttggat cctcttctgc cctctgcatg ttccaccccg cccagctccc tcttgcggtc
3241 ttacatagcc accggcatga ctcataacat cctttatgct ttgcccctct gcccttcctc
3301 ttgcccgttc tagcctctaa attctgggct ctgtattacc agtagatcca cgtaagagct
3361 tgcctttcct tttagaccgg tgtgctgtat tttggatact ggcgctacca gtttccttdd
3421 tacaggttga aaaacttgga gtcatctttg ttgtcccaga tctctcatgc agattaattt
3481 gacaaatgtt tattgagcct actccacgcc tgccgctgtg caaggttctg tggctccgcc
3541 cctggtggta tgtagctcac tgtgttcctg tttgcttgtt ttgctcctag tactctcatg
3601 gaggcctcgg tgcctccctc ctggacgcct tggtagtatg cttttcatag tttgatgcac
3661 caaactggtt atttggttat ttggggtgtg tgtttggctt ttactatagg ttcaaaatga
3721 gtcacccct cccaactcct gggttacaaa aggtggttgc atttagggtg ttgagctgtt
3781 ttctttgctt cgccctggca cctgtgagct ttttcaggtg tgacacactt tcctatagct
3841 gtgcttggca ttatcctagc acagaccctg ggcttgtctg ggatgagaca ggcctccctc
3901 gttcctctgc cctaggcttg ctttttaca tgttaaatca tgcggtggtg gggatccatg
3961 cagacaagcc atgctaacag ccagggcgtc tttaagaggg ggttgctgtg aaagcctgct
4021 gccgggttgg gagcaggtta aaaatgctat gcctgcttat tttaaatgct gttcatggaa
4081 caaaaatctg tgtagtgact ttgtgagaag ttgtgatgtt tatgttgtgt aactttgtgc
4141 aggaacactg cgtcttgcag tgggtgcaca gctctgagta gaaaccacct cttcatagga
4201 agcctgtggc cttaacacta ggcagtttaa gctttttaaat aataccagag ttactaacta
4261 gtgcagaagt gacatgcttt ttctttttc ctgctagaga ccatttgttt gtgactatga
4321 agggtgtaag tcttcccgtg aatcgtccaa atcttccaaa aagcacattc tgactcacac
4381 aggagaaaag ccgtttgtgt aagtagagac ctgtttttag gcttttgaag tgggttgtgt
4441 tgggcatata gacccagtaa gaagattgat gttaactcac gagatcagga atgtgaagcc
4501 tggcagggct cggtggctca tgcctgtaat cccagcactt tgggaggccg agatgggcag
4561 atcacttgaa cccaggagtt tgagacaaac ctgggcaaca tggtgaaacc ccgtatgtac
4621 aaaaatacaa aaattagtca gggatggtgg tttgtgcctg taatcctagc tacccaggag
4681 gctgagctaa cataaaatgc tcatgggtgg ggacaagcta aagtatatca acacaatggg
4741 ataccctaca gccaggaaaa tgaatgcaga tgctctctgc aaagccatga gaaaatcacc
4801 agggcacttt aattgaaaaa ccaaggtgca gaagagtcct ctttaggcta cttttatgtg
4861 tgtaaaaaag ctagggggta ggggagaggg tgagtagtgg gtgttgggta ggcaggaagc
4921 aactatattt gtatttgttc ctattttgta agaagtctta aaagttacat aacaaaacta
4981 aaaatgtcat ctgtttttgg agcagtgggg gatcctggcc aagtaggggg tggggatggt
5041 aggaaatgcc atgcaaccag gaactactgg acatgactct tccagctcat gatctaaccc
5101 agaccctgcc cctctttagc tgtagttccc cgtttcccac tgctcgctgg acagtgctac
5161 ttggctatct ctgtgtcttc ttaaattcca tgtggtaggc tgggtgtggt ggctcatgcc
5221 tgtaatccca gcactttgag aggctgaggt gggaggattg ctttgagtcc aggagttcag
5281 gctgggcaag atggtcaggt ccatctcta taaagaaata aataaataaa aaattccaca
5341 tggcccaaat ttgtcacagt caaactgagc tcacttttct gtttgatctt ctctcatgtt
5401 cttgtctgga gaggtggcct cgctgtctgt ccagtgaccc atagcaaaga taaggcagct
5461 ccctggactc tccattcttt ctcccatccc ttgcaacagg tgggttgcca gatcctgtaa
5521 ctgacccatc agatccagca gccactgtct tatctcggtc ccttcctctg gctggaatga
5581 cagtttgcag gccagccctc tcccccagtg ccctcccgtg tgcttccctt aaagctggtgc
5641 agtgctttca agcacggcct acatgtgaaa tccaggtttc aagtgtgtcc tacaatgacc
5701 tgcgtgattt agcccttttc tgcttatctt gccccatttg cttgacttgc aggcatgaag
5761 ctgtggtcca gctgtgctaa ctaaccagcc ccctctccaa gtgtgccggg gtctctcacg
5821 cccacttggg tcttgtcagg actcttcctg gcctgtcctc ctatcccata cccggttggg
5881 ttagatgcct gtgtcaggtt tagagtgaag aatggcagga accccagcac aagagatgct
5941 taaacaagat gggctctttg tcttgtgcga ctgaaataca gaaatacaga ggcaggagct
6001 ctggagcctc ttctgactgg tctctgccat cctcatcttg ggcttaacc tcactgtgat
6061 gcctgtttgg gcccatcgt cacataagca tgccactggc aggaaggagg aaagggcata
6121 agaggcatgc ccccttattt agagactttg tggggggttga gcaggatggg ctggactcag
6181 ccatgagccg ccctaattgc aggggagtgca ctttctgtcg gccacctgcc
6241 cagctaacac tcagcattct gtccctgcag ttaggggggc ttctagggtc tctgccacag
6301 cgcccctccc atttgtgggc ctctgtgctg tgcctcccat ggtcactgct ggcttgtttg
6361 tctctgcttg gccctaggaa tgggacagtg cctgcctcag ggttatcagt gagtgatggc
6421 taagattgag cctgggaaag gaagtcctgc ttcatccctc aagcttacga aggctcatca
6481 caagaggcac aaatttttctt ttgggaaaaa aaaaaaaaaa aaaggaaaag gctttgcaga
6541 ggattttagat cattcaaagc caagatgcca agataagggg aaccagaatg gcttggtaag
6601 ccagagaaca taatggttat ggttctgctc taagtatctg tttttacctct aatgataagc
6661 caagacaagt tttatggagg cctttctgga aatccagttc ataatgacat ctcaagcagc
6721 attaaggttg tcagattcta agctgagaat aatttgtctt aagcatgatt taggcctagt
6781 gtaggctttt gggactagtg tatttcacct tcccatctgc ccagtgtgta taaaagatga
6841 ctgatgtagt gtgtataatt tcagaagcct aatatgaaaa agcattttgt tacatgatag
6901 tcatcaggtt gagagtctat gtggtatggc ttaacactct ggaattcgct aagactattt
6961 tatagtatta ctattctttg gaagaattag cttctataaa gtaggaagat atatgtgtct
7021 taaaacttct tctcccttgg tttattaata ttttggttta tataacttct tacagttgtg
7081 cagccaatgg ctgtaagtct tccaaaaggt catccgagtc gtccgagaag catttttgaac
7141 gcaaacatga aaatcaacaa aaacaatata tagtaagtat gatttttatat gcttaaattt
7201 tttgagtatt tttacactta ctgcctatgt ttctgacatt ttcagccagg tgcggtggct
7261 caagcctata atcgtagctt gaggccagga atttgagacc agcctgggaa acatagtgaa
7321 atgctgtctc tgaaaaaaaa aaacaaaaac agaaaacaaa acaaaaaatt ttggggtaac
7381 agagaccctg tctctaaaaa ataaaagtga aaaataaagt tttcgtcaac caaatttttgt
7441 ctgccaaatg tctgaattta cttaatgcca tcataatgat aaaggttta atttggaagc
7501 agacattgtg caaattagtg tattgggaga ctattccaac tgaaacagtt ttgcttttc
7561 aaatgttata tgattcttca aaccttttg agataaagca gaattttaca gtaacaaaat
7621 gggtgaaagc agaaattta tacagtctcc aaaattgttt tatcttgagg attctgttac
```

```
 7681 gaactgttca ttttgttttg actttccata agactaacga gcctttacaa tttaacagtg
 7741 cagttttgaa gactgtcgct cctccaaaaa ctcgtccgag tcgtccaaaa ggcatcagtg
 7801 ccagcatacc aatgaacctc tattcaagta ggtacttcat gtggctgaaa atgcctggat
 7861 tctaggtgtg aataagattg gaaatgcaag ggtggtgttg agcattgttt catgtttttt
 7921 ggccatttgt atatcttctg agaaatgtct gttcatatcc tttgcccact tttcgatgga
 7981 ttgtttttttt cttgctgatc tgagttccct gtagatcctg gatatacatt ctttattgga
 8041 tgcataatgt gccagtattt tctcccactc tctgggttgt ctgtttactc tgctgattat
 8101 ttcttttgct gtgcagaagc tttttagttt aattaggtcc catttattta tttctatttt
 8161 tgttgcattt gctttcaggg ccttagtaag aattctttgc ctaggctgat gtccagaagt
 8221 ttttccaatg ttttcatttt gaatttttag tttcaggtca taaacttaat ttgagttgat
 8281 ttttgtataa ggtgagagat agggatccag tttttccagc accatttatt gaatagggag
 8341 tcctttcccc agtttacgtt tttatatgct ttgttgaaga tcgggtggct gtaagtattt
 8401 ggctttattt ctgttttgtt ccattggtct aagtgcctat ttttaaacca gtgccaccct
 8461 gttttggtaa ctgtagcctc gtagtataat ctgaagtctg gtcaaaggaa aagaagtcac
 8521 tatatgaaaa agacacatgc acacagtttt acagcagcac agttcacaat tgcaaataca
 8581 tggagccaat ttaagtgccc atcgaccaat gagtagataa agaaaacgtg atgtatatac
 8641 accatggaat actacacagc cataaaaggg aacaaaatga tgtcttttgc agcagcttgg
 8701 atggagctgg aggccattat tctcagtgaa gtaactcagg aatggaaaac caaataccat
 8761 agttttcact aagtgggcac taaactatga ggacaaaaag acacagtgat ttcataaact
 8821 ttggggactt ggggtgggga gtttggggag ggggtgagg gatgaaagac tacatattgg
 8881 gtacagtgta tgctgcttga gtgatggtgc gctaaaatct cagcaccact ataggattca
 8941 tccacgtaac gaaaaaacac ttgcaacccc aaaagccatt gaaatttaaa gcaacggtgg
 9001 gacaaatctt ctgaaagctt cctaatcaac attttttctgt taaaatgtac tgcatatgca
 9061 catttatata ttgggagcat tttaaaggtt tactttgctc tgaaagaaat atttaatgtg
 9121 tttcaaaata attttttgaga ttattctagt tgtggttaag cttaaaggct gagaaattac
 9181 ttaactattc aaatagagcc tgtgcaacta tatgaaaatgt cattatggag acactcatta
 9241 tgcttttcct gtagaacaaa acaagtagtt gggtttatct gcaattaggg tttttttgagg
 9301 aacgtgaggg tggctggaca agttgggtag acctgcaaaa gggccagcgg ctctctgcat
 9361 ggctctggcc atccggcact ttcccttgac ttgcacaggc tgccctgtgc cttggagttg
 9421 ctgcagtgac cttgcctgtc cttgcttgtg ggtctgctgc tgctgctttg ctgctgatgg
 9481 ctttagcaca gaggggggccc gtgcttttta ttgctcacca gaggcagatg catctactgc
 9541 tgtgctgtct cgcacacccc ctatgcagca tcattaggaa agctagacac aagtgattca
 9601 gaatggctta ggggtttatc taagccaagt cagataacct cttgaactat ctttttgtag
 9661 ccatgaaagc agagtatatt tccagaggta taaagatgaa aactgtttaa atgggtcaaa
 9721 aaaagtaacg tgactttttt ctccaacagt ttgtttttgtc ctaaagctgg tcaagtaact
 9781 tgaatctcac ctgtgatgag agctacattt taacatgggt ttggttatgg gaagaggcaa
 9841 gactttggtg ggagaaacag gacaaagtgc cattgacctt gagcggagtt ctctgtgaaa
 9901 atggattggc taatacctca tgtgttgcca atgcaggtgt acccaggaag gatgtcgcag
 9961 ctcccgtaaa tcttccgagt cgtccaaaga gcatgccaag gcccacgagg gtgtgtacgg
10021 atagcctggg tgtgctccga ggggatgcc aaatcctggg cgcctttgaa tctgttctgt
10081 gatcacgctg aaaagatggg aaccctgtga acagggaca ccatcctgct tatttgggtc
10141 ttacactctt gtccaaagag gcactgtata tgtctgtttt tccactaccg tatcattgct
10201 gttcacatgt aatgtgttgt ttgttcacaa caagcgcctg gttacacatt acactgacga
10261 atgtgctgat gctccagcca tggcttttgat gcttctgtca tttttaacct cttctattaa
10321 tatttactgc ctgtgccatt ctttttccttg ttggccattc acaaggcttg gataatcgtg
10381 tgacatttgt agagccatca gatgttacgt ttctcaaaaa aaaaaaaaaa agacttgatt
10441 atattaacta tttgaatcta tgatctgttt ccttgaggga tttttgctaa tctgtatttc
10501 aatttcccag gtcctagaat ttatgatttt ttttttttta agaggttagt agctaacagt
10561 gagaggcagc ctcattgttt ttagtttcta gttgggtgga actcagccct agtgttgtat
10621 acttattaat cccattttag tgctttgcac atatccattg ttattcagtg ttttttctctg
10681 ggtccttcca gtttattttc ttccttagct gtactctttt aaaaaaaaaa aacaaaaaaa
10741 aactttttttt tttttttttg tgataaagtt aaaatataat gtaccctact ttttttgtgc
10801 agtatgacac ttacaagatg gccagactag aggaagccag aggtgggcat ggtaacacta
10861 ctgaaaagtt ggtggtgtgc catggacaag ggaccgactg cagagtatgt ttgctgagga
10921 aaatagaggc gaggatagag caggcagggg aagggaaata agacatggag ataggaggtt
10981 aaaagcagttg ggagtccata cacagcctac ccaacttcct gagaactctt agagaggaaa
11041 aggcatcctt aggcatcctt cctgtgaagt ttgcctattc cgtgatcacg ctgagaagat
11101 gggaactctg aagtttgctt cacaggaagg taaaatcctt aaagggaggc accttgctgt
11161 gccactgttc agttttacta taacatcaat cttttttttag tttttattcc cacctcaaga
11221 ggctgagttg aatactatta ggcgggggaat ggaaaattat ataggcacct aagtttcctt
11281 tctagttatg gtcagtgttt acactgagta ttcatgacag acaatgcacc aatttttttta
11341 ataggctatg tatgtcaaaa aggatgtgca ttcgtggccg ccacctggac cgcactcctg
11401 ccccatgtga gagaaaccca taaagtaag gcaggcatga atggcaggca tggtgtaaat
11461 gtttgtcccc acagaactga tttagtgctt ttcaagagtg aaatgctgtg tgctttaaag
11521 taaaagggtt tctctatgat attttgtgaa gtgctgggta tgatgttgtt ggaaaggtga
11581 gcagagctgt gccaggtctc tgagccaccc caccatgcac aattagcatg ctgaaggcgg
11641 tggcaggtct gtagtgaaga atttcgggag gcactgctgt tctgtgggac cgcctgggaa
11701 acagtaccct gcatactggg ggacaaggaa ggacactggt ctgcttcatt ttctgtacct
11761 ccccacagtc accttcctga gagccctgcc tcttgcaag tgaacaatga ctgtgtggca
11821 tttaagaact tcagagaatt gagacaaact tcctaggtga taaaaactgg ggttgtttcc
11881 ttgggaattt ctgatttgta tatagtgatc aggtttcagg cactgaatgt tacttatata
11941 ttaggtatta attttttcta aatggtaata tctggggaaa tttgtgaaat ttgtctgtct
12001 gtcccaccag aggaaatact atgtgaagta tgcgcagcca cctttgccgc agccgactat
12061 ctcgcccagc acatgaaaac tcatgccccca gaaagggatg tatgtcgctg tccaagagaa
12121 ggctgtggcg ccaccgcaac aactgtgttt gccctcggcg cgcatatcct ctccttccat
12181 gaggaaagcc gcccttttgt gtgtgaacat gctggctgtg gcgccaccttt tgccatggcc
12241 gtaagcactc accctcatac tcatggtcct atagtctatg ctttcacaac atggttttca
12301 tattaatatt tcattaataa ctttctcttt cattgtagca ggcgctgacc gcacatgctg
12361 ttgtacatga tcctgacaag aagaaaatga agctcaaagt aagttgaaac tacttaggca
12421 agcttagttt tcaagtggaa attgtttaag gccagaagga gtctgtttgg aattctttttc
12481 acctgcttta ctgtttgagt ctgcactact gttgaagact ttacttcctc ataaagcaat
12541 gttgtacact atatctgctg gtacatatga ctatcgtaaa attaactcag acagttttga
12601 ttttgaattc taatcgtgtg tcttccttat tcccaaaggt caaaaaatct cgtgaaaaac
12661 ggagtttggc ctctcatctc agtggatata tccctcccaa aaggaaacaa gggcaaggct
```

— 344 —

```
12721 tatctttgtg tcaaaacgga gagtcaccca actgtgtgga agacaagatg ctctcgacag
12781 ttgcagtact tacccttggc taagaactgc actgctttgt ttaaaggact gcagaccaag
12841 gagcgagctt tctctcagag catgcttttc tttattaaaa ttactgatgc agaacatttg
12901 attccttatc atttcacatg gtctccttct tggaattaat tctgcatctg cctcttcttg
12961 tgggtgggaa gaagctccct aagtcctctc tccacaggct ttaagatccc tcggacccag
13021 tcccatcctt agactcctag ggccctggag accctacata aacaaagccc aacagaatat
13081 tccccatccc ccaggaaaca agagcctgaa cctaattacc tctccctcag ggcatgggaa
13141 tttccaactc tgggaattcc aatccttgct gggaaaatcc tgcagctcag gtgagatttc
13201 cggctgttgc agctggccag cagtccggag agagctggag aggagccgca ttctcaggta
13261 cctgaatcac acagccaagg gacttccaga gattcgggtg tctaggcttc aaatcaccct
13321 gtcctaactc tgcaacctga accagccact taacctatct atccaatggg gataggaatg
13381 tccaccacac atagggcatg tgagagaagg cctgacctcc atcagaggac ctcactcagc
13441 ccttggcaca gtgggcactt agtgaattct ggcttccttc aaccagtttc cagctgtttt
13501 atccccttcc attctctcag tgggtgaaat cgaagagact gaggacaata aagaacaagg
13561 aaccgaactg ccggacgtgg tggcatgcac ctgtaatcct accactttgc aaggccaagg
13621 tgagaggatc gcttgaaccc aggagttcca gagcaacctg ggcaacatag tgagatcctg
13681 tctctatttt ttaaaaaaga atgaaacata ggaataagat gtgggtgaag gactcacatg
13741 ccggcttggt cccactggtc tttgtggtga aggaggggag aggtgagagg tgggtaatcc
13801 ggaaagagaa aagcacccca tccctggatg aaggctcttc tggagagagt caaagacaaa
13861 taagggtggg gcgcagtggc tcatgcctgt tatcccaaca ctttgggagg ctgaggtggg
13921 aggaccactt gagcccacta gttcaagacc agcctgtgca acatgacaag accttgtttc
13981 tagaaaaaaa attaaagatt agtcaggtgt agtggtgcat gcctgtaatc ctagctcctc
14041 aggaggctga ggcaggagga tcactcaagc ccaggagttt gaggttacag taagctatga
14101 tcatgccact gtacccccgt ctgggtgaca gaacgagacc ctgtctcaaa aaaataataa
14161 ttccaaaaac aaatatggag acggaaattg agccccccta gactgggagc ccccactgag
14221 ttcggaaatt aggctttacc tccagccctg gggtgccagg caggagaaaa ccatgtggta
14281 ggctgagggg gtagggtgac ccattggggt gacctagata gggccttggg tcaccctctg
14341 cctcctccag cctgtggctg aaaagtcagcc atgaagtaat gggggacact gttactcatc
14401 ccagaagcac ccacacttac tcacttttgg gaaggggggac ctaaagtgtg aaaaaaaggt
14461 gaggattttc cgtctcaccc taaatgggac accctaagtg gggcatcggt ttttcctcct
14521 ccccagaact tcctggtgtt ttcaggcacc acaggctcct tcctgccatc cccatctctc
14581 tctaatattc tccccttctt tctccttcag cctcctccct tcagaccccca tgagccttga
14641 attaagctcc ttggaggaga agagttgact gtcgggtagg agacagagag gccttcaggc
14701 agctctaggg ggagaagtgc ggggcccctc caggcttcat tcctctgtca tgatagggggc
14761 ttactctgct gctgggcctt tctgagtggt gcttgctggg ctctgtaatg acccctctca
14821 ctgttgggggg gtacccaaga gaaaagagta tggtgcagag tctggttggg accatgtggc
14881 cctgaaaatc aggatgccta gagaagcttc ggagtttgag aagtccccct tcctcccacc
14941 ctccaactgg gctaatggtg gggcctggcc attcagaggc agggaggggg tgggacaggc
15001 agaccatcat ccctaggagc agaggccata cactgtgttg tgatgaattg tttcaagcaa
15061 ccagaagagt actgagaata tttaacccgc acccgtgcac ccaccctgaa ttaagacgtg
15121 tgtcgcaact cagcatcttt atcggcagca ctgaagcttt ccattcttta ttttcatcag
15181 gttcaaaatc aatttccaaa cagtctccta cattttcccc actgccatgg ggtcctgggc
15241 gtccgggccc ccaatattca cgcactcgca ccacgcactc atattccctc accccaccat
15301 cacggccca aagaaggtct tccctctcgc gaagtccacc atatcgqqgt gactgatgtt
15361 gacgtacacc ctctcgcccc tccggagctg caccaggccg ccgaacccca cgctcgtgta
15421 ccagagaggc ccgtaccctt gtctcctggc cgggtccagc actggagtca ccgtctcggc
15481 gccctcgagc agcagctcgg gagtgcccgg cccgtaggcg ccccccgccc ggtacagaga
15541 gctgcgcagc gtgaccgagc ggccctgggg gtccccgccg ccaggggggcg cccggccccg
15601 gtagccgacg agacagtaga ggtaatagag gccgtc
```

ABSTRACT

The Human Immunodeficiency Virus continues to claim lives across the planet. HIV embeds its genome in the nuclear DNA of human cells making the HIV virus difficult to root out and eradicate. An embedded DNA vaccine has been contrived utilizing the 5' and 3' sequences of a TNF alpha gene and the transcription sequence of a modified TFIIIA gene. When transcribed, this compounded gene will generate a mRNA molecule that will produce Transcription Factor IIIA proteins constructed specifically to target and neutralize the HIV genome.

METHOD TO SEMIPERMANENTLY BIND SYNTHETIC PROTEINS TO DNA

INDIVIDUALS REQUESTING PATENT: Dr. Lane B. Scheiber, ScD and Dr. Lane B. Scheiber II, MD

CITIZENSHIP: Both are United States Citizens

NUMBER OF DRAWINGS: 0

NUMBER OF CLAIMS: 3 Independent Claims

PATENT APPLICATION SPECIFICATION

TITLE OF THE INVENTION:

METHOD TO SEMIPERMANENTLY BIND SYNTHETIC PROTEINS TO DNA

CROSS-REFERENCE TO RELATED APPLICATIONS: None.

STATEMENT REGARDING SPONSORED RESEARCH OR DEVELOPEMNT: None.

REFERENCE TO SEQUENCE LISTING, A TABLE, OR COMPUTER LISTING COMPACT DISC APPENDIX: Not applicable.

BACKGROUND OF THE INVENTION

1. Field of the Invention

This invention relates to any method that involves synthetic proteins binding to a sequence of deoxyribonucleic acid.

2. Description of Background Art

[0001] A 'deoxyribose' is a deoxypentose ($C_5H_{10}O_4$) sugar. Deoxyribonucleic acid (DNA) is comprised of molecular subunits comprised of three basic elements: a deoxyribose sugar, a phosphate group and nitrogen containing bases. DNA is a macromolecule made up of two chains of repeating deoxyribose sugars linked by phosphodiester bonds between the 3-hydroxyl group of one and the 5-hydroxyl group of the next; the two chains are held antiparallel to each other by weak hydrogen bonds. DNA strands contain a sequence of nucleotides, these nucleotides are generally referred to by their nitrogenous bases, which include: adenine, cytosine, guanine and thymine.

[0002] Proteins are molecules comprised of a sequence of amino acids linked together. Asparagine, arginine, glutamic acid, and lysine are amino acids. Asparagine, arginine, glutamic acid, and lysine are among the twenty amino acids that are generally utilized to build proteins.

[0003] Definition of the term 'semipermanent': lasting or intended to last for a long time but not permanent. The term 'organic molecule' generally refers to molecules containing carbon atoms. Organic molecules generally constitute the majority of the substance of living organisms. Organic molecules and the bonds between organic molecules in Nature are generally not permanent. Most proteins are broken down at some point into individual amino acids, which such amino acids are then recycled into other proteins or in some instances, the amino acids comprising a protein are broken down to the individual elements that comprise the amino acid.

[0004] The term 'synthetic' is defined in this context as formed through a process by human agency; as opposed to by natural origin.

[0005] The term 'semipermanent' or 'semipermanently' is defined in this context as an amino acid binding to a nucleotide in a firm manner that has a low likelihood of becoming unbound during the remaining lifetime of the biologic cell where the amino acid is bound to a nucleotide.

[0006] Asparagine, arginine, glutamic acid, and lysine are among the twenty amino acids that are generally utilized to build proteins. Asparagine demonstrates a high affinity of tightly binding to the nucleotide adenine. Arginine demonstrates a high affinity of tightly binding to the nucleotide guanine. Glutamic acid demonstrates a high affinity of tightly binding to the nucleotide cytosine. Lysine demonstrates a high affinity of tightly binding to the nucleotide thymine. Creating a sequence of amino acids each with a high affinity of tight binding to the nucleotides comprising a specific sequence of nucleotides found in the DNA, creates a protein that semipermanently binds to the sequence of nucleotides in the DNA.

[0007] The Human immunodeficiency virus (HIV) embeds its genome into the human genome of a T-Helper cell.

[0008] The HIV genome (GenBank K03455.1) is comprised of a sequence of 9719 nucleotides. Nucleotides 431 to 455 exist between the TATA Box and the Transcription Start Site. The twenty-five nucleotides of the HIV genome that exist from 431 to 455 act as a unique identifier. The twenty-five nucleotides of the HIV genome that exist from 431 to 455 can be utilized as an inimitable target for a DNA target specific genetic pharmacology protein molecule to bind to in a semipermanent manner and prevent transcription of the HIV genome.

[0009] Some proteins found in Nature, bind to the DNA.

[0010] Transcription Factor IIIA (TFIIIA) molecule is a protein comprised of 365 amino acids. TFIIIA molecule binds to the DNA and assists in the initiation of the assembly of a transcription complex. TFIIIA molecule is associated with a transcription complex that utilizes a polymerase III molecule to transcribe DNA. The general construct of a TFIIIA molecule's amino acid sequence allows it to function in a manner whereby the TFIIIA molecule binds to the DNA upstream from a transcription start site, which assists in the initial assembly of a transcription complex, then the TFIIIA molecule releases from the DNA.

[0011] TFIIIA molecule is comprised of a sequence of 365 amino acids. The TFIIIA molecule is comprised of (1) a 5' end of the molecule or NH_2 end, (2) nine zinc fingers, (3) amino acid segments that separate each of the zinc fingers, and a 5' end or COOH end of the molecule. The TFIIIA molecule binds to the deoxyribonucleic acid of a genome and acts to facilitate the assembly of a transcription complex. As many as seventy different proteins assemble to form one transcription complex. Once fully assembled, the transcription complex transcribes the gene the transcription complex is attached to on the human genome.

[0012] The nine zinc fingers of a TFIIIA molecule each contain a binding loop where amino acids present in the loop bind to either nucleotides or amino acids in other proteins. Of the nine zinc fingers comprising the TFIIIA molecule, zinc fingers 1-5 bid to the nucleotides of the DNA, while zinc fingers 6-9 bind to other transcription factor protein molecules. The sequence of amino acids comprising zinc fingers 1-5 of the TFIIIA molecule dictates which segment of nucleotides along the DNA the TFIIIA molecule binds. Once a TFIIIA molecule has located and bound to a segment of DNA, other transcription factors bind to zinc fingers 6-9 of the bound TFIIIA molecule and assembly of the transcription complex is activated.

[0013] TFIIIA molecule gene (NC_000013) produces TFIIIA molecule is comprised of 365 amino acids.

[0014] The TFIIIA molecule is modified such that it remains comprised of 365 amino acids, but the amino acids constituting the binding sites of the TFIIIA molecule are altered so that the TFIIIA protein molecule is intended to bind semipermanently to the HIV genome when the TFIIIA protein molecule is in close proximity to the HIV genome, at a sequence of nucleotides to include nucleotides 431 to 455 of the HIV genome. The completed bonding described below includes nucleotides 431 to 460.

[0015] An example of the construct of a synthetic protein to bind to the DNA is provided as the construct of a modified TFIIIA protein as follows:

[0016] In the modified TFIIIA molecule, asparagine, the 48th amino acid in the 5' to 3' TFIIIA molecule, bonds to adenine, the nucleotide at position 431 in the 5' to 3' HIV genome.

[0017] In the modified synthetic TFIIIA molecule, arginine, the 51st amino acid in the 5' to 3' TFIIIA molecule, bonds to guanine, the nucleotide at position 432 in the 5' to 3' HIV genome.

[0018] In the modified synthetic TFIIIA molecule, glutamic acid, the 52nd amino acid in the 5' to 3' TFIIIA molecule, bonds to cytosine, the nucleotide at position 433 in the 5' to 3' HIV genome.

[0019] In the modified synthetic TFIIIA molecule, asparagine, the 55th amino acid in the 5' to 3' TFIIIA molecule, bonds to adenine, the nucleotide at position 434 in the 5' to 3' HIV genome.

[0020] In the modified synthetic TFIIIA molecule, arginine, the 58th amino acid in the 5' to 3' TFIIIA molecule, bonds to guanine, the nucleotide at position 435 in the 5' to 3' HIV genome.

[0021] In the modified synthetic TFIIIA molecule, glutamic acid, the 59th amino acid in the 5' to 3' TFIIIA molecule, bonds to cytosine, the nucleotide at position 436 in the 5' to 3' HIV genome.

[0022] In the modified synthetic TFIIIA molecule, lysine, the 78th amino acid in the 5' to 3' TFIIIA molecule, bonds to thymine, the nucleotide at position 437 in the 5' to 3' HIV genome.

[0023] In the modified synthetic TFIIIA molecule, arginine, the 81st amino acid in the 5' to 3' TFIIIA molecule, bonds to guanine, the nucleotide at position 438 in the 5' to 3' HIV genome.

[0024] In the modified synthetic TFIIIA molecule, glutamic acid, the 82nd amino acid in the 5' to 3' TFIIIA molecule, bonds to cytosine, the nucleotide at position 439 in the 5' to 3' HIV genome.

[0025] In the modified synthetic TFIIIA molecule, lysine, the 85th amino acid in the 5' to 3' TFIIIA molecule, bonds to thymine, the nucleotide at position 440 in the 5' to 3' HIV genome.

[0026] In the modified synthetic TFIIIA molecule, lysine, the 88th amino acid in the 5' to 3' TFIIIA molecule, bonds to thymine, the nucleotide at position 441 in the 5' to 3' HIV genome.

[0027] In the modified synthetic TFIIIA molecule, lysine, the 89th amino acid in the 5' to 3' TFIIIA molecule, bonds to thymine, the nucleotide at position 442 in the 5' to 3' HIV genome.

[0028] In the modified synthetic TFIIIA molecule, lysine, the 108th amino acid in the 5' to 3' TFIIIA molecule, bonds to thymine, the nucleotide at position 443 in the 5' to 3' HIV genome.

[0029] In the modified synthetic TFIIIA molecule, lysine, the 111th amino acid in the 5' to 3' TFIIIA molecule, bonds to thymine, the nucleotide at position 444 in the 5' to 3' HIV genome.

[0030] In the modified synthetic TFIIIA molecule, arginine, the 112th amino acid in the 5' to 3' TFIIIA molecule, bonds to guanine, the nucleotide at position 445 in the 5' to 3' HIV genome.

[0031] In the modified synthetic TFIIIA molecule, glutamic acid, the 115th amino acid in the 5' to 3' TFIIIA molecule, bonds to cytosine, the nucleotide at position 446 in the 5' to 3' HIV genome.

[0032] In the modified synthetic TFIIIA molecule, glutamic acid, the 118th amino acid in the 5' to 3' TFIIIA molecule, bonds to cytosine, the nucleotide at position 447 in the 5' to 3' HIV genome.

[0033] In the modified synthetic TFIIIA molecule, lysine, the 119th amino acid in the 5' to 3' TFIIIA molecule, bonds to thymine, the nucleotide at position 448 in the 5' to 3' HIV genome.

[0034] In the modified synthetic TFIIIA molecule, arginine, the 140th amino acid in the 5' to 3' TFIIIA molecule, bonds to guanine, the nucleotide at position 449 in the 5' to 3' HIV genome.

[0035] In the modified synthetic TFIIIA molecule, lysine, the 143th amino acid in the 5' to 3' TFIIIA molecule, bonds to thymine, the nucleotide at position 450 in the 5' to 3' HIV genome.

[0036] In the modified synthetic TFIIIA molecule, asparagine, the 144th amino acid in the 5' to 3' TFIIIA molecule, bonds to adenine, the nucleotide at position 451 in the 5' to 3' HIV genome.

[0037] In the modified synthetic TFIIIA molecule, glutamic acid, the 147th amino acid in the 5' to 3' TFIIIA molecule, bonds to cytosine, the nucleotide at position 452 in the 5' to 3' HIV genome.

[0038] In the modified synthetic TFIIIA molecule, lysine, the 150th amino acid in the 5' to 3' TFIIIA molecule, bonds to thymine, the nucleotide at position 453 in the 5' to 3' HIV genome.

[0039] In the modified synthetic TFIIIA molecule, arginine, the 151st amino acid in the 5' to 3' TFIIIA molecule, bonds to guanine, the nucleotide at position 454 in the 5' to 3' HIV genome.

[0040] In the modified synthetic TFIIIA molecule, arginine, the 170th amino acid in the 5' to 3' TFIIIA molecule, bonds to guanine, the nucleotide at position 455 in the 5' to 3' HIV genome.

[0041] In the modified synthetic TFIIIA molecule, arginine, the 173rd amino acid in the 5' to 3' TFIIIA molecule, bonds to guanine, the nucleotide at position 456 in the 5' to 3' HIV genome.

[0042] In the modified synthetic TFIIIA molecule, lysine, the 174th amino acid in the 5' to 3' TFIIIA molecule, bonds to thymine, the nucleotide at position 457 in the 5' to 3' HIV genome.

[0043] In the modified synthetic TFIIIA molecule, glutamic acid, the 177th amino acid in the 5' to 3' TFIIIA molecule, bonds to cytosine, the nucleotide at position 458 in the 5' to 3' HIV genome.

[0044] In the modified synthetic TFIIIA molecule, lysine, the 180th amino acid in the 5' to 3' TFIIIA molecule, bonds to thymine, the nucleotide at position 459 in the 5' to 3' HIV genome.

[0045] In the modified synthetic TFIIIA molecule, glutamic acid, the 181st amino acid in the 5' to 3' TFIIIA molecule, bonds to cytosine, the nucleotide at position 460 in the 5' to 3' HIV genome.

[0046] The molecular bonding as described represents a semi-permanent to permanent bonding of amino acids comprising the modified synthetic TFIIIA molecule bonding to designated nucleotides in the HIV genome to prevent transcription of the HIV genome, which if the HIV genome cannot be transcribed further infection by HIV is halted.

BRIEF SUMMARY OF THE INVENTION

[0047] The method whereby in constructing a protein to bind to the DNA the following is incorporated in the design of the molecule:

[0048] One amino acid asparagine binds semipermanently to each nucleotide adenine.

[0049] One amino acid arginine binds semipermanently to each nucleotide guanine.

[0050] One amino acid glutamic acid binds semipermanently to each nucleotide cytosine.

[0051] One amino acid lysine binds semipermanently to each nucleotide thymine.

DETAILED DESCRIPTION

[0052] The method whereby in constructing a protein to bind to the DNA the following is incorporated in the design of the molecule to create semipermanent binding of the protein to the DNA:

[0053] One amino acid asparagine binds semipermanently to each nucleotide adenine.

[0054] The amino acid asparagine binds semipermanently to the nucleotide adenine as a result of the asparagine donating a hydrogen to a nitrogen in adenine's molecule and an oxygen in the asparagine's molecule accepting a hydrogen from adenine.

[0055] One amino acid arginine binds semipermanently to each nucleotide guanine.

[0056] The amino acid arginine binds semipermanently to the nucleotide guanine as a result of the arginine donating one hydrogen to a nitrogen in guanine's molecule and another hydrogen to an oxygen in the guanine's molecule.

[0057] One amino acid glutamic acid binds semipermanently to each nucleotide cytosine.

[0058] The amino acid glutamic acid binds semipermanently to the nucleotide cytosine as a result of the cytosine donating a hydrogen to an oxygen in glutamic acid's molecule.

[0059] One amino acid lysine binds semipermanently to each nucleotide thymine.

[0060] The amino acid lysine binds semipermanently to the nucleotide thymine as a result of the lysine donating a hydrogen to an oxygen in thymine's molecule.

CONCLUSIONS, RAMIFICATIONS, AND SCOPE

[0061] Accordingly, the reader will see that the method described herein to construct synthetic proteins to bind to the DNA, represents a new and unique state of the art that has never before been recognized nor appreciated by those skilled in the art.

[0062] Although the description above contains specificities, these should not be construed as limiting the scope of the invention but as merely providing illustrations of some of the presently preferred embodiments of the invention.

NUMBER OF DRAWINGS: 0

CLAIMS

The terms and expressions which are employed here are used as terms of description and are not of limitation and there is no intention, in the use of terms and expressions, of excluding equivalents of the features presented, and described, or portions thereof, it being recognized that various modifications are possible in the scope of the invention or method as claimed.

What is claimed:

1. The method where when constructing a synthetic protein to semipermanently bind to a sequence of deoxyribonucleic acid, within the binding portion of said protein,

    (a) an asparagine is utilized to bind to each adenine when present,

    (b) an arginine is utilized to bind to each guanine when present,

    (c) a glutamic acid is utilized to bind to each cytosine when present, and

(d) a lysine is utilized to bind to each thymine when present,

whereby, in using these binding associations as described, protein molecules are created to semipermanently bind to segments of the DNA and block the transcription of viral genes to halt viral infections, block the transcription of oncogenes to halt or prevent the growth of cancer cells, block the transcription of lethal genes to treat lethal genetic disorders, and block the transcription of pathologic genes to treat diseases.

2. The method of constructing a synthetic protein to semipermanently bind to a sequence of deoxyribonucleic acid, within the binding portion of said protein, said protein comprising:

(a) providing an asparagine to bind to each adenine when present,

(b) providing an arginine to bind to each guanine when present,

(c) providing a glutamic acid to bind to each cytosine when present, and

(d) providing a lysine to bind to each thymine when present,

whereby, in using these binding associations as described, protein molecules are created to semipermanently bind to segments of the DNA and block the transcription of viral genes to halt viral infections, block the transcription of oncogenes to halt or prevent the growth of cancer cells, block the transcription of lethal genes to treat lethal genetic disorders, and block transcription of pathologic genes to treat diseases.

3. The method of constructing a synthetic protein to semipermanently bind to a sequence of deoxyribonucleic acid, comprising within the binding portion of said protein:

(a) providing an asparagine to bind to each adenine, where said adenine is present in said sequence of deoxyribonucleic acid,

(b) providing an arginine to bind to each guanine, where said guanine is present in said sequence of deoxyribonucleic acid

(c) providing a glutamic acid to bind to each cytosine, where said cytosine is present in said sequence of deoxyribonucleic acid and,

(d) providing a lysine to bind to each thymine, where said thymine is present in said sequence of deoxyribonucleic acid,

whereby, in using these binding associations as described, protein molecules are created to semipermanently bind to segments of the DNA and block the transcription of viral genes to halt viral infections, block the transcription of onco-genes to halt or prevent the growth of cancer cells, block the transcription of lethal genes to treat lethal genetic disorders, and block pathologic genes to treat diseases.

Abstract

The future of pharmacology will include the development of synthetic proteins to bind to specific segments of nuclear DNA in order to more effectively treat a wide variety of disease states. The method of constructing a synthetic protein to semipermanently bind to a sequence of deoxyribonucleic acid will include providing an asparagine to bind to each adenine when present, providing an arginine to bind to each guanine when present, providing a glutamic acid to bind to each cytosine when present, and providing a lysine to bind to each thymine when present. By utilizing these binding associations protein molecules are created to semipermanently bind to segments of the DNA and block transcription of pathologic genes to treat diseases.

GALLERY OF TERRA HOLOMETABOLOUS PROGRAMME

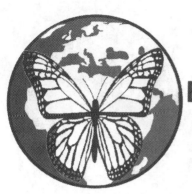 **ECOMETABOLOUS**

terra.holometabolous.programme

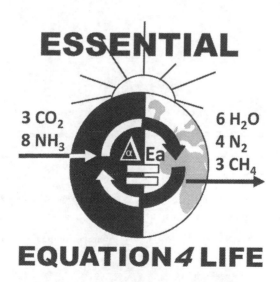

ESSENTIAL

$3\ CO_2$
$8\ NH_3$

$6\ H_2O$
$4\ N_2$
$3\ CH_4$

Δ Ea

EQUATION4 LIFE

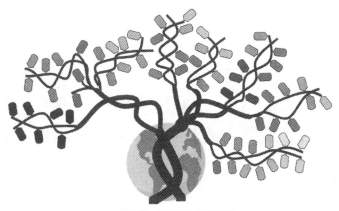

PRIME GENOME

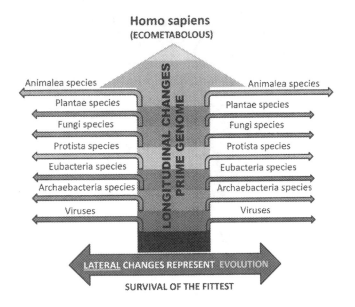

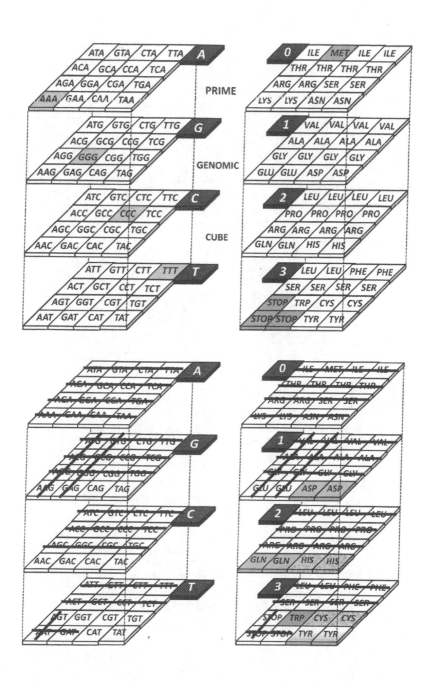

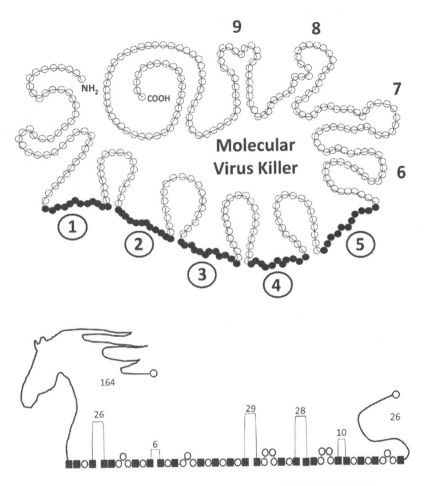

Molecular
Virus Killer

FOURTH GENERATION BIOLOGICS

EXECUTABLE GENE

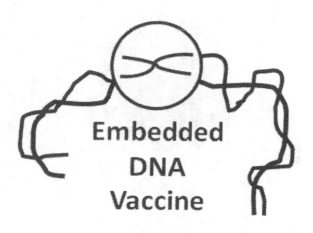

Embedded
DNA
Vaccine

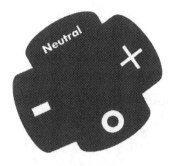

QUATRON

sub sub atomic particle

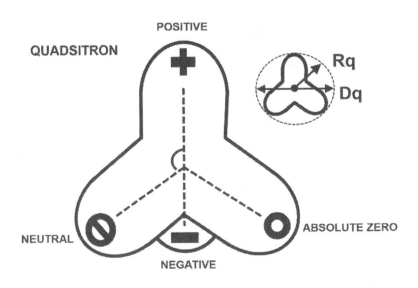

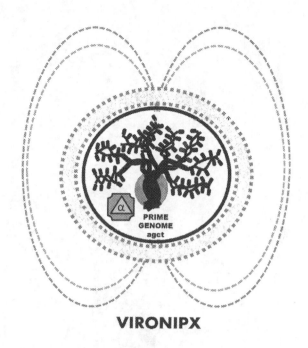

VIRONIPX

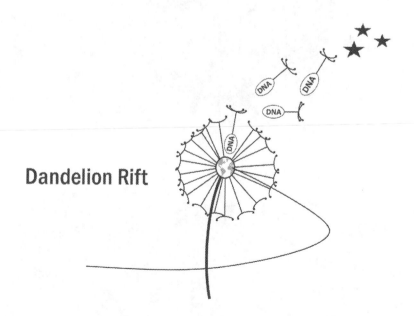

Dandelion Rift

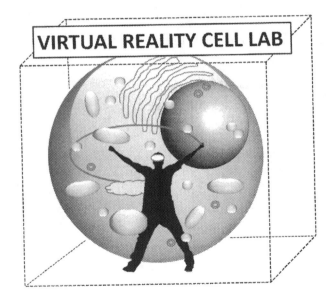

VIRTUAL REALITY CELL LAB

Presenting the design of a Courier gene
to defend cells against HIV
ESHG, Glasgow, Scotland 2015

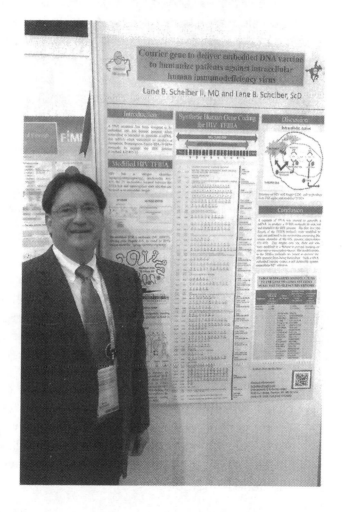

Optimizing data compression technique determined by decoding HIV-1 HXB2 DNA genome, assists in deciphering the means the human genome is transcribed and translated

An optimizing data compression technique involving multiple genes is revealed in analyzing HIV-1 HXB2 genome K03455.1. Understanding HIV's data compression assists in an expanded understanding of the human genome. The data compression technique ingeniously utilizes features of the codon code and nucleotide code to generate overlapping genetic information, which facilitates 8 segments of HIV's pre-mRNA code to be read twice producing differing mRNA sequences each time the pre-mRNA code is deciphered.

The HIV-1 HXB2 genome k03455.1, 9719 nucleotides, which produce 9 genes/master proteins designated as gag PRO_0000261216, gag-pol PRO_0000223620, vif PRO_0000042759, vpr PRO_0000085451, tat PRO_0000085364, rev PRO_0000085279, vpu PRO_0000085433, env PRO_0000239240, and nef PRO_0000038365.

Demonstrated in Table 1, is evidence of a frameshift involving each gene. There are 8 segments where the codon code overlaps, which facilitate the HIV genome to be 825 nucleotides shorter than if such a data compression technique were not utilized. Env, tat-2, rev-2 all share a 45 nucleotide sequence. This data compression technique represents a higher order complexity in the construct of the genome, beyond a simple linear read, facilitating the HIV genome to fit inside HIV virion.

HIV genome utilizes the same genetic cellular machinery as human genes; recognizing the microcosm of data compression present in HIV genome broadens the analysis regarding how the spliceosome and ribosome complexes interact with human DNA, which will inspire innovative human genetic therapies.'

Summary: The existence of the HIV genome, in the manner the viral DNA was constructed as shown above for HIV-1 HXB2, is conclusive testimony that at least in part, the genetics of life was designed with intent by an extraterrestrial intelligence.

Gene 1 Protein 1 Gene 2 Protein 2	Start-Stop Positions	Point of Frame Shift --- # Nucleotides that Overlap	Nucleotide Code at Point of Frame Shift	Codon Code at point of frame shift
GAG 261216 GAG-POL 223620	790 - 2292 --------- 2091 - 5096	2091 --------- 202	aat ttt tta ggg aag... ...agg gaa gat | 2091	NFLGK.... ...RED... ^ 2091
GAG-POL 223620 VIF 042759	2091 - 5096 --------- 5041 - 5619	5041 --------- 56	gat tat gga aaa cag... ......atg gaa aac aga | 5041	DYGKQ.... ....M(start)ENR ^ 5041
VIF 042759 VPR 085451	5041 - 5619 --------- 5559 - 5850	5559 --------- 61	gat aga tgg aac aag.... ...atg gaa caa gcc | 5559	DRWNK ....M(start)EQA ^ 5559
VPR 085451 TAT-1 085364	5559- 5850 --------- 5831 - 6049	5831 --------- 20	gca aga aat gga gcc... .....atg gag cca gta | 5831	ARNGA... ...M(start)EPV ^ 5831
TAT-1 085364 REV-1 085279	5831 - 6049 --------- 5970 - 6045	5970 --------- 80	ggc atc tcc tat ggc agg... ....atg gca gga | 5970	GISYGR ...M(start)AG ^ 5970
VPU 085433 ENV 239240 *33-856	6062 - 6310 --------- 6225 - 8795	6062 --------- 86	agt ggc aat gag agt... .....atg aga gtg | 6062	SGNES ....M(start)RV ^ 6062
ENV 239240 REV-2 085279	6225 - 8795 --------- 8379 - 8653	8379 --------- 275	tcg ttt cag acc cac... .....((a)ac) cca cct* | 8379 *combine 'a' from rev-1, 'ac' from rev-2	SFQTH ...(N)PP* ^ 8379 *combined 'aac' codon for 'N'
ENV 239240 TAT-2 085364	6225 - 8795 --------- 8380 - 8424	8380 --------- 45	ttt cag acc cac ctc... .....ccc acc tcc | 8380	FQTHL PTS ^ 8380
ENV 239240 NEF 038365	6225 - 8795 --------- 8797 - 9417	8797 --------- 0	att ttg cta taa... ...atg ggt ggc | 8797	ILL(stop).... ...MGG ^ 8797

Human Immunodeficiency Virus HXB2 Genome
(nucleotides 1-3720)

```
    1 tggaagggct aattcactcc caacgaagac aagatatcct tgatctgtgg atctaccaca
   61 cacaaggcta cttccctgat tagcagaact acacaccagg gccagggatc agatatccac
  121 tgacctttgg atggtgctac aagctagtac cagttgagcc agagaagtta gaagaagcca
  181 acaaaggaga gaacaccagc ttgttacacc ctgtgagcct gcatgggatg gatgacccgg
  241 agagagaagt gttagagtgg aggtttgaca gccgcctagc atttcatcac atggcccgag
  301 agctgcatcc ggagtactac aagaactgct gacatcgagc ttgctacaag ggactttccg
  361 ctggggactt tccaggggag gcgtggcctg ggcggactgg ggagtggcga gccctcagat
  421 cctgcatata agcagctgct ttttgcctgt actgggtctc tctggttaga ccagatctga
```

```
  481 gcctgggagc tctctggcta actagggaac ccactgctta agcctcaata aagcttgcct
  541 tgagtgcttc aagtagtgtg tgcccgtctg ttgtgtgact ctggtaacta gagatccctc
  601 agacccttt agtcagtgtg gaaaatctct agcagtggcg cccgaacagg gacttgaaag
  661 cgaaagggaa accagaggag ctctctcgac gcaggactcg gcttgctgaa gcgcgcacgg
  721 caagaggcga ggggcggcga ctggtgagta cgccaaaaat tttgactagc ggaggctaga
  781 aggagagaga tgggtgcgag agcgtcagta ttaagcgggg gagaattaga tcgatgggaa
```

GAG

GAG START ^

```
GAG        841 aaaattcggt taaggccagg gggaaagaaa aaatataaat taaaacatat agtatgggca
GAG        901 agcagggagc tagaacgatt cgcagttaat cctggcctgt tagaaacatc agaaggctgt
```

```
GAG       1021 ttatataata cagtagcaac cctctattgt gtgcatcaaa ggatagagat aaaagacacc
GAG       1081 aaggaagctt tagacaagat agaggaagag caaaacaaaa gtaagaaaaa agcacagcaa
GAG       1141 gcagcagctg acacaggaca cagcaatcag gtcagccaaa attaccctat agtgcagaac
GAG       1201 atccaggggc aaatggtaca tcaggccata tcacctagaa cttttaaatgc atgggtaaaa
GAG       1261 gtagtagaag agaaggcttt cagcccagaa gtgataccca tgttttcagc attatcagaa
GAG       1321 ggagccaccc cacaagattt aaacaccatg ctaaacacag tggggggaca tcaagcagcc
GAG       1381 atgcaaatgt taaaagagac catcaatgag gaagctgcag aatgggatag agtgcatcca
GAG       1441 gtgcatgcag ggcctattgc accaggccag atgagagaac caaggggaag tgacatagca
GAG       1501 ggaactacta gtacccttca ggaacaaata ggatggatga caaataatcc acctatccca
GAG       1561 gtaggagaaa tttataaaag atggataatc ctgggattaa ataaaatagt aagaatgtat
GAG       1621 agccctacca gcattctgga cataagacaa ggaccaaagg aacccttag agactatgta
GAG       1681 gaccggttct ataaaactct aagagccgag caagcttcac aggaggtaaa aaattggatg
GAG       1741 acagaaacct tgttggtcca aaatgcgaac ccagattgta agactatttt aaaagcattg
GAG       1801 ggaccagcgg ctacactaga agaaatgatg acagcatgtc agggagtagg aggacccggc
GAG       1861 cataaagcaa gagttttggc tgaagcaatg agccaagtaa caaattcagc taccataatg
GAG       1921 atgcagagag gcaattttag gaaccaaaga aagattgtta agtgtttcaa ttgtggcaaa
GAG       1981 gaagggcaca cagccagaaa ttgcagggcc cctaggaaaa agggctgttg gaaatgtgga
```

```
GAG/POL   2041 aaggaaggac accaaatgaa agattgtact gagagacagg ctaattttt agggaagatc
```

POL START ^

```
GAG/POL   2101 tggccttcct acaagggaag gccagggaat tttcttcaga gcagaccaga gccaacagcc
GAG/POL   2161 ccaccagaag agagcttcag gtctggggta gagacaacaa ctccccctca gaagcaggag
GAG/POL   2221 ccgatagaca aggaactgta tcctttaact tccctcaggt cactctttgg caacgacccc
GAG/POL   2281 tcgtcacaat aaagataggg gggcaactaa aggaagctct attagataca ggagcagatg
```

GAG STOP ^

```
POL       2341 atacagtatt agaagaaatg agtttgccag gaagatggaa accaaaaatg ataggggaa
```

POL transcription START ^

```
POL       2401 ttggaggttt tatcaaagta agacagtatg atcagatact catagaaatc tgtggacata
POL       2461 aagctatagg tacagtatta gtaggaccta cacctgtcaa cataattgga agaaatctgt
POL       2521 tgactcagat tggttgcact ttaaattttc ccattagccc tattgagact gtaccagtaa
POL       2581 aacaaagcca aggaatggat ggcccaaaag ttaaacaatg gccattgaca gaagaaaaaa
POL       2641 taaaagcatt agtagaaatt tgtacagaga tggaaaagga agggaaaatt tcaaaaattg
POL       2701 ggcctgaaaa tccatacaat actccagtat ttgccataaa gaaaaagac agtactaaat
POL       2761 ggagaaaatt agtagatttc agagaacttaa taagagaact caagacttc tgggaagttc
POL       2821 aattaggaat accacatccc gcagggttaa aaaagaaaaa atcagtaaca gtactggatg
POL       2881 tgggtgatgc atatttttca gttcccttag atgaagactt caggaagtat actgcattta
POL       2941 ccatacctag tataaacaat gagacaccag ggattagata tcagtacaat gtgcttccac
POL       3001 agggatggaa aggatcacca gcaatattcc aaagtagcat gacaaaaatc ttagagcctt
POL       3061 ttagaaaaca aaatccagac atagttatct atcaatacat ggatgatttg tatgtaggat
POL       3121 ctgacttaga aatagggcag catagaacaa aaatagagga gctgagacaa catctgttga
POL       3181 ggtggggact taccacacca gacaaaaaac atcagaaaga acctccattc ctttggatgg
POL       3241 gttatgaact ccatcctgat aaatggacag tacagcctat agtgctgcca gaaaaagaca
POL       3301 gctggactgt caatgacata cagaagttag tggggaaatt gaattgggca agtcagattt
POL       3361 acccagggat taaagtaagg caattatgta aactccttag aggaaccaaa gcactaacag
POL       3421 aagtaatacc actaacagaa gaagcagagc tagaactggc agaaaacaga gagattctaa
POL       3481 aagaaccagt acatggagtg tattatgacc catcaaaaga cttaatagca gaaatacaga
POL       3541 agcaggggca agggcaatgg acatatcaaa tttatcaaga gccatttaaa aatctgaaaa
POL       3601 caggaaaata tgcaagaatg aggggtgccc acactaatga tgtaaaacaa ttaacagagg
POL       3661 cagtgcaaaa aataaccaca gaaagcatag taatatgggg aaagactcct aaatttaaac
```

Human Immunodeficiency Virus HXB2 Genome
(nucleotides 3721-6600)

```
POL        3721 tgcccataca aaaggaaaca tggggaaacat ggtggacaga gtattggcaa gccacctgga
POL        3781 ttcctgagtg ggagtttgtt aataccccto cctagtgaa attatggtac cagttagaga
POL        3841 aagaacccat agtaggagca gaaacctcct atgtgaatgt ggcagctaac aggagacta
POL        3901 aattagggaa agcaggatat gttactaata gaggaagaca aaaagttgtc acctaactg
POL        3961 acacaacaaa tcagaagact gagttacaag caatttatct agctttgcag gattcgggat
POL        4021 tagaagtaaa catagtaaca gactcacaat atgcattagg aatcattcaa gcacaacag
POL        4081 atcaaagtga attaagagtta gtcaatcaaa taatagagca gttaataaaa aaggaaaagg
POL        4141 tctatctggc atgggtacca gcacacaaag gaattggagg aaatgaacaa gtagataaat
POL        4201 tagtcagtgc tggaatcagg aaagtactat ttttagatgg aatagataag gcccaagtg
POL        4261 aacatgagaa atatcacagt aattggagag caatggctag tgattttaac ctgccacctg
POL        4321 tagtagcaaa agaaatagta gccagctgtg ataaatgtca gctaaaagga gaagccatgc
POL        4381 atggacaagt agactgtagt ccaggaatat ggcaactaga ttgtacacat ttagaaggaa
POL        4441 aagttatcct ggtagcagtt catgtagcca gtggatatat agaagcagaa gttattccag
POL        4501 cagaaacagg gcaggaaaca gcatatttc ttttaaaatt agcaggaaga tggccagtaa
POL        4561 aaacaataca tactgacaat ggcagcaatt tcaccggtgc tacggttagg gccgcctgtt
POL        4621 ggtgggcggg aatcaagcag gaatttggaa ttccctacaa tccccaaagt caaggagtag
POL        4681 tagaatctat gaataaagaa ttaaagaaaa ttataggaca ggtaagagat caggctgaac
POL        4741 atcttaagac agcagtacaa atggcagtat tcatccacaa ttttaaaaga aaaggggggg
POL        4801 ttggggggta cagtgcaggg gaaagaatag tagacataat agcaacagac atacaaacta
POL        4861 aagaattaca aaaacaaatt acaaaaattc aaaattttcg ggtttattac agggacagca
POL        4921 gaaatccact ttggaaagga ccagcaaagc tcctctggaa aggtgaaggg gcagtagtaa
POL        4981 tacaagataa tagtgacata aaagtagtgc caagaagaaa agcaaagatc attagggatt
POL/VIF    5041 atggaaaaca gatggcaggt gatgattgtg tggcaagtag acaggatgag gattagaaca
```
^ VIF START   POL STOP ^

```
VIF        5101 tggaaaagtt tagtaaaaca ccatatgtat gtttcaggga agctaaggga tggttttat
VIF        5161 agacatcact atgaaagcc tcatccaaga ataagttcag aagtacacat cccactaggg
VIF        5221 gatgctagat tggtaataaa aacatattgg ggtctgcata caggagaaag agactggcat
VIF        5281 ttgggtcagg gagtctccat agaatggagg aaaaagagat atagcacaca agtagaccct
VIF        5341 gaactagcag accaactaat tcatctgtat tactttgact gtttttcaga ctctgctata
VIF        5401 agaaaggcct tattaggaca catagttagc cctaggtgtg aatatcaagc aggacataac
VIF        5461 aaggtaggat ctctacaata cttggcacta gcagcattaa taacaccaaa aaagggggga
VIF/VPR    5521 ccacctttgc ctagtgttac gaaactgaca gaggatagat ggaacaagcc ccagaagacc
```
^ VPR START

```
VIF/VPR    5581 aagggccaca gagggagcca cacaatgaat ggacactaga gcttttagag gagcttaaga
```
VIF STOP ^

```
VPR        5641 atgaagctgt tagacatttt cctaggattt ggctccatgg cttagggcaa catatctatg
VPR        5701 aaacttatgg ggatacttgg gcaggagtgg aagccataat aagaattctg caacaactgc
VPR        5761 tgtttatcca tttcagaat tgggtgtcga catagcagaa taggcgttac tcgacagagg
VPR/TAT-1  5821 agagcaagaa atggagccag tagatcctag actagagccc tggaagcatc caggaagtca
```
^ TAT-1 START   ^ VPR STOP

```
TAT-1      5881 gcctaaaact gcttgtaaca attgctattg taaaaagtgt tgctttcatt gccaagtttg
TAT-1/REV-1 5941 tttcataaca aagccttag gcatctccta tggcaggaag aagcggagac agcgacgaag
```
^ REV-1 START

```
TAT-1/REV-1 6001 agctcatcag aacagtcaga ctcatcaagc ttctctatca aagcagtaag tagtacatgt
```
REV-1 STOP ^   ^ TAT 1 STOP

```
VPU        6061 aacgcaacct ataccaatag tagcaatagt agcattagta gtagcaataa taatagcaat
```
^ VPU START

```
VPU        6121 agttgtgtgg tccatagtaa tcatagaata taggaaaata ttaagacaaa gaaaaataga
VPU/ENV    6181 caggttaatt gatagactaa tagaaagagc agaagacagt ggcaatgaga gtgaaggaga
```
^ ENV START

```
VPU/ENV    6241 aaatatcagca cttgtggaga tgggggtgga gatgggcac catgctcctt gggatgttga
VPU/ENV    6301 tgatctgtag tgctacagaa aaattgtggg tcacagtcta ttatggggta cctgtgtgga
```
^ VPU STOP

```
ENV        6361 aggaagcaac caccactcta ttttgtgcat cagatgctaa agcatatgat acagaggtac
ENV        6421 ataatgtttg ggccacacat gcctgtgtac ccacagaccc caacccacaa gaagtagtat
ENV        6481 tggtaaatgt gacagaaaat tttaacatgt ggaaaaatga catggtagaa cagatgcatg
ENV        6541 aggatataat cagtttatgg gatcaaagcc taaagccatg tgtaaaatta acccactct
```

Human Immunodeficiency Virus HXB2 Genome
(nucleotides 6601-9719)

```
ENV           6601 gtgttagttt aaagtgcact gatttgaaga atgataactaa taccaatagt agtagcggga
ENV           6661 gaatgataat ggagaaagga gagataaaaa actgctcttt caatatcagc acaagcataa
ENV           6721 gagataaggt gcagaaagaa tatgcatttt tttataaaact tgatataata ccaatagata
ENV           6781 atgataactac cagctataag ttgacaagtt gtaacacctc agtcattaca caggcctgtc
ENV           6841 caaaggtatc ctttgagcca attcccatac attattgtgc cccggctggt tttgcgattc
ENV           6901 taaaatgtaa taataagacg ttcaatggaa caggaccatg tacaaatgtc agcacagtac
ENV           6961 aatgtacaca tggaattagg ccagtagtat caactcaact gctgttaaat ggcagtctag
ENV           7021 cagaagaaga ggtagtaatt agatctgtca atttcacgga caatgctaaa accataatag
ENV           7081 tacagctgaa cacatctgta gaaattaatt gtacaagacc caacaacaat acaagaaaaa
ENV           7141 gaatccgtat ccagagagga ccagggagag catttgttac aataggaaaa atagggaata
ENV           7201 tgagacaagc acattgtaac attagtagag caaaatggaa taacacttta aaacagatag
ENV           7261 ctagcaaatt aagagaacaa tttggaaata ataaaacaat aatctttaag caatcctcag
ENV           7321 gaggggaccc agaaattgta acgcacagtt ttaattgtgg aggggaattt ttctactgta
ENV           7381 attcaacaca actgtttaat agtacttggt ttaatagtac ttggagtact gaagggtcaa
ENV           7441 ataacactga ggaagtgac acaatcacc tcccatgcag aataaaacaa attataaaca
ENV           7501 tgtggcagaa agtaggaaaa gcaatgtatg cccctcccat cagtggacaa attagatgtt
ENV           7561 catcaaatat tacagggctg ctattaacaa gagatggtgg taatagcaac aatgagtccg
ENV           7621 agatcttcag acctggagga ggagatatga gggacaattg gagaagtgaa ttatataaat
ENV           7681 ataaagtagt aaaaattgaa ccattaggag tagcacccac caaggcaaag agaagagtgg
ENV           7741 tgcagagaga aaaaagagca gtgggaatag gagctttgtt ccttgggttc ttgggagcag
ENV           7801 caggaagcac tatgggcgca gcctcaatga cgctgacggt actggccgca caattattgt
ENV           7861 ctggtatagt gcagcagcag aacaatttgc tgagggctat tgaggcgcaa cagcatctgt
ENV           7921 tgcaactcac agtctggggc atcaagcagc tccaggcaag aatcctggct gtggaaagat
ENV           7981 acctaaagga tcaacagctc ctggggattt gggttgctc tggaaaactc atttgcacca
ENV           8041 ctgctgtgcc ttggaatgct agttggagta ataaatctct ggaacagatt tggaatcaca
ENV           8101 cgacctggat ggagtgggac agagaaatta acaattacac aagcttaata cactccttaa
ENV           8161 ttgaagaatc gcaaaaccag caagaaaaga atgaacaaga attattggaa ttagataaat
ENV           8221 gggcaagttt gtggaattgg tttaacataa caaattggct gtggtatata aaattattca
ENV           8281 taatgatagt aggaggcttg gtaggtttaa gaatagtttt tgctgtactt tctatagtga
ENV/REV-2/TAT-2 8341 atagagttag gcagggatat tcaccattat cgtttcagac ccacctccca acccgagggg
```

START REV-2 ^^ TAT-2 START

```
ENV/REV-2/TAT-2 8401 gacccgacag gcccgaagga atagaagaag aaggtggaga gagagacaga gacagatcca
```

^ TAT-2 STOP

```
ENV/REV-2     8461 ttcgattagt gaacggatcc ttggcactta tctgggacga tctgcggagc ctgtgcctct
ENV/REV-2     8521 tcagctacca ccgcttgaga gacttactct tgattgtaac gaggattgtg gaacttctgg
ENV/REV-2     8581 gacgcagggg gtgggaagcc ctcaaatatt ggtggaatct cctacagtat tggagtcagg
ENV/REV-2     8641 aactaaagaa tagtgctgtt agcttgctca atgccacagc catagcagta gctgagggga
```

^ REV-2 STOP

```
ENV           8701 cagatagggt tatagaagta gtacaaggag cttgtagagc tattcgccac atacctagaa
ENV/NEF       8761 gaataagaca gggcttggaa aggattttgc tataagatgg gtggcaagtg gtcaaaaagt
```

ENV STOP ^ ^ NEF START

```
NEF           8821 agtgtgattg gatggcctac tgtaagggaa agaatgagac gagctgagcc agcagcagat
NEF           8881 agggtgggag cagcatctcg agacctggaa aaacatggag caatcacaag tagcaataca
NEF           8941 gcagctacca atgctgcttg tgcctggcta gaagcacaag aggaggagga ggtgggtttt
NEF           9001 ccagtcacac ctcaggtacc tttaagacca atgacttaca aggcagctgt agatcttagc
NEF           9061 cactttttaa aagaaaaggg gggactggaa gggctaattc actcccaaag aagacaagat
NEF           9121 atccttgatc tgtggatcta ccacacacaa ggctacttcc ctgattagca gaactacaca
NEF           9181 ccagggccag gggtcagata tccactgacc tttggatggt gctacaagct agtaccagtt
NEF           9241 gagccagata aggtagaaga ggccaataaa ggagagaaca ccagcttgtt acaccctgtg
NEF           9301 agcctgcatg ggatggatga cccggagaga gaagtgttag agtggaggtt tgacagccgc
NEF           9361 ctagcatttc atcacgtggc ccgagagctg catccggagt acttcaagaa ctgctgacat
```

NEF STOP ^

```
              9421 cgagcttgct acaagggact ttccgctggg gactttccag ggaggcgtgg cctgggcggg
              9481 actggggagt ggcgagccct cagatcctgc atataagcag ctgctttttg cctgtactgg
              9541 gtctctctgg ttagaccaga tctgagcctg ggagctctct ggctaactag ggaacccact
              9601 gcttaagcct caataaagct tgccttgagt gcttcaagta gtgtgtgccc gtctgttgtg
              9661 tgactctggt aactagagat ccctcagacc cttttagtca gtgtggaaaa tctctagca
```

Presenting Optimizing Data Compression Technique Utilized by HIV, ESHG, Copenhagen, Denmark 2017. Proof HIV Genome Designed.

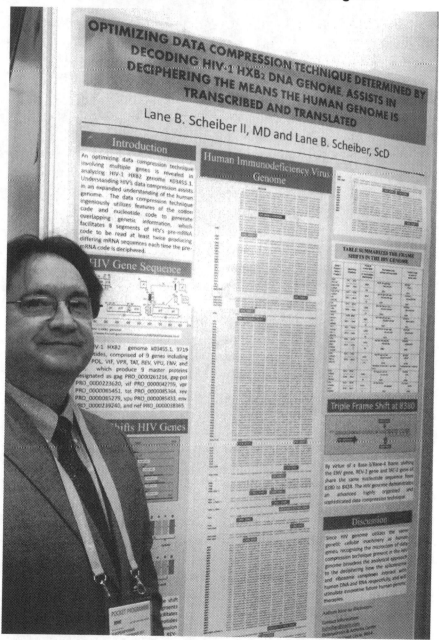

Printed in the United States
By Bookmasters